International Perspectives in Values-Based Mental Health Practice

W0043632

Drozdstoy Stoyanov · Bill Fulford
Giovanni Stanghellini · Werdie Van Staden
Michael TH Wong
Editors

International Perspectives in Values-Based Mental Health Practice

Case Studies and Commentaries

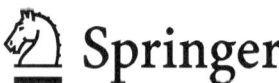 Springer

Editors
Drozdstoy Stoyanov
Medical University Plovdiv
Plovdiv, Bulgaria

Giovanni Stanghellini
Department of Psychological, Health &
Territorial Sciences
"G. D'Annunzio" University
Chieti Scalo, Italy

Michael TH Wong
Department of Psychiatry, Li Ka Shing
Faculty of Medicine
The University of Hong Kong
Hong Kong, China

Bill Fulford
St Catherine's College
University of Oxford
Oxford, United Kingdom

Werdie Van Staden
Centre for Ethics and Philosophy of Health
Sciences
University of Pretoria
Pretoria, South Africa

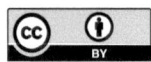

Preface: How the Book Came About[1]

This book has turned out to be an exercise in its own topic. Conceived originally as no more than a merely academic exploration of the impact of cultural values on mental health, the processes of co-writing by which the book has been realised, and our experiences in working together in this way have in themselves embodied the very changes towards which the book points.

The idea for the book came in part from a collaborative study between two of the editors, DS and KWMF, showing the importance of Balkan cultural values of pluralism as a resource for what was at the time a new skills-based approach to working with values in health care called 'values-based practice' (see chapter 1 'Surprised by Values: an Introduction to Values-based Practice and the Use of Personal Narratives in this Book'). Values-based practice had to that point been developed with a focus mainly on individual values. These are important across the board in mental health (e.g. in recovery, see chapters 22 'Three Points in Time: How Values and Culture Affected My Life, Madness and the People Around Me', 23 'Recovery and Cultural Values: on Our Own Terms (a Dialogue)', and 32 'Discovering Myself, a Journey of Rediscovery'). But the example of Balkan pluralism pointed to the potential importance also of cultural as well as individual values as resources for the further development of the field.

Thus arose the original academic project in cultural values and mental health. Once however we started to work on the project, it took on a life of its own. With the support of our editorial colleagues, we (DS and KWMF) approached a wide range of stakeholders in mental health from many different parts of the world, asking for narratives illustrating the roles of cultural values (positive and negative) in mental health. With past experiences in mind, we were fearful of a limited response. In the event we were overwhelmed! A glance down the contents pages of the book will show what a tremendously rich and diverse range of submissions we received.

But now we had what may be called the 'high class worry' of how to organise all these wonderful submissions into a coherent volume without losing the richness of their inherent diversity. Based on the established principles of values-based practice, we had planned a process of co-writing between the editors and individual

---

[1] **Authors**
   The editors with input from all contributors.

contributors. But co-writing like any other area of co-production depends critically on establishing an equality of voices. And the original editorial group, although indeed diverse, fell far short of the diverse perspectives represented by the full range of submitted materials. Yes, we (as editors) represented between us different parts of the world with very different cultural traditions and approaches to mental health. But we were all—to put it bluntly—white, male and psychiatrists.

So what to do? With a subgroup of contributors convened in London, we considered various options for balancing up the required perspectives. This proved to be a challenging and emotionally charged experience with views being expressed that in any other context might have been expected to result in multiple walkouts. But being held together as we were by the premise of mutual respect for differences of values underpinning values-based practice, we came to what we believe is an innovative approach to developing the book.

The essence of this approach was to use values-based practice itself to extend the principle of co-writing from individual chapters to the book as a whole. The process of co-writing thus established proved in practice to be labour intensive, and it presented a number of administrative and other challenges. We describe these in more detail in our concluding chapter (chapter 47 'Co-writing Values: What We Did and Why We Did It'). Of the merits of our co-writing approach, you, the reader, must be the judge. But at the very least it produced what none of us individually could have produced, a volume that opens up the rich resources available internationally to support the development of mental health care that is equally values-based as it is evidence-based.

Oxford, UK   Bill Fulford

Acknowledgements

We are grateful to The Collaborating Centre for Values-based Practice in Health and Social Care (St Catherine's College, Oxford), to the Centre for Ethics and Philosophy of Health Sciences, University of Pretoria (South Africa), to the Department of Psychological Sciences, Health and Territory, and to the Clinical Phenomenology Lab, both at "G. D'Annunzio" University (Chieti), and to the Scuola di Psicoterapia Fenomenologico-Dinamica, Firenze (Italy), for financial support: this support was crucial in allowing the book to be made available as an open access publication.

The book was developed in academic partnership with the Section of Philosophy and Humanities in Psychiatry of World Psychiatric Association, the Philosophy and Psychiatry section of the European Psychiatric Association, the Philosophy Special Interest Group in the Royal College of psychiatrists (UK) and the International Network for Philosophy and Psychiatry. We are grateful to each of these organizations for their gemerous academic support.

As editors and authors, we are grateful to each other for all the hard work and effort involved in sticking with the process of co-writing this book.

We are very grateful also to the Springer team for their encouragement and generous support for this process.

Contents

Contributors

Sola Adebiyi Director and Lead Facilitator, Narrative Mindfulness Ltd, London, UK

Temitope Ademosu Kings Global Health Institute, University of East London, London, UK

Hasanen Al-Taiar Oxford Health NHS Foundation Trust, Littlemore Mental Health Centre, Oxford, UK

Massimiliano Aragona Italian National Health System, Rome, Italy

Dialogues in Philosophy, Mental and Neuro Sciences, Rome, Italy

Jehannine Austin UBC Departments of Psychiatry and Medical Genetics, Vancouver, BC, Canada

Rosalind Austin Collaborating Centre for Values-Based Practice, St Catherine's College, University of Oxford, Oxford, UK

Michael Bennett The Professional Footballers Association, Manchester, UK

University of East Anglia, Norwich, UK

Asen Beshkov Department of Psychiatry and Medical Psychology, Medical University of Plovdiv, Plovdiv, Bulgaria

Steven Bettles General Osteopathic Council, London, UK

Meliha Bijedić Faculty of Special Education and Rehabilitation, Department of Behavioural Disorder, University of Tuzla, Tuzla, Bosnia and Herzegovina

Fiona Browne General Osteopathic Council, London, UK

Tamara Kayali Browne School of Medicine, Deakin University, Geelong, VIC, Australia

Simon Clarke Lead Coordinator of the Whiteness and Race Equality Network, St Catherine's College, University of Oxford, Oxford, UK

Stacey Clift General Osteopathic Council, London, UK

Diogo Telles Correia Clinica Universitária de Psiquiatria e Psicologia, Faculdade de Medicina da Universidade de Lisboa, Lisbon, Portugal

David Crepaz-Keay Applied Learning, Mental Health Foundation, London, UK
Mental Health Foundation, London, UK

Dennisa Davidson "Taunaki" Child and Adolescent Mental Health Service, Counties Manukau District Health Board, Auckland, New Zealand

Vincenzo Di Nicola Canadian Association of Social Psychiatry (CASP), World Association of Social Psychiatry (WASP), Department of Psychiatry and Addictions, University of Montreal, Montreal, QC, Canada
Department of Psychiatry and Behavioral Sciences, The George Washington University, Washington, DC, USA

Irma Dobrinjic Faculty of Special Education and Rehabilitation, Department of Behavioural Disorder, University of Tuzla, Tuzla, Bosnia and Herzegovina

Aida Duraković Faculty of Special Education and Rehabilitation, Department of Behavioural Disorder, University of Tuzla, Tuzla, Bosnia and Herzegovina

Julia Evangelista Centre for Cultural and Media Policy Studies, The University of Warwick, Coventry, UK

Bill Fulford Fellow, St Catherine's College, University of Oxford, Oxford, UK

William A. Fulford Faculty of Architecture and the Built Environment, The University of Westminster, London, UK

Michèle Gennart Centre de Recherches Familiales et Systémiques, Neuchâtel, Switzerland

Steven Gillard Social & Community Mental Health, Population Health Research Institute, St George's, University of London, London, UK

Caitlin Hick North Tec, Whangarei, New Zealand

Andrew Howie Whitiki Maurea Maori Mental Health and Addiction Service, Waitemata District Health Board, Auckland, New Zealand

Anna Hristova Institute of Mental Health and Development, Sofia, Bulgaria

Sik Hin Hung Centre of Buddhist Studies, University of Hong Kong, Hong Kong, China

Evette A. Hunkins-Hutchinson Faculty of Arts, Humanities and Cultures, University of Leeds, Leeds, UK

Justine Keen Service User, Bristol, UK

Colin King Lead Coordinator of the Whiteness and Race Equality Network, St Catherine's College, University of Oxford, Oxford, UK

Taryn Knox Bioethics Centre, University of Otago, Dunedin, New Zealand

Camillia Kong Institute for Crime and Justice Policy Research, School of Law, Birkbeck College, University of London, London, UK

Nermina Kravić Department of Child and Adolescent Psychiatry, Psychiatric Institution of Tuzla, Tuzla, Bosnia and Herzegovina

Lejla Kuralić-Čišić Faculty of Special Education and Rehabilitation, Department of Behavioural Disorder, University of Tuzla, Tuzla, Bosnia and Herzegovina

Janelle Lynne Kwee Master of Arts in Counselling Psychology Program, Faculty of Humanities and Social Sciences, Trinity Western University, Langley, BC, Canada

Ana Cristina Lopes Departamento de Psiquiatria, Centro Hospitalar de Entre o Douro e Vouga, Santa Maria da Feira, Portugal

Milena Mancini "G. d'Annunzio" University, Chieti, Italy

M. Y. Mantarkov Department of Psychiatry and Medical Psychology, Medical University of Plovdiv, Plovdiv, Bulgaria

Clinic of Psychiatry and Medical Psychology, University Multiprofile Hospital for Active Treatment "Sveti Georgi", Plovdiv, Bulgaria

Vanya Matanova Sofia University, Sofia, Bulgaria

Bulgarian Association of Clinical and Counseling Psychology and Bulgarian Association of Dyslexia, Sofia, Bulgaria

"Clinical Psychology in Action" Foundation, Sofia, Bulgaria

Institute of Mental Health and Development, Sofia, Bulgaria

Hillary Lianna McBride University of British Columbia, Vancouver, BC, Canada

Guilherme (G) Messas Department of Mental Health, Santa Casa de Sao Paulo School of Medical Sciences, São Paulo, Brazil

Postgraduate Program on Phenomenological Psychopathology, Santa Casa de São Paulo School of Medical Sciences, São Paulo, Brazil

I. Mitrev Department of Psychiatry and Medical Psychology, Medical University of Plovdiv, Plovdiv, Bulgaria

Clinic of Psychiatry and Medical Psychology, University Multiprofile Hospital for Active Treatment "Sveti Georgi", Plovdiv, Bulgaria

Michael Musalek Anton Proksch Institute, Vienna, Austria

Sadhana Natu Department of Psychology, Modern College, Ganeshkhind, Savitribai Phule Pune University, Pune, India

Disha Peer Support and Speak Out Group, Pune University, Pune, India

Neil Pickering Bioethics Centre, University of Otago, Dunedin, New Zealand

S. P. Popov Medical University, Plovdiv, Bulgaria

University Multiprofile Hospital for Active Treatment "Sveti Georgi", Plovdiv, Bulgaria

Mohammed Abouelleil Rashed Department of Philosophy, Birkbeck College, University of London, London, UK

Department of Philosophy, King's College London, London, UK

Waldo Roeg Central and North-West London Recovery and Wellbeing College, Central and North West NHS Foundation Trust, London, UK

Eisuke Sakakibara Department of Neuropsychiatry, The University of Tokyo Hospital, Tokyo, Japan

Oliver Scheibenbogen Department of Clinical Psychology, Anton Proksch Institute, Vienna, Austria

Richard J. Shaw Service User, Bristol, UK

Maria Julia (MJFR) Soares Postgraduate Program on Phenomenological Psychopathology, Santa Casa de São Paulo School of Medical Sciences, São Paulo, Brazil

Hospital do Servidor Público Estadual de São Paulo, São Paulo, Brazil

Dajana Stajić Department of Psychotherapy, Non-governmental Organization "Amica Educa", Tuzla, Bosnia and Herzegovina

Giovanni Stanghellini Department of Psychological, Health and Territorial Sciences, "G. D'Annunzio" University, Chieti Scalo, Italy

Drozdstoy Stoyanov Medical University Plovdiv, Plovdiv, Bulgaria

Tutiette Thomas South London and Maudsley NHS Foundation Trust, London Borough of Southwark, London, UK

Anna Todeva-Radneva Department of Psychiatry and Medical Psychology, Medical University of Plovdiv, Plovdiv, Bulgaria

Samuel Ujewe Canadian Institute for Genomics and Society, Toronto, ON, Canada

Werdie Van Staden Centre for Ethics and Philosophy of Health Sciences, University of Pretoria, Pretoria, South Africa

Jennifer Yim Shui Wa Tsz Shan Monastery Buddhist Spiritual Counselling Centre, Hong Kong, China

Tim Walker Former Chief Executive, General Osteopathic Council, London, UK

Lauren Weeks Mental Health Foundation, London, UK

Fiona Wilson Manaaki House Community Mental Health Centre, Auckland District Health Board, Auckland, New Zealand

Michael TH Wong Department of Psychiatry, Li Ka Shing Faculty of Medicine, The University of Hong Kong, Hong Kong, China

Kim Woodbridge-Dodd Faculty of Health, Education and Society, University of Northampton, Northampton, Northamptonshire, UK

Xiang Zou Department of Medical Humanities, Southeast University, Nanjing, China

Surprised by Values: An Introduction to Values-Based Practice and the Use of Personal Narratives in This Book

Bill Fulford

1.1 Introduction

Kim Woodbridge-Dodd, reflecting towards the end of this book with co-author Evette Hunkins-Hutchinson (chapter 44, 'Reflections on the impact of mental health ward staff training in race equality and values-based practice'), on their experience running a programme combining values-based practice with race equality training, expresses surprise at the difficulties they encountered:

- *I did not anticipate any difficulties. In addition to my earlier experience of staff members' positive attitude to change, I knew them all well—my office was just off the ward area and I spent much of my time either on the ward or nearby. Yet as described further below, a key learning point for me was my surprise at just how difficult for staff the training in this area proved to be.*

Kim was surprised by values. Values—the things *that matter or are important* to people—may seem obvious. But they have a disconcerting tendency to take us by surprise. Kim had many years experience working with values (she is the author of the original training manual for values-based practice, [1]) and she knew her ward staff well. Yet as she and Evette describe further in their chapter, she was much taken aback at the extent to which staff members, black and white, found their values challenged by the training.

It is the capacity of values to take us by surprise that motivates this book. Through a series of case narratives—many of them in the first person—we show how being

Authors
The editors with input from all contributors.

B. Fulford (✉)
St Catherine's College, University of Oxford, Oxford, UK

© The Author(s) 2021
D. Stoyanov et al. (eds.), *International Perspectives in Values-Based Mental Health Practice*, https://doi.org/10.1007/978-3-030-47852-0_1

surprised by values (notably cultural values) allows us to open up mental health to the resources needed to support person-centred clinical care.

We describe the structure and aims of the book in more detail below. First, what exactly are values?

1.2 Values

What are values? Philosophers, social scientists and others have found no quick or easy answer to this question. There are indeed deep theoretical challenges here to which Part II of this book is directed. But you can get a handle on the challenges by trying the following brief exercise.[1]

Write down three words (or very short phrases) that mean 'values' to you. Don't think too hard about this. Just write down the first three words that come into your head. Then compare what you wrote with the triplets of words in Table 1.1.

As Table 1.1 shows, people come up with very different triplets of words in this exercise. There are overlaps ('best interests' and 'principles', for example, both appear more than once). But no three words are the same. It is very likely that if you tried this for yourself, your three words were different again.

Table 1.1 Triplets of words from the 'three words' exercise in a training session for values-based practice

Figure 1.1—Example triplets of words in feedback from the 'three words' exercise	
Preferences	How we treat people
Needs	Attitudes
Best interests	Principles
Respect	Non-violence
Personal to me	Compassion
Difference … diversity	Dialogue
Beliefs	Responsibility
Right/wrong to me	Accountability
What I am	Best interests
Belief	What I *believe*
Principles	What makes me tick
Things held dear	What I won't compromise
Subjective merits	'Objective' core
Meanings	Confidentiality
Person-centred care	Honesty

---

[1] Kim Woodbridge-Dodd (co-author of chapter 'Reflections on the impact of mental health ward staff training in race equality and values-based practice') developed the three words exercise in the first training manual for values-based practice, 'Whose Values?' [1].

A first surprise from this exercise is thus the *diversity of meanings* people attach to the very word 'values'. A second surprise is that the word 'values' carries this diversity of meanings despite being familiar in everyday usage. Given this familiarity, it is natural we should suppose that we understand what 'values' means. Well, in a sense we do (we could all write down three words). But the surprise is that we all understand something *different* by 'values' (we all wrote down a different three words).

1.2.1 Values Are *What Matters or Are Important to Those Concerned*

The third surprise about values shown by this exercise is that notwithstanding its diversity of meanings there is a sense in which we can still agree what 'values' means. You can see this for yourself by looking again at the words listed in Table 1.1: Do you disagree with any of them? Most people answer 'no'. Most agree with everyone else's words.

An exception (that turned out to prove the rule) was Jim Smith's sausages.

*In a session on values-based surgical care for medical students, Jim Smith (not his real name), perhaps forewarned of the three words exercise, included 'sausages' in his triplet. 'Ah ah!' he said somewhat triumphantly at this point in the session, 'surely sausages have nothing to do with values!' But his colleagues quickly disabused him. 'Sausages', they pointed out, reminding him of his invariable choice of breakfast, 'have everything to do with **your** values!'*

Jim Smith's story strongly reinforces the key learning point from this exercise—the diversity of *individual* meanings attached to 'values'. But this brings us back to where we started. So, just what *are* values? In training sessions, focusing now on values in practice, participants come to see that for clinical purposes 'values' have to be understood as including *anything that matters or is important to those involved in a given situation.*

The clinical relevance of this broad use of the word 'values' is shown by the story of Mrs. Jones' knee.

1.2.2 Mrs. Jones' Knee[2]

Mrs. Jones (not her real name) was referred to an orthopaedic surgeon, Mr. Patel (not his real name), with painful arthritis in one of her knees. Mr Patel confirmed the diagnosis and told Mrs Jones they could go ahead with knee replacement surgery; she would need a period of physiotherapy; but 18 months from now she would in all likelihood be pain free.

---

[2]This story has been published in a number of places. As retold here, it is adapted from one of the case studies in [2].

As she got up to leave Mrs. Jones turned to Mr. Patel saying 'Thank you doctor, I'm so pleased I'll be able to garden again'. Mr. Patel asked her to tell him more. She explained that although her knee was indeed painful, what really mattered to her was that she could not bend it well enough to do her gardening. Mr. Patel then explained that while she would be pain free after the operation she would be no more mobile and possibly less so with the replacement knee joints currently available. So after further discussion they agreed to conservative management (physiotherapy and anti-inflammatories) in the first instance.

This worked well. Eighteen months later Mrs. Jones still had a painful knee but her mobility was restored and she was happily gardening again.

Mr. Patel knew from experience that pain relief was what mattered to most people with arthritic knees. This was the basis of his initial assumption about what mattered to Mrs. Jones. But had he not picked up on what *actually* mattered to her, the rather (in his experience) surprising value she placed on mobility (for gardening) over pain relief, Mrs. Jones would have ended up with a knee operation that although technically successful would have left her worse off (having now less mobility than before).

It is stories of this kind that explain the need for values-based practice as a partner to evidence-based practice in the delivery of contemporary person-centred clinical care.

1.3   An Introduction to Values-Based Practice

This section gives a brief introduction to values-based practice as a partner to evidence-based practice in clinical care.

1.3.1   Linking Science with People

In its partnership with evidence-based practice, values-based practice links science with people. As in the story of Mrs. Jones' knee, values-based practice links the science represented by evidence-based practice with the values of (with *what matters or is important to*) the individual patient involved in a given decision. The importance of this is illustrated by the following brief exercise. As with the 'three words' exercise, you may want to try this for yourself.

1.3.2   A Clinical Decision for You

In this exercise, you are asked to imagine yourself in the (clinically all too familiar) situation of being forced to choose between options neither of which is wholly satisfactory. Here, the situation is in imagination only. Even so, you may find it challenging.

You have developed early symptoms of a fatal disease. There are two possible treatments available and you can only choose one. Based on best current evidence,

- *TREATMENT A—gives you a guaranteed period of remission but no cure.*
- *TREATMENT B—gives you a 50:50 chance of 'kill or cure'.*

Now for your decision:

- *How long a period of remission would you want from Treatment A to choose that treatment rather than going for the 50:50 'kill or cure' from Treatment B?*

Remember the decision is about you. It is the *you* at *your* current age and in *your* current life situation, that is relevant, not what people in general would decide, still less what in some theoretical sense the 'right' answer would be.

Most people find this a difficult exercise—this is one of its learning points. But the main learning point is *how differently people react when faced with the same choice*. Everyone is offered the same options backed by the same evidence. Yet as Fig. 1.1 illustrates, people decide very differently.

The range of responses shown in Fig. 1.1 is typical. So where did you come in the range? And why did you choose the period you did? In discussion following this exercise, participants in training sessions come to see that they have made very different decisions solely because *their values* (the things *that matter or are important to them*) are very different. One person may choose, say, 20 years because they have a young family and want enough time to see them safely grown up; for another, their priority is to travel and for this a year would be enough to 'live life to the full'.

Fig. 1.1 Range of remission times required for choosing Treatment A over B

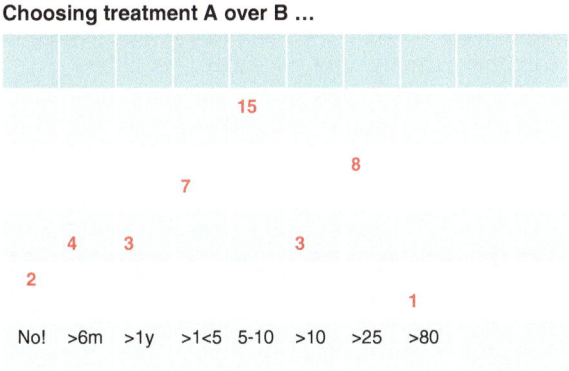

Choosing treatment A over B …

No! >6m >1y >1<5 5-10 >10 >25 >80

1.3.3   Zoe Barber's Surprise

A further surprise from this exercise for many people is just how differently *people they think they know really well* react from the way they expect. This was Kim Woodbridge-Dodd's surprise in the training sessions she recalled at the start of this chapter. It was the same surprise that Zoe Barber, a trainee surgeon, experienced. She recalls:[3]

The forced choice exercise [as above] *was a 'light bulb moment' for me. I was sitting next to my partner of 6 years who is also a trainee surgeon and from a similar background to mine. We often discuss difficult clinical decisions and I feel that we share similar outlooks and ambitions. However, his 'value for choosing treatment A' (18 months) compared to mine (25 years) completely astounded me.*

Once he explained his answer, I fully understood and agreed with it: his 18 months had to do with finishing his doctorate whereas my 25 years was tied up with starting a family. But at the time it was a big surprise. If I could misjudge the values of the man I share my life with so profoundly, just how wrong might I be in assuming that I know what is important to my patients? So this made me realize that unless we ask, we will never know what matters to our patients.

1.3.4   An Outline of Values-Based Practice

The message from the forced choice exercise can be summed up in the equation

$$\text{Same evidence} + \text{Different values} = \text{Different decisions}$$

So, as Zoe Barber realised and as Mr. Patel (above) discovered from experience, we cannot just assume we know what is important to other people. This is why the first and foundational skill for values-based practice is raised awareness of the surprising diversity of individual values. As long as we assume that we know what is important to other people, values-based practice, of the kind with which this book is concerned, simply can't get started.

Getting started, however, is no more than, well, getting started. Many other skills—communication skills, for example—are required for understanding the values in play in a given situation. And the sheer diversity of values involved brings all kinds of balancing complications into play. Hence, besides raising awareness, many further elements are required for successful implementation of values-based clinical care. These elements are shown diagrammatically in Fig. 1.2 and spelled out briefly in Table 1.2. Supported by a premise of mutual respect, ten process elements of values-based practice together support its outputs in balanced dissensual clinical decisions made within locally defined frameworks of shared values.

We return to these various elements of values-based practice in more detail in later chapters of the book (see especially the introductory chapters to each Part).

---

[3] This material is adapted from Zoe Barber's account of her experience published in [3].

Fig. 1.2 A summary flow diagram of values-based practice

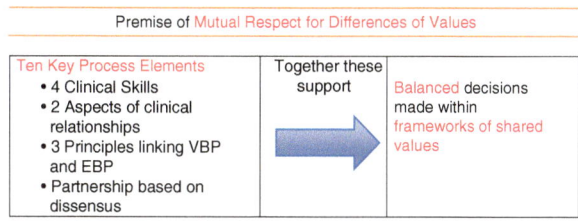

Table 1.2 Brief definitions of the elements of values-based practice

Values-based practice	Brief definition
Premise	
Mutual respect	Mutual respect for differences of values
Ten process elements	
Four clinical skills	
1. Awareness	Awareness of values and of the surprising diversity of individual values
2. Knowledge	Knowledge retrieval and its limitations
3. Reasoning	Used to explore the values in play rather than to close down on 'right answers'
4. Communication	Especially for eliciting values and of conflict resolution
Two aspects of clinical relationships	
5. Person-values-centred care	Care centred on the actual rather than assumed values of the patient
6. The extended MDT	MDT (multi-disciplinary team) role extended to include values as well as knowledge and skills
Three principles linking VBP and EBP	
7. Two-feet principle	All decisions are based on the 2 feet of values and evidence, including decisions about diagnosis
8. Squeaky wheel principle	We notice values when they cause difficulties (like the squeaky wheel) but (like the wheel that doesn't squeak) they are always there and operative. (with counterpart implications for evidence)
9. Science-driven principle	Advances in medical science drive the need for VBP (as well as EBP) because they open up choices and with choices go values
Shared clinical decision-making	
10. Shared clinical decision-making based on evidence and values	Shared clinical decision-making between clinician and patient or service user based on bringing together the relevant evidence with the values of those concerned
Outputs	
Locally defined frameworks of shared values	Values shared by those concerned in a given decision-making context (e.g. a GP practice) and within which balanced decisions can be made on individual cases
Balanced dissensual decisions within frameworks of shared values	Balanced decisions made within the relevant locally defined framework of shared values according to the circumstances presented by the case in question—The framework of shared values remains in play to be balanced sometimes one way and sometimes in other ways according to the particular circumstances presented by each case
Values tool kit	
Ethics	
Law	
Health economics	

1.3.5   Limitations

Values-based practice faces many challenges when it comes to implementation. Some of these are specific to particular circumstances. Other challenges, however, are built into the very fabric of the approach. Chief among these is what the political philosopher, Isaiah Berlin, writing in middle years of the Twentieth Century, in the shadow of National Socialism, identified as the challenge of values pluralism [4]. Our default, Berlin pointed out, when it comes to values, is monism: people want answers not options, they want to know or be told what is the right thing to do rather than having to make judgement calls. In the terms of this book, it is values monism not values pluralism that is our characteristic cultural 'value of values' as a species.

Well, values-based practice as we have described in this chapter is from top to toe pluralistic. It is all about the skills and other elements needed to support making judgement calls where complex and conflicting values are in play. Correspondingly, it has faced the challenge of pluralism when it comes to implementation (see Part VI). We return to the challenge of pluralism later in the book. As we will see cultural values although at the heart of the challenge of pluralism also provide many resources with which to respond to it (see, for example, chapter 20, 'Living at the Edge of Compromise: Balkan Pluralism as a Resource for Balanced Decision-Making' on Balkan pluralism and chapter 21, '"Thinking Too Much": A Clash of Legitimate Values in Clinical Practice Calls for an Indaba Guided by African Values-Based Practice' on the African indaba).

Values-based practice, moreover, besides facing many and deep-rooted challenges, is no panacea. It is, indeed, just one tool among others in what may be called the 'values tool kit' of health care. Other tools in the tool kit, as Table 1.2 indicates, include ethics, law, and health economics. We give further examples in Part IV, Science, with the roles respectively of African indabas (chapter 29, 'Policy-Making Indabas to Prevent "Not Listening": An Added Recommendation from the Life Esidimeni Tragedy'), transcultural ethics (chapter 30, 'Covert Treatment in a Cross-Cultural Setting') and anthropology (chapter 31, 'Discouragement Towards Seeking Health Care of Older People in Rural China: The Influence of Culture and Structural Constraints'), in the values tool kit. Values-based practice adds to the tool kit a particular focus on the uniqueness of individual values and a skills-based approach to resolving the difficulties this presents in coming to balanced decisions. This is important clinically as the contributions to this book illustrate. But values-based practice, to repeat, is just one tool among many others in the values tool kit.

1.4   Values-Based Practice and This Book

The chapters that follow in this book are organised broadly according to the above outline of values-based practice as summarised in Table 1.2.

Part I: Exemplars, sets the scene with three worked examples (stories respectively about anorexia, abnormal body experiences and psychosis) illustrating the role of cultural values (positive and negative) in the causes and presentation of mental health issues.

Part II: Theory, illustrates the range of additional resources for the theory supporting values-based practice that is opened up by engaging with cultural values. Values-based practice has thus far been based on the resources mainly of the ordinary language tradition of analytic philosophy (see below, Sect. 1.4.1, 'Why Now?'). Additional resources opened up by engaging with cultural values range from aesthetics and phenomenology through qualitative social science methods to African and Asian traditions of thought and practice.

Part III: Practice, is concerned with the practical resources that cultural values bring to the development and delivery of values-based mental health services. We focus in this Part on 'person-values-centred care', on the 'extended multidisciplinary team', on 'dissensus' and its role in shared clinical decision-making and on the contributions of these and other elements of values-based practice to recovery-oriented service provision.

Part IV: Science, covers the role of cultural values in influencing the impact of science on practice. In this regard, values-based practice links science with people. Contributing chapters thus examine the three principles of values-based practice of particular importance in this and the complementary roles of other resources from the wider values tool kit.

Part V: Training, explores the additional training demands of a culturally enriched form of values-based practice and the additional resources for training that is made available by it. Contributing chapters cover the four key skills areas of values-based practice: awareness, knowledge, reasoning and communication skills.

Part VI: Reflections, deals with the *RealPolitik* of implementing values-based practice. The three chapters in this section report on their authors' respective experiences of implementing values-based practice 'for real' in their respective contexts. Their shared message about implementing values-based practice can be summed up in one word—*difficult.*

Each part of the book thus illustrates the rich resources for values-based practice opened up by extending its scope from individual to cultural values. So rich, indeed, are these resources, it is natural to ask why values-based practice has taken so long (some 20 years in fact) to fully wake up to the importance of cultural values.

1.4.1 Why Now?

The answer to this question brings us to yet another surprise. For the answer is that it is a result of values-based practice itself having been blind to its own inherent values! There is irony in this surprise, in that, as noted above, values-based practice starts from and places particular emphasis on the importance of raised awareness of values.

With hindsight, it is clear that there are at least two reasons for the values blindness of values-based practice, one theoretical, one practical. The theoretical reason has to do with the origins of values-based practice in ordinary language philosophy

[5]. Interestingly, ordinary language philosophy grew out of insights into what may be called the cultural nature of language. We learn how to use words, these insights suggested, not from definitions (by looking them up in dictionaries for example) but through shared use in a social context.

When it came to applying this insight in practice, however, those concerned, consistently with the mores of their day, remained firmly individualistic in focus. J.L. Austin, for example, a founder figure in ordinary language philosophy [5], worked on the excuses made by individuals in legal court cases [6]. It is from Austin's ordinary language philosophy, applied first to the language of values [8], and then, in turn, to the language of medicine [10], that values-based practice is derived. This has proven to be a fruitful approach. Ordinary language philosophy lies behind many of the elements of values-based practice: its premise, many of its training exercises and its distinctive dissensual model of balanced decision-making [9]. All the same this was and remains an individual-centred approach.

The practical reason for the blindness of values-based practice to its own individualistic values has to do with its embedding in the equally individualist values of contemporary Western health care. The philosopher Sridhar Venkatapuram was the first to point this out [7]. Drawing on growing evidence of the importance of population-level factors as determinants of disease, he encouraged values-based practice to engage similarly at a cultural rather than merely individual level. This book thus owes its existence in part to Sridhar's acute observations.

1.5   The Role of Personal Narratives

In this book, each main chapter is grounded in personal narratives of one kind or another: some chapters start with conventional case histories, others are autobiographical, and still others take the form of dialogues.

1.5.1   Personal Narratives in This Book

In adopting this approach, we draw on deep historical and anthropological roots. Cave paintings at Lascaux in France depicting hunting scenes date from 20,000 years ago. Similar paintings recently discovered in Indonesia have pushed the origins of storytelling back still further to over 40,000 years [11]. Storytelling, indeed, as professional storyteller, Olusola Adebiyi, and co-authors, described in chapter 11, 'Madness, Mythopoetry and Medicine' has a strong track record throughout recorded human history as a resource both for teaching and for healing.

It is on this track record that we rely here. In whatever form they take, the personal narratives in this book convey, immediately and vividly, the values in play of those concerned in the stories they tell.

1.5.2   Personal Narratives and Evidence-Based Practice

In grounding the book in this way on personal narratives, it might seem that we are pitting ourselves against the received medical wisdom of the day as embodied in evidence-based practice. Personal narratives, after all, come right at the bottom of the evidence hierarchy.

There are, however, dissenting voices even within evidence-based medicine. The Oxford primary care clinician, Trish Greenhalgh, for example, has called for narratives to be brought back into evidence-based medicine alongside the standardly employed quantifications [12]. Here, we extend this approach by, in effect, inverting the evidence hierarchy, turning it right-upside-down.

This is shown diagrammatically in Fig. 1.3. The idea is that just as randomised controlled trials (aggregated by robust statistical methods) are among the best ways to learn about evidence (and thus come out at the top of the evidence hierarchy), so personal narratives are among the best ways to learn about values (thus coming out at the top of the values hierarchy).

1.5.3   Values in Evidence-Based Practice

That learning about values through personal narratives is very far from pitting ourselves against evidence-based practice is shown by the (perhaps surprising) extent to which values are themselves intertwined with evidence in evidence-based practice.

This intertwining is evident in many ways: in the embedded values guiding science—this is touched on by professional researcher, Steven Gillard, in chapter 46, 'Beyond the Color Bar: Sharing Narratives in Order to Promote a Clearer Understanding of Mental Health Issues across Cultural and Racial Boundaries' of this book; in the early days of evidence-based practice;[4] in the implementation of contemporary evidence-based practice—the UK's NICE,[5] for example, includes in

Fig. 1.3 Turning the evidence hierarchy of evidence-based practice upside down in values-based practice

Top of Hierarchy

RCTs for evidence … Personal narratives for values

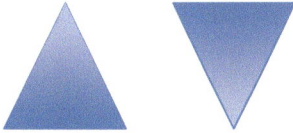

---

[4] David Sackett, in his role as first Director of Oxford's Centre for Evidence-based Medicine, defined evidence-based medicine as combining best research evidence with clinical experience and patients' values [13, p. 1].

[5] National Institute for Health and Care Excellence, the body responsible for producing evidence-based guidelines for the UK National Health Service.

the Preface to each of its evidence-based guidelines an explicit requirement that in employing their guidelines clinicians should 'take into account the individual needs, preferences and values of their patients or service users';[6] and in medical law—a recent decision from the UK's Supreme Court, the *Montgomery* judgement, makes consent dependent on a model of shared decision-making that brings together the clinician's knowledge of the evidence with the values of the individual patient concerned [2].

1.5.4 Individual and Cultural Values

In adding cultural values to the traditional focus of values-based practice on individual values, we should be careful to avoid swinging to the opposite extreme, focusing on cultural values at the expense of the individual. When it comes to values, as one of us has put it elsewhere [14], 'everyone is an *n* of 1'.

But here, too, personal narratives of the kind privileged in this book have a role to play. For in exploring cultural values through personal narratives, the person or persons with their individual values at the heart of each story, and their often surprising and uniquely individual ways of reacting within their respective cultures, remain very much at the front of our minds.

1.6 Conclusions

This chapter has provided an introduction to the book.

- *Section 2* described the key features of values relevant to understanding their role in health care—in this context (and correspondingly in values-based practice), values include *anything that matters or is important to those concerned in a given situation.*
- *Section 3* gave an overview of the framework elements of values-based practice. As summarised in Table 1.2, these elements cover, skills, service model, links between values and evidence, and shared clinical decision-making based on dissensual balancing within frameworks of shared values.
- *Section 4* outlined the structure of the book indicating how this reflects the framework elements of values-based practice while extending its scope from individual to cultural values.
- *Section 5* explained the prominence given to personal narratives in this book: personal narratives, we suggested, offer a powerful way of exploring values much as randomised controlled trials offer a powerful way of exploring evidence.

---

[6] See for example: National Institute for Health and Care Excellence (2015/2017) Suspected cancer: recognition and referral: NICE guideline NG12 (published date: June 2015. Last updated: July 2017) at: https://www.nice.org.uk/guidance/ng12 [and scroll down the page to the statement 'Your Responsibility'].

A theme running through this chapter has been the many surprises thrown by values: Kim Woodbridge-Dodd's surprise at the values revealed by mental health staff in a training exercise; Mr. Patel's surprise at Mrs. Jones' preference for mobility over pain relief in the treatment of her arthritic knee; Zoe Barber's surprise at her partner's values revealed by the 'forced choice' exercise; our own surprise that values-based practice had remained for so long blind to the influence of its own innate values of individualism; and surprises all round at the elevation of personal narratives from the bottom of the evidence hierarchy to the top of the values hierarchy.

And values have still one more surprise to spring, rather a pleasant surprise in fact, a surprise we will call the 'mental health first' surprise. But we will have more to say about that at the end of the book in our concluding chapter.

1.7   Guide to Further Information

For more on values-based practice including developments in values-based surgical care, please see the website for the Collaborating Centre for Values-based Practice in Oxford at: valuesbasedpractice.org.

The website includes a special section of its bespoke 'wikiVBP library' dedicated to the links and other materials indicated in the Guides to Further Information included in the chapters of this book.

References

1. Woodbridge K, Fulford KWM. 'Whose values?' A workbook for values-based practice in mental health care. London: The Sainsbury Centre for Mental Health; 2004.
2. Herring J, Fulford KWM, Dunn D, Handa A. Elbow room for best practice? Montgomery, patients' values, and balanced decision-making in person-centred care. Med Law Rev. 2017;25(4):582–603. https://doi.org/10.1093/medlaw/fwx029. https://academic.oup.com/medlaw/advance-articles.
3. Handa IA, Fulford-Smith L, Barber ZE, Dobbs TD, Fulford KWM, Peile E. The importance of seeing things from someone else's point of view. BMJ Careers on-line Journal (Published in hard copy as 'Learning to talk about values'). 2016. http://careers.bmj.com/careers/advice/The_importance_of_seeing_things_from_someone_else's_point_of_view.
4. Berlin I. Two concepts of liberty. Oxford: Clarendon Press; 1958.
5. Fulford KWM, van Staden W. Values-based practice: topsy-turvy take home messages from ordinary language philosophy (and a few next steps). Chapter 26. In: Fulford KWM, Davies M, Gipps R, Graham G, Sadler J, Stanghellini G, Thornton T, editors. The Oxford handbook of philosophy and psychiatry. Oxford: Oxford University Press; 2013. p. 385–412.
6. Austin JL. A plea for excuses. Proc Aristotelian Soc. 1956–1957;57:1–30. Reprinted in White AR, editor. The philosophy of action. Oxford: Oxford University Press; 1968. p. 19–42.
7. Hare RM. The language of morals. Oxford: Oxford University Press; 1952.
8. Fulford KWM. Moral theory and medical practice. Cambridge: Cambridge University Press; 1989, reprinted 1995 and 1999.

9. Fulford KWM. Living with uncertainty: a first-person-plural response to eleven commentaries on values-based practice. Chapter 13. In: Loughlin M, editor. Debates in values-based practice: arguments for and against. Cambridge: Cambridge University Press; 2014.
10. Venkatapuram S. Values-based practice and global health. Chapter 11. In: Loughlin M, editor. Debates in values-based practice: arguments for and against. Cambridge: Cambridge University Press; 2014.
11. New Scientist report (14 Dec 2019, p. 19) The earliest story tellers, citing. Nature. https://doi.org/10.1038/s41586-019-1806-y.
12. Greenhalgh T, Hurwitz B. Narrative based medicine: dialogue and discourse in clinical practice. London: BMJ Books; 1998.
13. Sackett DL, Straus SE, Scott Richardson W, Rosenberg W, Haynes RB. Evidence-based medicine: how to practice and teach EBM. 2nd ed. Edinburgh: Churchill Livingstone; 2000.
14. Fulford KWM, Peile E, Carroll H. A smoking enigma: getting and not getting the knowledge. Ch 6. In: Fulford KWM, Peile E, Carroll H, editors. Essential values-based practice: clinical stories linking science with people. Cambridge: Cambridge University Press; 2012. p. 65–82.

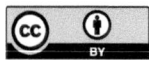

Bill Fulford

The narratives on which the three chapters included in this first Part are based all involve migration. Many other scenarios are explored in later chapters. But as the contributions to this part illustrate, scenarios involving migration helpfully exemplify a number of aspects of the significance of cultural values in mental health.

In this chapter, we start by briefly introducing the migration narratives as told in full in their respective chapters. We then draw out four common themes about cultural values exemplified by these narratives, indicating how they play out across the book as a whole.

2.1 The Migration Narratives

We open with a narrative from the New World, specifically Canada. In his case study of eating disorders across cultures (chapter 3, 'Antonella: 'A Stranger in the Family'—A Case Study of Eating Disorders Across Cultures'), psychiatrist Vincenzo Di Nicola relates the story of *a 24-year-old woman (Antonella)* who was referred to him with a pre-existing eating disorder after she migrated to Canada from Italy to join her partner. Antonella remains, as Vincenzo graphically puts it, 'a stranger in the family' until she connects emotionally with the Canadian wilderness and finds cross-species identification as a breeder of husky dogs.

In the next chapter (chapter 4, 'The Role of Culture, Values and Trauma in Shaping Abnormal Bodily Experience in Migrants'), Italian philosopher-psychiatrist Massimiliano Aragona examines the role of culture, values and trauma in shaping

Authors
The editors with input from the contributors to Part I.

B. Fulford (✉)
St Catherine's College, University of Oxford, Oxford, UK

abnormal bodily experiences in migrants. Massimiliano draws on four contrasting narratives from his extensive experience as a clinician working with migrants: a *30-year-old Bangladeshi man (MD)* who emigrated to Italy after a natural disaster at home leaving his wife and sons in Bangladesh; *a 40-year-old Pakistani woman (Shafia)* who arrived at a migrant reception centre in Italy with her two sons after being abandoned by her husband; *a 43-year-old Ugandan woman (Pretty)* who presented in a neuropsychiatry outpatient clinic with persistent and unexplained headache; and *a 23-year-old Nigerian man (Godwin)* who had fled to Italy when his father died to avoid taking up his preordained role in his home village as a fetish priest.

With the final chapter in this Part (chapter 5, 'Premorbid Personality and Expatriation as Possible Risk Factors for Brief Psychotic Disorder: A Case Report from Post-Soviet Bulgaria'), we move from Italy to post-Soviet Bulgaria, with psychiatrists, Stefan Popov and Mladen Mantarkov's exploration of the interactions between premorbid personality and expatriation in the aetiology of brief psychotic disorder. They present the story of *a 29-year-old single Bulgarian woman (Alice)* who developed psychotic symptoms while living and working alone in Germany. Like many others, Alice had migrated to Germany after the fall of the Soviet regime in Bulgaria in the hope of finding a better life. Once she settled back in Bulgaria, her psychotic symptoms resolved. Popov and Mantarkov speculate on the possible wider significance of the protective Bulgarian cultural values from which Alice benefitted in recovering her mental health.

2.2   Common Theme 1: Cultural Values May Have a Negative Role Acting as Factors in the Causes and Presentation of Mental Health Issues

Cultural factors are widely recognised to be important in the causes and presentation of mental health issues. With eating disorders, as Vincenzo Di Nicola notes in chapter 3, this recognition extends to the role specifically of cultural *values*. The prevalence of eating disorders, as he describes, varies widely between cultures (arguably) corresponding with variations in cultural values—the cultural importance of 'fashionable slimness', for example, has been identified with the greater prevalence of eating disorders among women in industrialised societies. Not only that, but the form these disorders take appears to vary between cultures. Vincenzo Di Nicola has coined the term 'anorexia multiforme' to capture the extent of this culturally driven variation in clinical presentations of anorexia.

With many other mental health issues, however, while the importance of cultural factors has been recognised, the impact specifically of cultural *values* has by and large been overlooked. Massimiliano Aragona (chapter 4) makes this point in respect of somatisation disorders. The roles of trauma and culture in shaping these disorders, he suggests, are well recognised, but, again, the role specifically of cultural values has been relatively neglected. The four narratives he presents are aimed at remedying this neglect for somatisation disorders. Chapter 5 makes a similar point in respect of brief psychotic episodes. Stefan Popov and Mladen Mantarkov's story of Alice brings out the hitherto neglected role of cultural and other values interacting with personality and life events in provoking psychotic breakdowns.

Taken together therefor the narratives presented in the three chapters of Part I illustrate the impact not just of culture but specifically of cultural values on the causes and presentation of three representative kinds of mental health issue. The importance of cultural values these narratives thus suggest is not limited to a narrow group of 'culture-bound disorders'. It is generic. Other chapters in the book extend the range of conditions that are demonstrably impacted by cultural values still further: eating disorders and psychosis continue to figure strongly in the book, but to these are added, in Part III alone, for example, identity disorders in adolescence (chapter 16, 'Cross-Cultural Factors and Identity in Adolescence'), depression and infanticide (chapter 17, 'Multidisciplinary Teamwork and the Insanity Defence: A Case of Infanticide in Iraq') and alcoholism (chapter 19. 'Alcohol Use Disorder in a Culture that Normalizes the Consumption of Alcoholic Beverages: The Conflicts for Decision-Making'). Many other examples are to be found elsewhere in the book.

2.2.1   A Note on Diagnostic Categories

In noting the role of cultural values across these diagnostic categories, we should not be taken as endorsing the categories in question, still less the supposedly 'value free' descriptive terms by which they are standardly defined. To the contrary, a number of chapters later in the book illustrate the role of cultural and other values in delineating the boundary between health and illness: chapters 13, 'Spiritual, Religious and Ethical Values in a Suicidal Individual' and 14, 'Cultural Values, Religion and Psychosis: Five Short Stories', for example, are concerned with the boundary between mental disorder and spiritual experience, and chapter 17, 'Multidisciplinary Teamwork and the Insanity Defence: A Case of Infanticide in Iraq' is concerned with the scope of the 'insanity defence'.

We return below to the relationship between cultural values and mental health science as reflected in contemporary descriptive classifications of mental health issues (see common theme 3). But our point here as we have said is not to endorse (nor indeed to critique) current diagnostic categories. It is rather to note that once we start looking for them, prompted as we have been by the migration narratives presented in this Part, we find cultural values evident across the board in mental health.

2.3 Common Theme 2: Cultural Values May Also Play Positive Roles Acting as Protective Factors for Mental Health

The news about cultural values, though, is, as they say, 'not all bad'. Yes, cultural values may be important in provoking and shaping mental health issues: Massimiliano Aragona's four narratives in chapter 4 illustrate these negative influences all too well. But cultural values may also exert positive influences.

These positive influences are evident in the protective roles of cultural values exemplified particularly by the narratives in the other two chapters in this Part. Vincenzo Di Nicola's Antonella (chapter 3) was only able to move towards recovery when she found a sense of identity in her role as a breeder of Husky dogs in the Canadian wilderness. Stefan Popov and Mladen Mantarkov (chapter 5) note that Alice's sustained recovery from her psychotic symptoms once she was allowed to leave Germany and return home, may well have resulted from the positive and supportive work environment prevailing in her native Bulgaria. They speculate that similar cultural values may have wider significance as protective factors in mental health.

As with the negative influences of cultural values, their positive roles are reflected across the book as a whole. There is no scope for romanticism here. Cultural values may have highly negative effects. The recovery narratives with which Part III concludes (chapters 22, 'Three Points in Time: How Values and Culture Affected My Life, Madness and the People Around Me' and 23, 'Recovery and Cultural Values: On Our Own Terms (A Dialogue)') illustrate these negatives influences all too well. But these same narratives also show that cultural values may have positive impacts as well. This mix of positive and negatives is also evident elsewhere in the book. African cultural attitudes for example may be responsible for male suicide (chapter 10, 'African Personhood, Humanism, and Critical Sankofaism: The Case of Male Suicide in Ghana') but African Mythopoetry (chapter 11, 'Madness, Mythopoetry and Medicine') heals; Brazilian values may normalise problem drinking (chapter 19, 'Alcohol Use Disorder in a Culture that Normalizes the Consumption of Alcoholic Beverages: The Conflicts for Decision-Making') but Brazilian carnival liberates (chapter 18, 'Colonial Values and Asylum Care in Brazil: Reclaiming the Streets through Carnival in Rio de Janeiro') and so on.

2.3.1 Balancing Positives and Negatives

Balancing positives and negatives is important. It is natural that clinicians should focus on the negatives—it is after all with the negatives of problem situations that clinicians are concerned day-to-day. But in mental health, understanding the balance of positives and negatives is important to effective care: Roz Austin's two contrasting narratives (chapter 34, 'Values-Based Practice When Engaging with Voice-Hearers'), of Paul and Mary, make the point about the need for balance in relation to voice hearing. When it comes to recovery in mental health, furthermore, it is the positives that are often key. This is true for example in the three autobio-graphical recovery narratives in this book (chapters 22, 'Three Points in Time: How Values and Culture Affected My Life, Madness and the People Around Me', 23 'Recovery and Cultural Values: On Our Own Terms (A Dialogue)' and 32, 'Discovering Myself, a Journey of Rediscovery'). The importance in recov-ery of the StAR values of values-based practice (Strengths, Aspirations and Resources) is correspondingly recognised in UK good practice guidance.[1]

Again, the point exemplified by the narratives in this Part is about balance. Cultural values may be inimical to recovery but they may be the key to recovery as well. The challenge is to recognise both kinds of influence and to balance them in a way that works for the individual concerned. It is to this challenge that the resources for training in values-based practice illustrated by the contributions to Part V are centrally directed.

2.4 Common Theme 3: Narrative Understanding of Cultural Values

The importance of narrative understanding of cultural values—the third theme exemplified by the contributions to Part I—was anticipated by what we said about inverting hierarchies in our introduction to values-based practice in chapter 1, Sect. 1.5.3.[2] Where narratives, as we put it, come at the bottom of the evidence hier-archy, they come at the top of the corresponding hierarchy for values.

The rationale for this inversion of hierarchies is evident in the contributions to Part I. Each of the narratives presented speaks to us directly. The validity of Antonella's story for example (chapter 3, 'Antonella: 'A Stranger in the Family'—A Case Study of Eating Disorders Across Cultures') does not depend on the availabil-ity of a randomised controlled trial of the impact of the Canadian wilderness on personal identity (still less does it depend on there being available a meta-analysis of multiple such trials). In the context of her story, this speaks to us directly. We understand *Antonella*. We understand her as one human being understands another. This is the power of narrative.

It is the need for narrative understanding that underpins the importance of many of the philosophical resources explored in Part II of this book. Aesthetics (chap-ter 7, 'The Will to Beauty as a Therapeutic Agent: Aesthetic Values in the Treatment of Addictive Disorders') and phenomenology (chapters 8, 'Anorexia as Religion: Ocularcentrism as a Cultural Value and a Compensation Strategy in Persons with Feeding and Eating Disorders' and 9, 'Ethos, Embodiment, and Psychosis: Losing One's Home—Identity Stakes') are both directly concerned with understanding as distinct from explanation. So, too, is hermeneutics, with its intriguing links with the

---

[1] The StAR values of values-based practice were derived from co-produced guidance on best prac-tice in mental health assessment sponsored by the UK Department of Health [1].

[2] See especially Fig. 3, chapter 1, 'Surprised by Values: An Introduction to Values-Based Practice and the Use of Personal Narratives in this Book'.

Critical Sankofaism of African philosophy (chapter 10, 'African Personhood, Humanism, and Critical Sankofaism: The Case of Male Suicide in Ghana'). The storytelling tradition of African Mythopoetry (chapter 11, 'Madness, Mythopoetry and Medicine') directly exemplifies the power of narrative understanding. All these resources furthermore come together to good effect in exploring specific aspects of the role of cultural values in mental health: the impact of cultural values on body image for example (chapter 12, 'Inside and Out: How Western Patriarchal Cultural Contexts Shape Women's Relationships with Their Bodies') and their role in delineating psychopathological and spiritual experiences (chapters 13, 'Spiritual, Religious and Ethical Values in a Suicidal Individual' and 14, 'Cultural Values, Religion and Psychosis: Five Short Stories').

Our selection of topics in Part II, as with other areas of the book, is far from exhaustive. There are whole areas of contemporary philosophy that deserve mention. From the history of ideas, for example, we could have included Karl Jaspers' distinction between meaningful understanding and causal explanation [2] and how this became one of the building blocks of his seminal General Psychopathology [3]. Relevant too are whole areas of the philosophy of mind: work on 'other minds' for example is all about our capacity for understanding what is going on in someone else's mind. The latter, furthermore, reinforcing the theme of partnership, is one of the many areas of contemporary philosophy where psychopathology informs philosophy as well as philosophy psychopathology[3] (for examples, see [4]).

So understood, the importance of narrative understanding of values is an aspect of the essential partnership between values-based practice and evidence-based practice outlined in chapter 1.[4] It is to the importance of this partnership as reflected in the contributions to this book that we turn next.

2.5   Common Theme 4: The Partnership Between Cultural Values and Mental Health Science

Whereas the first three themes exemplified by the contributions to Part I have all been evident in what was said, the fourth theme is evident in what has not been said. It is evident in the fact that in drawing out the importance of cultural values in mental health, the contributors to Part I have said nothing against the importance of science in mental health.

Well, some may respond, they would say that, wouldn't they! The authors of the three chapters making up Part I are all psychiatrists, and psychiatry is committed to a scientific view of mental health issues. But that is precisely our point. Yes, psychiatry—along with other mental health disciplines such as psychology—is committed to a scientific understanding of mental health. This is indeed one of the key

---

[3] See, for example, work on theory of mind and autism [4] and on deafness [5] and, for a different view [6].

[4] See in particular the first part of Sect. 3, chapter 1, 'Surprised by Values: An Introduction to Values-Based Practice and the Use of Personal Narratives in this Book'.

cultural values of psychiatry as a medical discipline. In the terms of chapter 1, 'Surprised by Values: An Introduction to Values-Based Practice and the Use of Personal Narratives in this Book', science *matters or is important to* psychiatry as a medical discipline. The authors of the chapters in Part I are in this respect well placed to represent the cultural values of psychiatry: Vincenzo Di Nicola is indeed a leading international figure in the medical scientific discipline of transcultural psychiatry.

Our point therefor, the point of the final theme to be taken from the contributions to Part I, is that there is no contradiction between, on the one hand, recognising the importance of cultural values in mental health and, on the other hand, recognising the importance equally of mental health science.

This 'no contradiction' conclusion is consistent with the partnership model of the relationship between values and science in values-based practice described in chapter 1.[5] The contributions to Part IV, Science, later in this book, fill out this partnership model. The early chapters of Part IV between them illustrate the impact of cultural values on the three principles of values-based practice by which (as described in chapter 1) its relationship with evidence-based practice is characterised: the Two Feet principle (chapter 25, 'A Cross-Cultural Values-Based Approach to the Diagnosis and Treatment of Dissociative (Conversion) Disorders'), the Squeaky Wheel principle (chapters 26, 'Treatment of Social Anxiety Disorder or Neuroenhancement of Socially Accepted Modesty? The Case of Ms. Suzuki' and 27, 'Nontraditional Religion, Hyper-Religiosity, and Psychopathology: The Story of Ivan from Bulgaria') and the Science Driven principle (chapter 28, 'Journey into Genes: Cultural Values and the (Near) Future of Genetic Counselling in Mental Health'). These three principles together characterise how values-based practice 'links science with people'. The remaining chapters in Part IV reflect the importance of the wider 'values tool kit'[6] of healthcare in linking science with people, illustrated respectively by the African indaba (chapter 29, 'Policy-Making Indabas to Prevent "Not Listening": An Added Recommendation from the Life Esidimeni Tragedy'), transcultural ethics (chapter 30, 'Covert Treatment in a Cross-Cultural Setting') and anthropology (chapter 31, 'Discouragement Towards Seeking Health Care of Older People in Rural China: The Influence of Culture and Structural Constraints').

Migration narratives, to return to the focus of this Part, provide a case in point of the Squeaky Wheel principle. It is through migration that cultural values are most likely to come into conflict and it is where values come into conflict that they are drawn to our attention—it is when they come into conflict that in the metaphor of the Squeaky Wheel, the values in question 'squeak'. This is why migration narratives of the kind presented in this Part are particularly helpful in drawing out and making explicit the operation of cultural values in mental health. But to extend the

---

[5] See footnote 4 above.

[6] See the final part of Sect. 3, and Table 2, chapter 1, 'Surprised by Values: An Introduction to Values-Based Practice and the Use of Personal Narratives in this Book'.

Squeaky Wheel metaphor, just as the wheel is still there and important even when it is not squeaking, so, too, are cultural values there and important across the board in mental health.

2.6   Conclusions

We have discussed four themes about the role of cultural values in mental health exemplified by the migration narratives described in the three chapters making up Part I of this book. Taken together, these narratives indicate (1) that cultural values have a *negative role* in mental health, impacting as they do on the causes and presentation of mental health issues well beyond the limits of traditionally defined 'culture-bound' syndromes; (2) that cultural values also have a *positive role* as protective factors, notably in contributing to recovery in mental health; (3) that *narrative understanding* is as important for understanding values as randomised controlled trials and other empirical resources are important for understanding evidence; and (4) that the relationship between values (cultural and otherwise) and science in mental health is best understood as one of *partnership*.

We have indicated how these four themes play out across and are further developed in later parts of the book. The importance of narrative understanding is reflected in the diverse contributions to Part II, Theory. The impact (positive as well as negative) of cultural values on mental health is reflected particularly in Part III, Practice. The partnership between values and science is reflected in Part IV, Science. And, lest it be thought we have neglected Part V, Training, it was with the training tasks presented by all four themes in mind that we gave our introduction to that Part (chapter 33), the title 'Training for Task'.

We recognise that a partnership model of the relationship between values and science is far from universally accepted. There are many, we openly acknowledge, who from adverse personal experiences reject outright any role whatsoever for science in mental health. There are many others, we also recognise, who in defence of what they take to be a scientific perspective, reject outright any role whatsoever for values in mental health. The partnership model adopted here will satisfy neither of these extremes. It is however consistent with the framing of values within values-based practice as 'linking science with people'. And it is through this frame, we believe, it is through the frame of values as linking science with people that a deeper understanding of cultural values will contribute to improvements in mental health care.

References

1. National Institute for Mental Health in England (NIMHE) and the Care Services Improvement Partnership. 3 Keys to a shared approach in mental health assessment. London: Department of Health; 2008. Also available as a free full-text download from the Collaborating Center for Values-based Practice at http://valuesbasedpractice.org/More-about-VBP/Full-text-downloads.

2. Jaspers K. Causal and meaningful connexions between life history and psychosis. Ch. 5. In: Hirsch SR, Shepherd M, editors. Themes and variations in European psychiatry. 1974. Bristol: John Wright and Sons Ltd; 1913. p. 80–93.
3. Jaspers K. Allgemeine Psychopathologie. Berlin: Springer; 1913. (Trans. Hoenig J, Hamilton MW. General psychopathology. Chicago: University of Chicago Press; 1963. New edition (two volumes, paperback), with a Foreword by Paul R McHugh, Baltimore: The Johns Hopkins University Press; 1997.
4. Avramides A. Other minds. London: Routledge; 2000.
5. Peterson CC, Siegal M. Insights into theory of mind from deafness and autism. Ch 5. In: Coltheart M, Davies M, editors. Pathologies of belief. Oxford, Blackwell Publishers; 2000.
6. Hobson RP. Against the 'theory of mind'. Br J Dev Psychol. 1991;9:33–51.

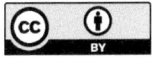

Antonella: 'A Stranger in the Family'—A Case Study of Eating Disorders Across Cultures

3

Vincenzo Di Nicola

3.1 Introduction

Eating disorders are a potentially fruitful area of study for understanding the links between values—in particular cultural values—and mental distress and disorder. Eating disorders show widely different prevalence rates across cultures, and much attention has been given to theories linking these differences with variations in cultural values. In particular, the cultural value placed on 'fashionable slimness' in the industrialised world has for some time been identified with the greater prevalence of eating disorders among women in Western societies [1]. Consistently with this view, the growing prevalence of eating disorders in other parts of the world does seem to be correlated with increasing industrialisation [2, 3]. In my review of cultural distribution and historical evolution of eating disorders, I was so struck by its protean nature and its variability of clinical presentations of anorexia nervosa that I renamed this predicament 'anorexia multiforme' [4, 5].

The story of Antonella that follows illustrates the potential importance of contemporary theories linking cultural values with eating disorders though also some of their limitations.

V. Di Nicola (✉)
Canadian Association of Social Psychiatry (CASP), World Association of Social Psychiatry (WASP), Department of Psychiatry and Addictions, University of Montreal, Montreal, QC, Canada

Department of Psychiatry and Behavioral Sciences, The George Washington University, Washington, DC, USA
e-mail: vincenzodinicola@gmail.com

3.2   Case Narrative: Antonella's Story

Ottawa in the early 1990s. Antonella Trevisan, a 24-year-old woman, was referred to me by an Italian psychiatrist and family therapist, Dr. Claudio Angelo, who had treated her in Italy [6]. When Antonella came to Canada to live with a man she had met through her work, Dr. Angelo referred her to me. Antonella's presenting problems concerned two areas of her life: her eating problems, which emerged after her emigration from Italy, and her relationship with her partner in Canada.

3.2.1   Antonella's Predicament

My initial psychiatric consultation (conducted in Italian) revealed the complexities of Antonella's life. This was reflected in the difficulty of making an accurate diagnosis. Her food-related problems had some features of eating disorders, such as restriction of intake, the resulting weight loss, and a history of weight gain and being teased for it. What was missing was the 'psychological engine' of an eating disorder: a drive for thinness or a morbid fear of fatness. Her problem was perhaps better understood as a food-related anxiety arising from a 'globus' sensation (lump in the throat) and a learned avoidance response that generalized from one specific situation to eating in any context.

Although it was clear that her weight gain in late adolescence and the teasing and insults from her mother had sensitized her, other factors had to be considered. Antonella showed an exquisite rejection sensitivity that both arose from and was a metaphor for the circumstances of her birth and adoption. Her migration to Canada also seemed to generate anxieties and uncertainties, and there were hints of conflicts with her partner. Was she also re-enacting another, earlier trauma? In the first journey of her life, she was given up by her birth mother (or taken away?) and left on the steps of a foundry. In the first year of her life, Antonella had shown failure to thrive and developmental delays. And she had, at best, an insecure attachment to her adoptive family, predisposing her to lifelong insecurities.

3.2.2   A Therapeutic Buffet

After my assessment, we faced a choice: whether to treat the eating problem concretely, in purely behavioral terms, or more metaphorically, with some form of psychotherapy. Given the stabilization of her eating pattern and her weight and the larger context of her predicament, we negotiated to do psychotherapy. There were several components to her therapy. Starting with a psychiatric consultation, three types of therapy were negotiated, with Antonella sampling a kind of 'therapeutic buffet' over a period of some 2 years: individual therapy for Antonella, couple therapy for Antonella and Rick, and brief family therapy with Antonella's adoptive family visiting from Italy.

The individual work with Antonella was at first exploratory, getting to know the complex bicultural world of the Italian Alps, how she experienced the move to Canada, examining her choices to move here and live with Rick. Sessions were conducted in a mix of Italian and English. At first, the Italian language was like a 'transitional object' in her acculturation process; slowly, as she gained confidence in her daily life, English began to dominate her sessions. Under stress, however, she would revert to Italian. I could follow her progress just by noting the balance of Italian and English in each session. This does not imply any superiority of English or language preferences; rather, it acknowledges the social realities of culture making its demands felt even in private encounters. This is the territory of sociolinguistics [7, 8]. Like Italian, these individual sessions were a secure home base to which Antonella returned during times of stress or between other attempts to find solutions.

After some months in Canada and the stabilization of her eating problems, Antonella became more invested in examining her relationship to Rick. They had met through work while she was still in Italy. After communicating on the telephone, she daringly took him up on an offer to visit. During her holiday in Canada, a romance developed. After her return to Italy, Antonella made the extraordinary decision to emigrate, giving up an excellent position in industry, leaving her family for a country she did not know well. Rick is 22 years her senior and was only recently separated from his first wife.

In therapy she not only expressed ambivalence about her situation with Rick but enacted it. She asked for couple sessions to discuss some difficulties in their relationship. Beyond collecting basic information, couple sessions were unproductive. While Rick was frank about his physical attraction to her and his desire to have children, Antonella talked about their relationship in an oddly detached way. She could not quite articulate her concerns. As we got closer to examining the problems of their relationship, Antonella abruptly announced that they were planning their wedding. The conjoint sessions were put on hold as they dealt with the wedding arrangements.

Her parents did not approve of the marriage and boycotted the wedding. Her paternal aunt, however, agreed to come to Canada for the wedding. Since I was regarded by Antonella as part of her extended family support system, she brought her aunt to meet me. It gave me another view of Antonella's family. Her aunt was warm and supportive of Antonella, trying to smooth over the family differences. A few months later, at Christmas time, her parents and sister visited, and Antonella brought them to meet me. To understand these family meetings, however, it is necessary to know Antonella's early history.

3.2.3 A Foundling Child

Antonella was a foundling child. Abandoned on the steps of a foundry in Turin as a newborn, she was the subject of an investigation into the private medical clinics of Turin. This revealed that the staff of the clinic where she was born was 'paid off to hide the circumstances of my birth.' As a result, her date of birth could only be presumed because the clinic staff destroyed her birth records. She was taken into care by the state and, as her origins could not be established, she was put up for adoption.

Antonella has always tried to fill in this void of information with meaning that she draws from her own body. She questions me closely: 'Just look at me. Don't you think I look like a Japanese?' She feels that her skin tone is different from other Italians, that her facial features and eyes have an 'Asian' cast. With a few, limited facts, and some speculation, she has constructed a personal myth: that she is the daughter of an Italian mother from a wealthy family (hence her hidden birth in a private clinic) and a Japanese father (hence her 'Asian' features). It is oddly reassuring to her, but also perhaps a source of her alienation from her family.

At about 6 months of age, Antonella was adopted into a family in the Italian Alps, near the border with Austria. This is a bicultural region where both Italian and German are spoken and services are available in both languages (much like Ottawa, which is bilingually English and French). Her father, Aldo, who is Italian, is a retired FIAT factory worker. Annalise, her mother, who is a homemaker, had an Italian father and an Austrian mother. About her family she said, 'I had a wonderful childhood compared to what came afterwards.' Years after her adoption, her parents had a natural child, Oriana, who is 15.

She describes her mother as the disciplinarian at home. Her mother, she said, was 'tough, German.' When she visited her Austrian grandmother, no playing was allowed in that strict home. Her own mother allowed her 'no friends in the house,' but her father 'was my pal when I was a kid.' Although she had a good relationship with her father, he became 'colder' when she turned 13. Her parents' relationship is remembered as cordial, but she later learned that they had many marital problems. Mother told her that she married to get away from home, but in fact she was in love with someone else. Overall, the feeling is of a rigid family organization. Her father is clearly presented by Antonella as warmer and more sociable. She experiences her mother as being 'tough'. But she is crying all the time, feeling betrayed by everybody.

3.2.4   A Family Visit from the Italian Alps

When her family finally came to visit, Antonella brought them to see me. At first, the session had the quality of a student introducing out-of-town parents to her college teacher. They were pleased that I spoke Italian and knew Dr. Angelo, who they trusted. I soon found that the Trevisans were hungry to tell their story. Instead of a social exchange of pleasantries, this meeting turned into the first session of an impromptu course of brief family therapy.

Present were Antonella's parents, Aldo and Annalise, and her sister, Oriana. Annalise led the conversation. Relegating Aldo to a support role. Oriana alternated between disdain and agitation, punctuated by bored indifference. Annalise had much to complain about: her own troubled childhood, her sense of betrayal and abandonment, heightened by Antonella's departure from the family and from Italy.

I was struck by the parallel themes of abandonment in mother and daughter. Mother clearly needed to tell this story, so I tried to set the stage for the family to hear her, what narrative therapists call 'recruiting an audience' [9]. I used Antonella, who I knew best, as a barometer of the progress of the session, and by that indicator, believed it had gone well.

When I saw them again some 10 days later, I was stunned by the turn of events. Oriana had assaulted her parents. The father had bandages over his face and the mother had covered her bruises with heavy make-up and dark glasses. Annalise was very upset about Oriana, who was defiant and aggressive at home. For her part, Oriana defended herself by saying she had been provoked and hit by her mother. Worried by this dangerous escalation, I tried to open some space for a healthy standoff and renegotiation.

Somehow, the concern had shifted away from Antonella to Oriana. Antonella was off the hook, but I waited for an opening to deal with this. I first tried to explore the cultural attitudes to adolescence in Italy by asking how the Italian and the German subcultures in their area understood teenagers differently. What were Oriana's concerns? Had they seen this outburst coming? The whole family participated in a kind of sociological overview of Italian adolescence, with me as their grateful audience. The parents demonstrated keen insight and empathy. Concerned about Oriana's experience of the session, I made a concerted effort to draw her into it. Eventually, the tone of the session lightened. Knowing they would return to Italy soon, I explored whether they had considered family work. Since they had met a few times with Dr. Angelo over Antonella's eating problems, they were comfortable seeing Dr. Angelo as a family to find ways to understand Oriana and her concerns and for Oriana to explore other, nonviolent ways to be heard in the family. I agreed to meet them again before their departure and to communicate with Dr. Angelo about their wishes. On their way out, I wondered aloud about the apparent switch in their focus from Antonella to Oriana. The parents reassured me that they were ready to let Antonella live her own life now.

When they returned to say goodbye, we had a brief session. Oriana and Antonella were oddly buoyant and at ease. The parents were relieved. Antonella had offered the possibility of Oriana returning to spend the summer in Canada with her. I tried to connect this back to the previous session, wondering how much the two sisters supported each other. I was delighted, I said emphatically, by the family's apparent approval of Antonella's marriage to Rick. It was striking that, even from a distance of thousands of miles away, Antonella was still a part of the Trevisan family. And Rick was still not in the room.

3.3   Discussion

In this section, I will consider the impact of cultural and other values on Antonella and those around her and then look briefly at the wider implications of her story for our understanding not only of eating disorders but of mental distress and disorders in general.

3.3.1   Antonella: Life Before Man

The key to understanding Antonella's attachments was her passion for her Siberian huskies. In the language of values-based practice, it was above all her huskies that mattered or were important to her. And it is not hard to see why. From the beginning of her relationship with Rick, she used her interest in dogs as a way for them to be more socially active as a couple, getting them out of the house to go to dog shows, for example. As her interests expanded, she wanted to buy bitches for breeding and to set up a kennel. Rick was only reluctantly supportive in this. Nonetheless, they ended up buying a home in the country where she could establish a kennel. Her haggling with Rick over the dogs was quite instrumental on her part, representing her own choices and interests and a test of the extent to which Rick would support her.

Yet the importance to Antonella of her huskies rests I believe on deeper cultural factors, both negative and positive. As to negative factors, these are evident in the fact that from the first days of her life, Antonella was rejected by her birth parents, literally abandoned and exposed, and later adopted by what she experienced as a non-nurturing family. Positive cultural factors, on the other hand, are evident in the way that having thrown her net wider afield, she looked initially to Canada, and to Rick, for nurturance and for identity. Then, finding herself only partly satisfied, she turned to the nonhuman world for the constancy of affection she could not find with people. Her huskies gave her pleasure, a task, and an identity. She spent many sessions discussing their progress, showing me pictures of her dogs and their awards. As it happened, my secretary at the time was also a dog lover who raised Samoyed dogs (related to huskies) and the two of them exchanged stories of dog lore.

As to positive factors, again, is there something, too, in the mythology of Canada that helps us understand Antonella? Does Canada still hold a place in the European imagination as a 'New World' for radical departures and identity makeovers? Or does Canada specifically represent the 'malevolent North,' as Margaret Atwood [10] calls it in her exploration of Canadian fiction? Huskies are a Northern animal, close to the wolf in their origins and habits. Bypassing the human world, Antonella finds her identity within a new world through its animals. If people have failed her, then she will leave not only her own tribe (Italy), but skip the identification with Canada's Native peoples, responding to the 'call of the wild' to identify with a 'life before man' (to use another of Atwood's evocative phrases, [11]), finding companionship and solace with her dogs.

3.3.2   Wider Implications of Antonella's Story

Antonella may seem on first inspection something of an outlier to the human tribe. Orphaned from her culture of origin, she finds her place not in another country but by identification with another and altogether wilder species, her husky dogs. Yet, understood through the lens of values-based practice Antonella's story has, I believe, wider significance at a number of levels.

First, Antonella's story is significant for our understanding of the role of values – of what is important or matters to the individual concerned – in the presentation and treatment of eating disorders, and, by extension, of perhaps many other forms of mental distress and disorder. Specifically, her story provides at least one clear 'proof of principle' example supporting the role of cultural values.

As noted in my introduction, much attention has been given in the literature to the correlations between the uneven geographical distribution of eating disorders and cultural values. Correlations are of course no proof of causation. But in Antonella's story at least the role of cultural values seems clearly evident. They were key to understanding her presenting problems. And this understanding in turn proved to be key to the cultural family therapy [12] through which these problems were, at least to the extent of her presenting eating disorder, resolved.

The cultural values involved, it is true, were not those of fashionable slimness so widely discussed in the literature. But this takes us to a second level at which Antonella's story has wider significance. For it shows that to the extent that cultural values are important in eating disorders, their importance plays out at the level of individually unique persons. In this sense, social stresses and cultural values are played out in the body of the individual suffering with an eating disorder, making her body the 'final frontier' of psychiatric phenomenology [13]. Yes, there are no doubt valid cultural generalisations to be made about eating disorders and mental disorders of other kinds. And yes, these generalisations no doubt include generalisations about cultural values—about things that matter or are important to this or that group of people as a whole. Yet, this does not mean that we can ignore the values of the particular individual concerned. It has been truly said in values-based practice that as to their values, everyone is an 'n of 1' [14]. Antonella, then, in the very idiosyncrasies of her story, reminds us of the idiosyncrasies of the stories of each and every one of us, whatever the culture or cultures to which we belong.

Antonella's identification with animals, furthermore, to come to yet another level at which her story has wider significance, was a strongly positive factor in her recovery. As with other areas of mental health, it is with the negative impact of cultural values that the literature has been largely concerned: the pathogenetic influences of cultural values of slimness being a case in point in respect of eating disorders. Antonella's story illustrates what has been clear for some time in the 'recovery movement', that positive values are often the very key to recovery. Not only that, but as Antonella's passion for her husky dogs illustrates, the particular positive values concerned may, and importantly often are, individually unique.

Not, it is worth adding finally, that Antonella's values were in this respect entirely unprecedented. Animals, after all, are widely valued, positively and negatively, and for many different reasons, in many cultures [11]. Their healing powers are indeed acknowledged. Just how far these powers depend on the kind of cross-species identification shown by Antonella, remains a matter for speculation. But, again, her story even in this respect is far from unique. Elsewhere, I have described the story of a white boy with what has become known as the 'Grey Owl Syndrome', wishing to be native [12, chapter 5]. Similarly, in *Bear*, Canadian novelist Marion Engel [15] portrays Lou, a woman who lives in the wilderness and befriends a bear. Lou seeks her identity from him: 'Bear, make me comfortable in the world at last. Give me your skin' [15, p. 106]. After some time with the bear, the woman changes: 'What had passed to her from him she did not know.... She felt not that she was at last human, but that she was at last clean' [15, p. 137]. It was perhaps to some similarly partial resolution that Antonella came.

3.4   Conclusions

Antonella's story as set out above goes to the heart of the importance of cultural values in mental health. Her presenting eating disorder develops when, displaced from her culture of origin in Italy, and in effect rejected by her birth family, she finds healing only through cross-species identification with the wildness of husky dogs in her adoptive country of Canada. Although somewhat unusual in its specifics, her story illustrates the importance of cultural values at a number of levels in the presentation and management of eating and other forms of mental distress disorder.

And Antonella? I met her again in a gallery in Ottawa, rummaging through old prints. She was asking about prints of dogs; I was looking for old prints of Brazil where my father had made a second life. How was she, I asked? 'Well …,' she said hesitantly. Was that a healthy 'well' or the start of an explanation? 'Me and Rick are splitting up,' she said without ceremony, 'but I still have the huskies.' For each of us, the prints represented another world of connections.

Acknowledgements The story of Antonella was first published in reference [12] (pp. 214–220) and presented at the Advanced Studies Seminar of the Collaborating Centre for Values-based Practice in Health and Social Care at St Catherine's College, Oxford in October 2019. The names and other details of the case have been altered to maintain confidentiality. Parts of the discussion are adapted from that publication and the Oxford seminar. I am grateful to the publishers for permission to reproduce these materials here and to Professor Fulford and the members of the Advanced Studies Seminar for their stimulating exchanges. The subheading to the discussion of Antonella's story ('Life before Man') was inspired by Margaret Atwood's novel, *Life Before Man* [11].

3.5   Guide to Further Sources

For a more extended treatment of the role of culture in eating disorders and family therapy see:

- Di Nicola VF (1990a) Overview: Anorexia multiforme: Self-starvation in historical and cultural context. I: Self-starvation as a historical chameleon. *Transcultural Psychiatric Research Review, 27(3):* 165–196.
- Di Nicola VF (1990b) Overview: Anorexia multiforme: Self-starvation in historical and cultural context. II: Anorexia nervosa as a culture-reactive syndrome. *Transcultural Psychiatric Research Review, 27(4):* 245–286.
- Di Nicola, V (1997) *A Stranger in the Family: Culture, Families, and Therapy.* New York & London: W.W. Norton & Co.
- Nasser M and Di Nicola, V. (2001) Changing bodies, changing cultures: An intercultural dialogue on the body as the final frontier. In: Nasser M, Katzman M A, and Gordon R A, eds. *Eating Disorders and Cultures in Transition.* East Sussex, UK: Brunner-Routledge, pp. 171–193.

References

1. Makino M, Tsuboi K, Denerson L. Prevalence of eating disorders: a comparison of Western and non-Western countries. MedGenMed. 2004;6(3):49. Published online 2004 Sep 27 at: https://www.ncbi.nlm.nih.gov/pubmed.
2. Erskine HE, Whiteford HA, Pike KM. The global burden of eating disorders. Curr Opin Psychiatry. 2016;29(6):346–53.
3. Selvini Palazzoli M. Anorexia nervosa: a syndrome of the affluent society. Transcult Psychiatr Res Rev. 1985;22(3):199–205.
4. Di Nicola VF. Overview: anorexia multiforme: self-starvation in historical and cultural context. I: self-starvation as a historical chameleon. Transcult Psychiatr Res Rev. 1990;27(3):165–96.
5. Di Nicola VF. Overview: anorexia multiforme: self-starvation in historical and cultural context. II: anorexia nervosa as a culture-reactive syndrome. Transcult Psychiatr Res Rev. 1990;27(4):245–86.
6. Andolfi M, Angelo C, de Nichilo M. The myth of atlas: families and the therapeutic story. Edited & translated by Di Nicola VF. New York: Brunner-Routledge; 1989.
7. Douglas M. Humans speak. Ch 11. In: Implicit meanings: essays in anthropology. London: Routledge & Kegan Paul; 1975. p. 173–80.
8. Crystal D. The Cambridge encyclopedia of language. Cambridge: Cambridge University Press; 1987.
9. Parry A, Doan RE. Story re-visions: narrative therapy in the postmodern world. New York: Guilford Press; 1995.
10. Atwood M. Strange things: the malevolent north in Canadian literature. Oxford: Oxford University Press; 1995.
11. Atwood M. Life before man: a novel. New York: Anchor Books; 1998.
12. Di Nicola VF. A stranger in the family: culture, families, and therapy. New York: W.W. Norton & Co.; 1997.
13. Nasser M, Di Nicola V. Changing bodies, changing cultures: an intercultural dialogue on the body as the final frontier. Ch 9. In: Nasser M, Katzman MA, Gordon RA, editors. Eating disorders and cultures in transition. East Sussex: Brunner-Routledge; 2001. p. 171–93.
14. Fulford KWM, Peile E, Carroll H. A smoking enigma: getting and not getting the knowledge. Ch 6. In: Fulford KWM, Peile E, Carroll H, editors. Essential values-based practice: clinical stories linking science with people. Cambridge: Cambridge University Press; 2012. p. 65–82.
15. Engel M. Bear: a novel. Toronto: Emblem (Penguin Random House Books); 2009.

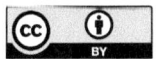

The Role of Culture, Values and Trauma in Shaping Abnormal Bodily Experience in Migrants

4

Massimiliano Aragona

4.1 Introduction

In most cultures, somatization is a common idiom of distress. However, the way somatization is expressed varies between persons and across cultures. Psychologically, there are theories linking somatization symptoms to cognitive biases in selecting information or to deeper problems in symbolization. Many researchers believe that traumatic experiences have causal power in determining neurocognitive modifications. Largely unexplored, however, is exactly how culture, values and trauma interact to shape abnormal bodily experiences.

It is this shaping that I explore in this chapter through four brief ideal-typical (and carefully anonymized) clinical narratives. Taken together, these show that such shaping may occur in different ways, facilitating, genetic, plastic and interpretive.

4.2 Narrative Histories

1. *MD was a 30-year old Bangladeshi man. He emigrated to Italy after a natural disaster leaving his wife and sons in Bangladesh. He presented with worries about economic issues affecting his parents and sons. He did not talk about himself, complaining only of bodily symptoms, in particular a sense of burning in his stomach. A gastroenterologist found no pathophysiological reason for these symptoms. Worries, difficulty in concentration and learning, sleep difficulty, weakness and low mood, were other symptoms that were later found to have been present. It was only with time, when he started to trust the doctor and to understand that he would not be judged negatively for his symptoms, that he*

M. Aragona (✉)
Italian National Health System, Rome, Italy

Mental and Neuro Sciences, Rome, Italy
e-mail: email.aragona@gmail.com

© The Author(s) 2021

D. Stoyanov et al. (eds.), *International Perspectives in Values-Based Mental Health Practice*, https://doi.org/10.1007/978-3-030-47852-0_4

started talking about the other phenomena. It then became clear that his symptoms had started with a loss of energy consequent on nocturnal emission. His initial response to this was an acute anxiety reaction, with tachycardia, sweating, and related symptoms. His first idea was about something morally wrong, but soon he focused on the medical symptoms (see discussion below on culture for the effect of semen loss on bodily energy). *He felt exhausted but unable to sleep. Starting from this first episode, he developed enduring weakness and loss of appetite. Then when he tried to eat something he felt burning pain in the stomach, and this was the main initial symptom presented to the physician.*

Transcultural psychiatrists would easily recognize here a typical culture-bound syndrome (the so-called Dhat), typical of the South-Asian regions. This patient (as is usually the case) failed to admit the full array of symptoms on his first visit, complaining only of the burning pain.

2. *Shafia was a 40-year old Pakistani woman. She was dressed in typical clothes, and arrived crying. A staff member of the migrant reception center where she was housed together with two sons (aged 11 and 14) accompanied her. In her face sadness and hopelessness were easy to detect. She had a severe headache and was unable to find the energy to talk. During the interview, she made no eye contact and remained with her head reclined on the shoulder of the person accompanying her. She had arrived 2 months earlier to rejoin her husband who had been in Italy for 10 years. In Pakistan she had lived with her husband's family where she felt loved by her mother-in-law as well as by her husband's brothers. She worked as a kindergarten teacher and felt herself to be well regarded by the members of her community. Her husband regularly sent money to Pakistan, where he periodically returned to visit his family. During the last visit he was confronted by his mother who told him it was time to take responsibility for his family: he had either to definitively return to Pakistan or take his family to Italy with him. In the end he decided to activate the procedure for family reunion. But when his wife and sons arrived in Italy, they discovered he was living with another woman. He segregated them in a room, without permission to go out, and started beating his wife for trivial reasons. After 1 week he abandoned them near the airport, where days later they were found by a police officer and taken to a centre for women victims of family violence.*

Clinically, Shafia had major depression with secondary headache. She was treated with antidepressants but these had little effect. With time, a different picture emerged: despite depression, Shafia was exemplary in the way she cleaned and ordered her room, as well as in the education of her children. Nevertheless, when she had to be active in order to find a job or to follow the procedure for the renewal of the permission of stay, lack of energy and abulia (lack of will) became incapacitating. In discussing this difference of energy depending on context, it became clear that for Shafia wellbeing was a matter of being in the right social role in the right way. She was ready to understand that in a reception center cleaning the room and doing services was valued, but had no idea that in Italian society you are expected to become active in order to receive what you deserve. With time, she understood the difference and became more flexible, with self-determined activation to reach what she needed. That she had become flexible enough to orient herself in the new society became clear when she, a Pakistani woman, asked an Indian male friend for information and support about a job. Correlatively, her depression and headache had disappeared.

3. *Pretty was a 43-year old Ugandan woman. She presented with a very severe headache recurring over 3 years. Several physicians had visited her, a Nuclear Magnetic Resonance and an EEG were negative, and the diagnosis was still undetermined. Several therapies had had little or no effect. During the interview, it was clear that although her headache was the presenting problem, many other symptoms were present as well: intrusive post-traumatic thoughts and memories, hyper-arousal, negative ideas about herself, with regrets and depression, difficulty in sleeping, nightmares with a post-traumatic content, etc. Eventually it emerged that in her home country Pretty had discovered and reported corruption in the school where she was a teacher. She had subsequently been kidnapped, beaten and sexually abused before managing to escape and leave the country. Unfortunately, like many other migrants coming from the Sub-Saharan regions, she had to cross Libya, where she was again kidnapped and sexually abused several times.*

   It was after her arrival in Italy that Pretty' headaches and the post-traumatic symptoms began. The headache episodes were typical. They occurred in therapy when she was asked to remember the traumatic events in her past and were associated with changes in her facial expression: retracted lips, teeth clenched, brow lowered, eyes part-closed, weeping. All these symptoms including her headache disappeared within a few minutes, leaving only a sense of feebleness, when Pretty was reassured that she did not have to talk about her experiences there and then (they could be picked up it in another session, or perhaps not at all), with the focus of the session shifting to practical issues in her everyday life.

4. *Godwin was a 23-year old Nigerian man. His father was a fetish priest, a traditional priest with the role of mediating between the spirit world and the living, particularly in health matters. In this role, Godwin's father had to perform rituals sometimes including violence against other people. When he died, Godwin was required by the law of the village to take his place (fetish priests are often selected from specific families 'possessed' by the god). He refused, but this was not accepted because it could have caused misfortunes to the community. As a consequence Godwin was threatened with death. He left the village, and, in turn, being afraid he would be found in other cities, the country. In Libya he was kidnapped, tortured and sold as a slave. In that period he became constantly watchful, afraid of everything, and unable to sleep because the memories of his horrifying experiences of violence continuously came to his mind.*

On arrival in Italy Godwin experienced initial relief of his symptoms. After a while, however, intrusive thoughts about the Libyan experiences returned and he experienced further sleep disturbance. He took 2 or 3 h to fall asleep, because of intrusive memories of the Libyan experience, with rumination and hyper-arousal. When he was finally able to sleep, he suffered recurrent dreams, starting with the image of his father offering fruits, and then changing with an increase of

emotional tension and the feeling that undefined persons were touching him, try-
ing to throttle him. When asked about his own interpretation of this, Godwin said
that it was the spirit of his father persecuting him because he had refused to take
the place he was born for. The fruit (in his dream) was an invitation to rejoin the
group, and the attack was because of his refusal. The people touching him in his
dream were perhaps the other members of the sect in the village. He knew that
all this could not be real but at the same time believed that someone in his village
may have made a ritual to recall his father's spirit and that this was the reason
for his suffering. He had come to Europe in the hope that the distance would be
enough to prevent the magic influence touching him: but sadly he had found that
its power was strong enough to be effective even at this distance.

4.3   Discussion

In this discussion, the role of trauma, values and culture will be considered. There
is of course an overlap between culture and values. The latter, interpreted generally
as what is important for or matters to the person, are clearly part of culture. But the
reverse does not always apply. If we consider as cultural everything that has a meaning (a signification), then values refer only to those aspects of culture that are significant (that matter, that have importance) to the person concerned. Thus, values
are a subset of all cultural items. Traumas may appear as something more objective,
but they have a psycho-traumatic role depending on the way they are personally
experienced.

Clearly, all three factors, trauma, values and culture, are important in any given
case. In this discussion, however, I will focus on values. This is partly for reasons
of space and partly because of the relative neglect of values in earlier
publications.

Trauma. All cases experienced at least one severe traumatic experience in their
life. However, they were different. In case 1, it was a natural disaster that acted as a
migration push factor adding to already precarious economic conditions; in case 2,
it was a matter of intra-familial violence and abandonment in a foreign country; in
cases 3 and 4, we have the (unfortunately typical) severe, long-lasting and repeated
interpersonal violence in Libya, but also torture and sexual abuses in the subject's
own country (case 3), while in case 4 in the country of origin, there were menaces
and threats to life albeit without direct physical violence.

These cases together illustrate the established finding in the literature that traumatic experiences may have different roles and clinical effects depending on the
kind of trauma, the contextual situation, the characteristics of the person involved,
the possibility or impossibility of giving meaning to the experience and so on. In our
cases, the traumatic events have a pathogenetic role in cases 2, 3 and 4, although
only in 3 and 4 do we find a typical post-traumatic reaction that takes the form of
PTSD. This means that the pathogenetic effect of traumatic experience is often but
not always typical; in some cases (like case 2), it causes other kinds of reactions,
depending on other factors involved that will be discussed below.

Values. The values permeating these four stories are potentially infinite. The following selection is based on my own perception of their relevance for the cases under discussion. Other selections are of course possible but I hope these—and in particular the conflicts of values they illustrate—will indicate the important though neglected role of cultural values in the aetiology, presentation and management of somatizations in different reactive mental disorders.

In case 1 (the Bangladeshi man with a sense of burning in the stomach following nocturnal emission), there is a conflict between ethical and religious duties on the one side, which give value to sexual purity and restraint, hence forbid sexual relationships outside marriage, and, on the other side, the fact that a young man who remains alone for a long time normally has sexual needs that can explain nocturnal emission. In this case, the value conflict was largely implicit—the patient had the initial ephemeral idea of a moral conflict with consequent anxiety and guilt but this was soon replaced by a preoccupation with bodily functioning. Here, we can say that the value conflict has a pathogenetic role, because it is one of the causes from which the phenomenon arises: i.e. nocturnal emission is the key experience that makes possible the following onset of the Dhat syndrome, a necessary although not sufficient cause (cultural factors are also required).

In case 2, there are several conflicts of values, two of which seem particularly relevant in this context. The first is the conflict we imagine took place in Shafia's husband. For years, he lived a double life, husband and father working abroad on one side, while on the other side he was the partner of another woman in Italy. The first life is in line with traditional values that are common in Pakistan; the latter could be normal in the Western country in which he is living but clashes with the values of his country of origin and must be kept secret. In fact, nobody in his family would understand and accept his "Italian" behaviour. The balance achieved (a public identity and a secret one) fails when he feels forced by his mother to accept his wife and sons joining him in Italy. We can never be sure, but both the violence and the unplanned abandonment of the family at the airport suggest he was totally unable to find a way to manage his internal conflict, i.e. only impulsive acts were available to discharge the tension. This first conflict of value, in Shafia's husband, has no direct pathogenetic effect but it is what makes it possible to delineate a contextual situation in which interpersonal violence emerges as a possible way to escape the tension.

The second conflict of values emerging in this case is that between traditional, society-centred identity and individuation. Shafia will react to what happened according to her culture (see below) but in the new context, where a more direct activation is required, this way of behaving is not appropriate. It is around this conflict of values (i.e., "Do I stay in my place or do I activate to have what I need?") that psychotherapy will contribute to help Shafia to change her stance in order to be able to act in ways more useful for her life in Italy.

In case 3, the values initially clashing are Pretty's honesty against a social context where corruption is frequent and shared by many actors. A second conflict is between universal rights that guarantee to victims of violence like Pretty the right to request asylum in Europe, and the European political pragmatic agreements with

Libya that condemn hundreds of sub-Saharan migrants to sexual abuse, torture and other forms of re-traumatization. If Pretty had been allowed to arrive in Europe directly from a sub-Saharan state, instead of crossing Libya, at least the second part of her terrible experience could have been avoided.

Finally, there is the conflict between the interviewer's need to know her history (that *must* be presented to the territorial commission entitled to decide about her asylum request), and Pretty's need to avoid such memories. In this last case, the values involved in the pre-migration context and in Libya are those that contribute to create a social environment in which such extreme forms of interpersonal violence can take place. They have no direct pathogenetic role (the traumatic experiences are those responsible for the onset of PTSD), but it is clear that in different social contexts, this story would probably not begin at all. The third one, instead, i.e. the conflict between socially construed expectations that she has to tell in detail what she experienced, and her distress in trying to do so, has a direct pathogenetic role in the emergence of headache as a conflict solution, allowing the patient and the interviewer to stop the enquiry into distressing memories.

In case 4, there is the conflict between, on the one side, the traditional spiritual beliefs of a society and the social roles stemming from them, and, on the other side, the individual refusal by the patient to take up these roles. There are parallels with the previous case: the conflict of values has no direct pathogenetic role but creates the contextual preconditions for the story; and there is the traumatic experience in Libya with the same conflict of values arising. Finally, there is in this case an interesting conflict within the patient himself: on one side, he rejects traditional values and does not accept his inheritance of his father's role; on the other side, his interpretation of his symptoms is based on traditional beliefs like those he had refused. It was not possible to investigate this conflict more deeply during our meetings, so I will refrain from speculating about the role of this deep internal conflict in the pathogenesis of his problems.

Culture. Case 1, the Bangladeshi man with Dhat, is an example of a typical culture-bound syndrome in which culture has a clear pathogenetic effect. In case 2 (of Shafia, the woman beaten by her husband), culture has a pathoplastic role, i.e. it is not at the origins of the psychopathological reaction but it shapes the symptoms according to the cultural background. This is why she showed no improvement with antidepressants but did improve (slowly) when she started to reflect about her attitude and came to accept the idea that in Italy a woman must be active in pursuing her goals. In the case of Pretty (case 3), culture does not have a primary role, the symptoms (including the headache) being typical reactions to severe interpersonal violence. Her headache for example has to be seen as part of an avoidance mechanism that is frequent and phenomenally similar in many traumatized patients, often independently from country, ethnicity and culture of origin.

Finally, Godwin (case 4), the man who refused to be a fetish priest, presents yet another way in which culture may enter into the construction of mental symptoms, namely in a modality we could call "pathointerpretation." Godwin presents the full range of typical post-traumatic symptoms, including sleep disorder and nightmares, but he reads them through the cultural glasses of magic influences. Godwin's interpretation thus has a significant role in shaping what medical anthropologists call the "illness," i.e. the subjective experience of being ill, the disease as seen from the standpoint of the patient. This is again important for the effectiveness of treatment Only if the "illness" experienced by the patient is in accordance with the "disease" as the physician sees it from his professional standpoint, will good collaboration and compliance be possible.

4.4   Conclusion

This chapter discusses four narratives where trauma, culture and values contribute in different ways to how bodily experiences are shaped. These factors may be patho-facilitating (creating a social context which is necessary for the experience to take place), pathogenetic (taking a causal role in the onset of the psychopathological reaction), pathoplastic (shaping the form such a psychopathological reaction takes) or pathointerpretive (different interpretation of the same symptoms depending on the patient's beliefs).

While previous accounts have recognized the roles of trauma and culture, the four narratives presented in this chapter illustrate the importance also of values, including cultural values, in the aetiology, presentation and management of somatization disorders. As a consequence, the therapeutic approach in any given case has to be adjusted depending on the particular way all three factors interact in the patient's construction of their mental distress.

Acknowledgements Dr. Aragona wrote this chapter as an independent researcher (formal communication at his home institution, Protocol No. 2131 dated 11 April 2019).

4.5   Guide to Further Sources

Please see the following for further reading on the links between culture and trauma:

- Ali F, Chemlali A, Andersen MK, Skar M, Ronsbo H, Modvig J. Consequences of torture and organized violence. Libya needs assessment survey. Copenhagen: DIGNITY Publication Series; 2015.
- Aragona M, Catino E, Pucci D, Carrer S, Colosimo F, Lafuente M, et al. The relationship between somatization and posttraumatic symptoms among immigrants receiving primary care services. J Trauma Stress. 2010; 23:615 622.

- Aragona M, Geraci S, Mazzetti M. Quando le ferite sono invisibili. Vittime di tortura e di violenza: strategie di cura [When wounds are invisible. Victims of torture and violence: healing strategies.]. Bologna: Pendragon; 2014.
- Tseng W-S. Handbook of cultural psychiatry. San Diego, CA: Academic Press; 2001.

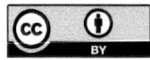

Premorbid Personality and Expatriation as Possible Risk Factors for Brief Psychotic Disorder: A Case Report from Post-Soviet Bulgaria

5

S. P. Popov and M. Y. Mantarkov

5.1 Introduction

After the collapse of communist rule in 1989, democratic changes occurred in Bulgaria. These involved renewal not only of freedom of speech but also of freedom of movement of people to other European countries. Over one million people left the country either permanently or as temporary workforce resulting in the greatest demographic collapse in Bulgarian history. Initially those who left the country were proud to taste freedom and live the western dream. At that time, few thought about the difficulties with cross-cultural adaptation and the price they would have to pay…

We report the case of a young Bulgarian woman, who lived and worked in Germany for 10 years before she presented with symptoms of brief psychotic disorder. Her story is based on that of a real person but with her name and other biographical details changed to protect confidentiality. It illustrates the possible contribution of cultural values interacting with her premorbid personality and experiences of expatriation as risk factors in the etiology of the condition.

5.2 Alice's Story

At the time of her emergency admission to an inpatient psychiatric facility in Cologne, Germany, Alice (not her real name) was a 29-year-old single Bulgarian woman with no prior psychiatric history. Her family and general medical history were unremarkable and she had no unhealthy lifestyle habits other than smoking about 5 cigarettes a day. Although she was born with signs of perinatal asphyxia, Alice reached all major developmental milestones as expected.

S. P. Popov (✉) · M. Y. Mantarkov
Department of Psychiatry and Medical Psychology, Medical University, Plovdiv, Bulgaria

University Multiprofile Hospital for Active Treatment "Sveti Georgi", Plovdiv, Bulgaria
e-mail: stefan_popov@yahoo.com; mantarkov@gmail.com

Alice was brought up in a family with a dominant, authoritarian father and a passive, submissive mother. She went to a German language school in Bulgaria from which she graduated with top marks. She was also a keen basketball player. Ten years prior to her admission Alice moved to Germany and obtained a master's degree in finance while working in a number of part-time jobs. After she finished her studies she worked simultaneously as a stock analyst and a private tutor. A year and a half before the admission she started work as an event organizer for a catering company because she could not find a job in her field of competence. At that time she enjoyed a good standard of living. Her family described Alice as "active, enterprising and independent."

About a week prior to her admission Alice became increasingly tense and irritable. According to her housemate she worked more than 12 h a day and hardly got any sleep. On the morning of the admission she became visibly agitated and emotionally unstable and confided that she had sensations of electricity passing through her body. She felt that she could connect with her colleagues through this electricity. When an ambulance was called she became aggressive, threw apples at the medical staff and bit her housemate's arm. At the hospital she was diagnosed with brief psychotic disorder with marked stressors. She was treated with Perphenazine 4 mg t.i.d. and discharged in 6 days with a marked reduction of psychotic symptoms.

After the discharge Alice went back to her family in Plovdiv, Bulgaria. She adhered to treatment for about 10 days after which she discontinued the medication because she could not obtain a timely resupply. In a matter of days she grew tense and verbally aggressive to her family. She insisted her mother helped her "chase away the Devil." She left her home, switched off her mobile phone and went to the city's ancient amphitheater where she scattered her belongings and stuck advertising stickers on the stones. She talked about Bulgarian traditions, ancient rituals and attributed symbolic meanings to current events. She was admitted to the university psychiatric clinic in Plovdiv where laboratory work-up and a CT brain scan showed no clinically significant findings. The patient was treated with Olanzapine 10 mg q.d., consequently tapered to 5 mg q.d. due to sedation. The psychotic symptoms resolved relatively quickly and the patient was discharged calm, free of psychotic symptoms and with good insight.

In view of the importance of personality disorders in brief psychotic disorder upon resolution of psychotic symptoms the patient was referred for psychological assessment and testing. Schmieschek's personality accentuation test showed signs of accentuation of the demonstrative and pedantic type, a tendency for accentuation of the suspicious and emotive type, and a significant accentuation of the hyperthymic and anxious and fearful type. Psychological exploration identified the patient's habitually excessive level of activity as a coping mechanism to deal with negative thoughts and feelings. A strong drive for independence coexisted with a low level of emotional differentiation. The patient returned to her premorbid level of functioning but refused to go back to Germany.

However, her father thought Alice must work and prosper in Germany. He himself had dreamt of a good life in Germany during his youth and had tried to escape from Bulgaria to Germany via Yugoslavia but was detained and arrested. The dream *should be realized at any cost. He refused to recognize that Alice had really been ill and was convinced "it was just too much stress; she is a brave girl and will make it." At her father's insistence Alice went back to Germany and tried to begin work there. Despite strict medication adherence, every time she started a new job, her condition worsened with depressed mood, ideas of reference and vague persecutory ideation associated with her superiors and colleagues. A year later she moved home to Sofia, Bulgaria and started a job as a financial auditor. She continued her treatment with Olanzapine 5 mg q.d. for a year. Three years ago she was tapered off her medication by her psychiatrist and has had no mental health problems since.*

5.3   Discussion

Brief Psychotic Disorder is a transient, sometimes recurrent, psychotic disorder in which symptoms persist for at least 1 day and resolve in less than a month with a return to the former level of functioning [1]. The condition is uncommon, typically occurs in adolescence or young adulthood and is twice as frequent in women as in men. In the majority of cases, brief psychotic disorder is precipitated by marked stressors that overwhelm the individual's coping skills. Thus, both acute and chronic stress, underdeveloped social skills, isolation and lack of social support may increase the risk for brief psychotic disorder. According to the DSM-5, the presence of a personality disorder is also a recognized risk factor [1].

Traveling and living abroad have long been recognized as risk factors for psychotic disorders. In view of the established association between stress and brief psychotic disorder, it is not surprising the disorder has often been described in relation to travel stress. It is hypothesized that the isolation of long-distance travel, jet lag, alcohol and substance misuse, and insomnia may contribute to its occurrence in some cases [2]. In Alice's story, however, it seems that a key factor was the interaction between her premorbid personality and the particular constellation of cultural and other values associated with her expatriation.

5.4   The Values Impacting on This Story

The principal value held by Alice throughout the story is *work*. She always attached excessive importance to her job and regarded it as a primary source of self-satisfaction. Her excessive preoccupation with work in the week prior to her first hospital admission can be seen as a futile attempt to respond to chronic stress and feelings of low self-esteem and dissatisfaction with her job. Her desire for independence was hindered by lack of emotional differentiation, fearful avoidance of social contacts, and excessive anxiety in professional interactions. This may explain her inability to return to her level of functioning in the year after her psychotic episode when she tried to live and work in Germany. Arguably, she lacked the personality resources and coping skills to live, work, and manage the chronic stress of acculturation in a foreign country. The return to Bulgaria allowed for a return to premorbid interpersonal and occupational functioning. So, another value that arose for Alice in the aftermath of the brief psychotic disorder was *security*. The patient needed a more stable and predictable environment in order to function professionally and interpersonally.

Crucial also to Alice's story was the value her father placed on *living the Western dream.* He discounted his daughter's illness and put additional pressure on her "to make it" in Germany. His value was at conflict with her need for security resulting in relapses of her condition.

5.5   The Cultural Influences on Alice's Story

Interacting with the values operative in a given case, cultural and personality factors may be important from an etiological perspective. Travel often entails an encounter with a new culture that necessitates adjustment to different customs, lifestyle, and languages. Acculturation is particularly essential when traveling for a long period (such as during expatriation or migration). Cultural change can cause persistent distress in some individuals—this has been termed "culture shock" [3]. It is important to recognize that acculturation is more stressful when as in the case of Alice the expatriate lacks sufficient social support from friends and family [4].

It is also notable that her psychotic episode developed after a significant overburden in a job for which she was clearly overqualified. Occupational dissatisfaction and lack of opportunities for long-term professional development were arguably a major source of chronic stress for a person who had invested significant time and effort in her education and career abroad. Not surprisingly, some of the delusional themes during the psychotic episode that also resurfaced during the first year of follow-up involved persecutory ideation and delusions of influence associated with her colleagues and superiors. Alice's return to Bulgaria was marked by a culture-specific shift of delusional content to themes of indigenous traditions and ancient rituals.

Differences in cultural practices and values between Bulgarian society and those of other European countries revealed in a recent comparative [5] study may be relevant to Alice's story. The study established a distinctive profile of Bulgaria's societal culture in terms of practices and value orientations and compared these data to EU (European Union) average scores. Three cultural factors identified in the study stand out as being of potential relevance to Alice's story, "uncertainty avoidance," "performance orientation," and "assertiveness." We will look briefly at these before coming to our conclusions.

Uncertainty avoidance is the degree to which members of society try to avoid uncertainty by relying on social norms, rituals, or bureaucratic practices. In the above study, Bulgarian society scored much lower on practices and much higher on values of "uncertainty avoidance." This is understandable. In comparison to the EU average, Bulgarian society in the post-communist era is a society of transformation and its members have learned to accept uncertainty as its inherent characteristic. However, they have developed a preference for order and discipline as a way of dealing with the chaos and ambiguities in their new social, political, and economic life. Arguably, *security,* the second value that became important in Alice's story overlaps to a substantial degree with uncertainty avoidance. Alice needed a stable and predictable environment to remain symptom-free.

The next two factors, performance orientation and assertiveness, may be considered together in their impact on Alice's story. Performance orientation reflects the extent to which a society encourages or rewards group members for innovation, high standards, excellence, and performance improvement. The Bulgarian behaviors score in the study on performance orientation was lower than the average EU score due to a communist era heritage of planned economy. Assertiveness is the extent to which individuals in a society are assertive, provocative, or aggressive in their social relationships. In the study, the Bulgarian score on assertiveness was lower than the average EU countries' score on practices, maybe due to family bonds, favoritism, friendliness, and kindness, all deeply rooted in Orthodox traditions.

It may be speculated that the company with which Alice ended up working in Sofia (when she remained symptom-free) scored as in the study lower on practices of performance orientation and assertiveness than the companies in which she worked in Germany. On a practical level, this would mean that she experienced in Sofia an informal, subtle, and non-judgmental style of communication in the workplace and an emphasis on cooperation, people and relationships, equality, solidarity, tradition, and experience. Any or all of these factors may have contributed positively to Alice's sustained recovery once she returned home. If so, the possibility that as cultural values they may have wider significance as protective factors against the development of mental disorders would be worth further investigation.

5.6 Conclusions

A number of factors appear to have contributed to the emergence, development, and resolution of Alice's condition. Expatriation, insufficient support from friends and family, occupational dissatisfaction, and lack of prospects for professional development escalated into a brief psychotic disorder in a young woman whose preoccupation with her job led her to work for more than 12 h a day hardly getting any sleep at all. Preoccupation with work determined the delusional content of her psychotic disorder while living in Germany, comprising mainly persecutory ideation associated with her superiors and colleagues. Interestingly, a return to Bulgaria saw a dramatic shift in the content of her delusions, now mainly concerning religious themes, ancient rituals, and local traditions. Her need for security was at odds with her father's insistence that she should return to Germany and make a success of her career. Alice's low levels of emotional differentiation, avoidance of social contact, and excessive anxiety in professional interactions were responsible for the consequent paranoid and depressive exacerbations of her disorder. With a final return to Sophia, Bulgaria's capital, Alice was able to find a job that corresponded with her qualifications and she has subsequently remained symptom and medication free.

The findings of a recent comparative study of the cultural values and practices of Bulgaria and other EU countries may be relevant to understanding Alice's story.

Compared with other EU countries, including Germany, Bulgaria scored higher on values of uncertainty avoidance and lower on those of performance orientation and assertiveness. These cultural values, operating in Alice's final work environment back in Sophia, are likely to have contributed positively to her recovery. It may well be that they have wider significance as protective factors for individuals at risk of mental disorder.

5.7   Guide to Further Sources

Wikipedia, the free encyclopedia. Bulgarian diaspora. https://en.wikipedia.org/wiki/Bulgarian_diaspora

ExpatFocus. How To Look After Your Mental Health In Bulgaria. https://www.expatfocus.com/bulgaria/health/how-to-look-after-your-mental-health-in-bulgaria-5708

Cornelius N. Grove (2005). Worldwide Differences in Business Values and Practices: Overview of GLOBE Research Findings. http://www.grovewell.com/pub-GLOBE-dimensions.html

References

1. Diagnostic and statistical manual of mental disorders: DSM-5, 5th ed. Arlington, VA: American Psychiatric Association; 2013.
2. Airault R, Valk TH. Travel-related psychosis (TrP): a landscape analysis. J Travel Med. 2018;25(1):tay054.
3. Macionis J, Gerber L. Chapter 3—Culture. In: Sociology. 7th ed. Toronto: Pearson Canada Inc.; 2010. 54. Print.
4. Hombrados-Mendieta I, Millán-Franco M, Gómez-Jacinto L, Gonzalez-Castro F, Martos-Méndez MJ, García-Cid A. Positive influences of social support on sense of community, life satisfaction and the health of immigrants in Spain. Front Psychol. 2019;10:2555.
5. Bobina M. Bulgaria and the European Union: cultural differences and similarities. Bulg Stud J. 2018;2:5–25.

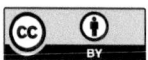

Theory First: An Introduction to Part II, Theory

Bill Fulford

Why theory? Or as a contributor to one of our writing workshops put it, why did we put not just theory but philosophical theory first in the book? This is a good question to which we have no unassailable answer. Certainly, it was not in hopes of the popular vote—in an age of "18-character 'tweets'" a book approaching 180,000 words could hardly be accused of courting popularity. Neither was it out of any assumed priority of theory over practice. We were not buying into the traditional idea that philosophy is, as it has sometimes been said to be, 'the queen of the sciences', a necessary ground-clearing preliminary for the heavy lifting of empirical science.

6.1 Widening the Theory Base

True, the practice of values-based practice (including its principle elements and their enactment through training in clinical care) was derived originally as we described in Chap. 1,[1] from work in ordinary language philosophy. True, also, our book was motivated, in part, though importantly, by recognition that the further development of values-based practice required a widening of its philosophical base to encompass philosophies that are less individual focused than was ordinary language philosophy. That is why our book is about *cultural* values. It is also why the philosophies included in this first part of the book are predominantly from the traditions of Continental Europe and Africa. Elsewhere in the book, we extend these

[1] See Sect. 1.4.1 in Chap. 1.

Authors
The editors with input from the contributors to Part II.

B. Fulford (✉)
St Catherine's College, University of Oxford, Oxford, UK

© The Author(s) 2021
D. Stoyanov et al. (eds.), *International Perspectives in Values-Based Mental Health Practice*, https://doi.org/10.1007/978-3-030-47852-0_6

sources still further to include, for example, those of South East Asia and Brazil. All these philosophies, as their respective chapters illustrate, reflect the relational more than individual character of human values.

6.1.1 Building on Two-Way Partnerships

But all that being said, perhaps the real reason that we put theory first was to emphasise the fact that values-based practice, and the wider movement in philosophy and mental health from which it is derived,[2] were from the very start conceived as building on *partnerships* between theory and practice. The partnerships in question, moreover, were conceived, again from the very start, essentially as *two-way* partnerships. That is to say, whilst in such partnerships theory does indeed inform practice, so practice also informs theory. That is why the interdisciplinary field from which values-based practice was derived is a 'Philosophy *and* ... discipline' not a 'Philosophy *of*... discipline'.

The conjunction 'and' says it all. There are, nowadays, in today's pragmatically justified academic world, many philosophies *of* this or *of* that practical area (*of* psychology, *of* physics, *of* politics and so forth). The idea perhaps is that philosophy is somehow justified by its contributions to the practical disciplines in question. However, the field from which values-based practice was derived is and has been from the start very definitely a 'philosophy *and* ... discipline', a discipline based on a two-way partnership between philosophy in all its richness and the no less-rich disciplines of mental health practice.[3]

6.2   Theory as a Resource for Practice

As indicated in the Table 6.1, the two-way partnership between theory and practice is explored in this Part mainly from the side of theory, drawing in particular on sources in the philosophy of values.

Thus, in Chap. 7, Oliver Scheibenbogen and Michael Musalek draw on cultural history and aesthetics in their description of a novel application of the 'will to beauty' (experienced by most human beings) as a therapeutic agent in the treatment of addictive disorders. The next two chapters together illustrate the power of phenomenology to draw out and make explicit the otherwise taken for granted (and hence largely invisible) cultural values that are important in shaping psychopathology, respectively, in eating disorders (Giovanni Stanghellini and Melena Mancini, Chap. 8), and in psychosis secondary to trauma (Michèle Gennart, Chap. 9).

---

[2] The work in philosophical value theory from which as described in Chap. 1 values-based practice is derived was one of five main strands of work in the 'new' philosophy and psychiatry that emerged in parallel with the 'new' neurosciences in the last decade of the Twentieth Century [1].

[3] See Guide to Further Information below for examples and sources.

Table 6.1 Annotated table of contents for Part II, Theory

Other philosophies may be illuminating in quite different ways. African philosophy is represented here first (in chap. 10 by Camillia Kong's exploration of Critical Sankofaism for working with conflicting values. Temitope Ademosu and her colleagues (chap. 11) then explore the importance of story telling within the African tradition. There are further examples of the role of African philosophy later in the book.

Finally in this section, Janelle Kwee and Hilary McBride (Chap. 12), drawing on a (disguised) narrative of anorexia from their own practice, show how feminist theory not only illuminates the cultural values driving psychopathology but may directly guide forms of therapy motivated by the aim of restoring the agency of the person concerned.

6.3   Practice as a Resource for Theory

With the remaining two chapters in this Part (Chaps. 13 and 14) we turn from the role of theory in illuminating practice to the other side of the two-way partnership, the role of practice in illuminating theory. Both chapters explore the boundary between mental disorder and spiritual or religious experience. The richly nuanced and complex nature of the boundary as illuminated by their respective narrative materials illustrates the importance of embedding philosophical analysis (in this case of the concept of mental disorder) in the details of the stories of real people rather than relying (as philosophers still all too often rely) on generalisations based on a restricted range of 'canonical' cases.

The conceptual issues arising in mental health—including radically different views on how the very concept of mental disorder should be understood—are of course wide ranging and matters of on-going debate. We do not have space to explore these issues in detail.

One such issue, however, to which the grounding of these two chapters in the experiences of real people, makes a distinctive contribution, is the role of values in defining mental health issues. There is much to be said even on this restricted aspect of the debate about mental disorder: it is a case in point after all of the is-ought debate of general ethical theory [2]. As to the boundary problem, furthermore, one view might be that, to the extent that the boundary involves values, it is really rather well defined: pathology, this view might suggest, is characteristically a *negative and disempowering* experience, whilst spiritual and religious experiences are characteristically *positive and empowering*. Yet as the stories in these two chapters, respectively, about suicidal behaviour (Chap. 13) and psychotic experiences (Chap. 14), make clear, the boundary of pathology can prove surprisingly difficult to draw along these lines, with both positive and negative aspects sitting side-by-side in the complexity of particular cases.

Again, the conceptual issues raised by these two chapters are deep indeed. Their bottom line, though, consistently with the bottom line of the three exemplar chapters in Part I, is that in whatever way the wider conceptual boundary is drawn, cultural and other values play an irreducible role in shaping the presentation and management of mental health issues.

6.4   Other Areas of Philosophy

Although we have focussed in this Part on philosophy of values, there are similarly rich two-way connections to be found in many other areas of philosophy—philosophy of mind, for example, and of science, are self-evidently cases in point. With our aim of extending values-based practice to cultural values, it was natural that philosophies of value would be our first port of call. But even with this limited aim in mind, we could have included a number of other sources. Within analytic philosophy, for example, the philosopher Anna Bergqvist, who leads the Theory Network in the Collaborating Centre for Values-based Practice in Oxford, is working on evaluative perception [3]; and the lead for the Centre in North America, Nancy Potter, has an on-going research programme on the nature of 'uptake' and its links with such key areas of mental health practice as co-production and recovery [4].

Again, there are other philosophies not standardly part of moral theory with potential for two-way exchange with mental health practice: political philosophy, for example, and hermeneutics. We return to the potential role of political philosophy in the introduction to our concluding Part VI (see Chap. 43). Hermeneutics has a proven track record in application to mental health [5], with, as Camillia Kong notes (Chap. 10 conclusions), intriguing links to the Critical Sankofaism of African philosophy. Other examples are provided by the philosophy of mind. The nature of personal identity, for example, is a key topic in this area of philosophy directly relevant to understanding the relationship between individual and cultural values [6].

Therefore, the scope is wide indeed. But for now, and for this book, we hope our selection is sufficient to indicate the potential for two-way exchange that exists between philosophical theory and mental health practice.

6.5 An Endorsement from Practice

In the early days of the Oxford Collaborating Centre for Values-based Practice, we received endorsement for this partnership model of the relationship between theory and practice from an unexpected but at the same time very welcome source. Over this period, the Centre was generously supported by an Advisory Board made up of senior members of many of the key organisations responsible for practical implementation of health care in the UK through the NHS (National Health Service). One might be forgiven for expecting that such a practically focused group would resist the Centre's proposed inclusion of a strong commitment to theory. But quite to the contrary, the Advisory Board welcomed it. Theory, they said, was our one defence against the everyday pressures of 'dumbing down' to which so many initiatives in the NHS had fallen prey. Evidence-based medicine (to which we return in Part IV) was a case in point.[4] Theory is in itself no guarantee that values-based practice will not suffer a similar fate. But absent theory, the Advisory Board said, and a similar fate is more or less guaranteed.

6.6 Conclusions

The contributions to this Part illustrated some of the many ways in which a culturally enriched form of values-based practice may draw to good effect on an enlarged theoretical base. Building on its origins in the ordinary language tradition of analytic philosophy, contributions to the Part explore the roles in values-based practice, respectively, of aesthetics, of phenomenology, of African philosophy, and of feminist philosophy. Elsewhere in the book as we have indicated, these resources are extended still further, to those of Buddhism and of Brazilian philosophy. We have noted that our selection is far from exhaustive even of the resources of analytic philosophy. We have emphasised the two-way nature of the partnership between theory and practice, with practice informing theory just as theory informs practice. The role of practice in informing theory is illustrated in the last two chapters in this Part by an exploration of the conceptual boundary between psychopathology and religious experience.

We concluded with an endorsement of the role of theory from the very practical perspective of the Advisory Board for the Collaborating Centre for Values-based Practice in Oxford. The richness of the contributions to this Part of the book, we believe, amply justify our Advisory Board's endorsement of the importance of theory as a partner to practice in the delivery of mental health care. The richness of the contributions to the book as a whole amply justifies our claim that the relationship between theory and practice is one of two-way partnership. Theory first, then, we conclude, but certainly not last.

---

[4] Evidence-based medicine is nowadays widely regarded as being just about best evidence. Yet over 20 years ago, one of the founders of evidence-based medicine, David Sackett, defined it as being about combining best research evidence with clinical experience and patients' values [7, p. 1].

6.7　Guide to Further Information

The Oxford book series, *International Perspectives in Philosophy and Psychiatry* (IPPP) includes many volumes illustrating both the contributions of theory to practice and the contributions of practice to theory (for comprehensive selections of materials, see for example, [8, 9]).

These and many other resources are indicated in the website of *The Collaborating Centre for Values-based Practice* in Oxford (valuesbasedpractice.org—see especially the section 'More about VBP') and that of *The International Network for Philosophy and Psychiatry* (INPPonline.com—this includes free-to-download materials from *The Oxford Textbook of Philosophy and Psychiatry*, [9]).

References

1. Fulford KWM, Morris KJ, Sadler JZ, Stanghellini G, editors. Nature and narrative: an introduction to the new philosophy of psychiatry. Oxford: Oxford University Press; 2003.
2. Fulford KWM. Moral theory and medical practice. Cambridge: Cambridge University Press; 1989, reprinted 1995 and 1999.
3. Bergqvist A, Cowan R. Evaluative perception. Oxford: Oxford University Press; 2018.
4. Potter NN. In the spirit of giving uptake. Philos Psychiatr Psychol. 2003;10(1):33–5.
5. Widdershoven G, Widdershoven-Heerding I. Understanding dementia: a hermeneutic perspective. Chapter 6. In: Fulford KWM, Morris KJ, Sadler JZ, Stanghellini G, editors. Nature and narrative: an introduction to the new philosophy of psychiatry. Oxford: Oxford University Press; 2003. p. 103–12.
6. Wilkes KV. Real people: personal identity without thought experiments. Oxford: Clarendon Press; 1988.
7. Sackett DL, Straus SE, Scott Richardson W, Rosenberg W, Haynes RB. Evidence-based medicine: how to practice and teach EBM. 2nd ed. Edinburgh: Churchill Livingstone; 2000.
8. Fulford KWM, Davies M, Gipps R, Graham G, Sadler J, Stanghellini G, Thornton T. The Oxford handbook of philosophy and psychiatry. Oxford: Oxford University Press; 2013.
9. Fulford KWM, Thornton T, Graham G. The Oxford textbook of philosophy and psychiatry. Oxford: Oxford University Press; 2006.

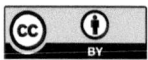

The Will to Beauty as a Therapeutic Agent: Aesthetic Values in the Treatment of Addictive Disorders

Oliver Scheibenbogen and Michael Musalek

7.1   Introduction

The cultural values of the post-war generation in Austria are often rooted in the many deprivations they experienced during the War and the scarcity of resources in the subsequent post-war years of reconstruction. The values that were formed during these years continue to have a powerful effect and influence how values are experienced, and how interactional situations are evaluated and interpreted down to the present day.

At the same time, for Austrians in general and for those who live in eastern Austria in particular, a rich and rewarding life has always been a central life goal and this is defined not just as a good and successful life, but above all as a life rich in pleasure [1].

The following study (which is presented in four parts) describes the shift in the values of a woman to whom, in her own words, fate had always been cruel, who had always had a harder time than others and whose efforts had always been directed to being able to keep up with others and not towards self-fulfilment. At the same time, there is an interaction between the patient's initial adverse and existentially threatening circumstances and cultural and pathological determinants. The 'healing process' is to a large extent also influenced by the shift in values prompted by the therapy.

O. Scheibenbogen (✉)
Department of Clinical Psychology, Anton Proksch Institute, Vienna, Austria
e-mail: oliver.scheibenbogen@api.or.at

M. Musalek
Anton Proksch Institute, Vienna, Austria
e-mail: michael.musalek@api.or.at

© The Author(s) 2021
D. Stoyanov et al. (eds.), *International Perspectives in Values-Based Mental Health Practice*, https://doi.org/10.1007/978-3-030-47852-0_7

7.2 Case History (Part I): The Loss of Beauty

Frau S. is a 73-year-old woman who for 15 years has been undergoing regular treatment for her addiction at the Anton Proksch Institute. The Anton Proksch Institute is Europe's largest addiction clinic and treats approximately 2000 inpatients and 8000 outpatients per year. In addition to treating addictions to substances such as alcohol, medicines, illegal drugs and tobacco, the Institute has for approximately 10 years treated non-substance addiction disorders, i.e. addictive behaviours such as pathological gambling, and addictions to computer games, shopping and work.

The patient suffers from an alcohol dependency against the background of a multiple post-traumatic stress disorder and a depressive disorder. The patient comes from a very modest family background, grew up in Meidling, a part of Vienna with a high proportion of working-class residents, and she herself worked as a building caretaker, sales assistant and in the hospitality industry. Despite a very intensive and regular employment history, the patient was often at risk of poverty. Her childhood was dominated by the existential anxieties of her mother who, because of her own occupation, was only able to provide limited resources for raising her daughter. Until the age of 12, the patient lived alone with her mother whom she cared for until the latter's death despite a very ambivalent relationship. The identity of her father is still unknown. Her mother's second husband, and here financial considerations probably played a role in the decision to get married again, abused the patient physically and sexually over a period of several years. At the age of 16, the patient moved in with an acquaintance of her mother to escape the violence. Although the patient confided to her mother that she had been sexually abused by her stepfather, her mother either did not believe her or did not want to believe her due to fear of the drastic existential consequences this would have. 'Nothing can happen that isn't supposed to happen' the patient remarked many years later during her therapy. The mother's lack of understanding exacerbated the patient's feelings of guilt and shame. As only money and financial security were considered to bestow a certain degree of social prestige and status, the matter was not discussed further within the family. As a result, it became a family secret that only came to light decades later during therapy. From a psychological-therapeutic perspective, the fact that the daughter cared for her mother until the latter's death, despite the lack of support she received to end the sexual assaults and the mistrust and contempt the mother showed for her daughter, are of central importance. The ambivalence this produced in the patient of approach-and-avoidance feelings—this is my biological mother accompanied by simultaneous feelings of hatred and death wishes directed against her mother and herself—persisted for many years even after the mother had died. For example, it is only in the last few years that the patient has been able to visit her mother's grave. Due to a lack of alternative possibilities caused by the fact that at the same time she was solicitously caring for her mother on a daily basis, the patient redirected the negative destructive feelings she had towards her mother towards herself. In addition to self-harming and massive episodes of intoxication as

*well as periods of gambling in an effort to improve her financial situation, her atti-
tude to religion and to humanity as such also underwent a massive change.*

*One aspect of the patient's biography that has not been mentioned so far is her
homosexuality. In Roman Catholic post-war Vienna and among her working-class
friends, homosexual people often faced hostility, mockery and discrimination.
Moreover, her love for another woman developed at a time when her future partner
was still in a relationship with a man. He stalked her in later years calling her out
as an adulteress.*

*In 2002, the patient first sought professional help to tackle her addiction. Her
decision was triggered by an acute coronary syndrome combined with major physical impairments caused by chronic alcohol abuse. When her doctors told her she
would not have much longer to live if she did not change her ways it prompted her
to begin treatment for her addiction. The patient was admitted to the Anton Proksch
Institute for the first time for an 8-week course of treatment as an inpatient. As she
repeatedly said of herself afterwards, she had not really been able to engage with
the therapy at the time; nevertheless, following treatment she was abstinent for
approximately 1 year. After suffering a relapse during a moderately severe depressive episode, she was readmitted for further in-patient treatment. Unlike her previous stay, the patient this time came into contact with the newly introduced Orpheus
programme of treatment.*

7.3   Digression: The Concept Behind the Orpheus Treatment Programme

In Greek mythology, Orpheus was an inspired singer. When Orpheus and the
Argonauts were sailing in search of the Golden Fleece, they came across the sirens,
the notorious bird-women of antiquity whose sweet and seductive song promised
passing sailors beauty and pleasure, but instead brought death and destruction.
Anyone who hears the sirens is lost. It was said that those who heard them were
burned up with passion and indeed it was the case that everything around them
turned to dust and ashes.

However, there were at least two famous ancient heroes who succeeded in passing the sirens unscathed. Odysseus and our Orpheus. Odysseus had his men tie him
to his ship's mast and ordered the crew to seal their ears with wax in order to resist
the temptation. Orpheus chose a different method that would enable him to pass the
sirens with lust and pleasure and that would allow him to live a full and rewarding
life. When he and the Argonauts sailed past the sirens, he took his lyre and sang so
beautifully that he drowned out the sound of their singing—he played the better music.

This ancient myth forms of the basis of the Orpheus programme of treatment at
the Anton Proksch Institute. The therapeutic goal of abstinence is often associated
with such negative attributes as self-denial, sacrifice and compulsory life-time

abstinence, and is, therefore, often seen by those concerned as unattractive and not worthwhile. In the Orpheus programme, abstinence is only presented to individuals suffering from an addiction disorder as an opportunity for a transformation process within the scope of the therapy; the actual goal is autonomy and a full and rewarding life. This therapeutic goal has enormous motivational and volitional power, however, for many patients, including Frau S., it means totally reorienting their lives and ultimately also learning to manage their own lives. In addition to the mindfulness and cosmopoesis (or new design for life) modules in the Orpheus Programme, it is above all the elements focusing on experiencing pleasure and exploring what is beautiful that induces a change in values and attitudes that is effected by the patient himself (e.g.: learning to enjoy social interactions again).

7.4   Case History (Part II): Recovering the Beautiful

In this way, Frau S. was gently led back to the beautiful. During her after-treatment and continuing treatment as an outpatient following her second course of residential treatment, the patient was gradually able to perceive beauty more frequently and more intensively again. This is certainly not something that can be taken for granted, given that addiction in itself, but also the comorbidities such as post-traumatic disorder and depression also often lead to a loss of beauty. Subsequently in the face of beauty the patient was once more able to perceive first emotional stirrings, a feeling of being infused and a longing for the beauty in herself. With increasing frequency she reported having had stirring experiences of nature, such as extraordinarily beautiful plants and encounters with animals (e.g. birds) that moved her and inspired her to reflection; later on, she described beautiful encounters with other people. Someone to whom 'fate has been so cruel' is extremely negative, contemptuous and hostile towards themselves. Typical cognitions in this context are 'I don't deserve this', 'I'm not entitled to it', and many individuals prefer to remain trapped in the suffering that is familiar to them than to embark on new, perhaps much more beautiful, but uncertain paths.

The patient's recovery process and the shift in values associated with it was not one of steady progress; on the contrary, she suffered repeated relapses. Her core assumption that 'fate was cruel to her' was experientially confirmed many times in a dysfunctional form and led the patient to even greater passivity and into a victim role. Thus for example, on the day she was released from her second period of residential treatment, the patient, who had been diagnosed with claustrophobia, got stuck in the lift when she came home and a short time later was robbed in an underpass during which she received a minor injury to her arm. This list could be continued almost ad infinitum and the reader would indeed begin to develop a similar view of the patient (that fate was cruel to her), but this case study is instead concerned with describing work with aesthetic values. To this end, the therapeutic process began with a reflection on the experience of pleasure in an inpatient setting, but above all during the after-care Frau S. received as an outpatient.

7.5 The Values Arising in This Story

Spiritual values, which had formerly been a resource, were largely lost as a result of the way those around her dealt with the traumatisation. 'A God who lets that go unpunished, is not a God I can believe in'. Subsequently, as is typical for trauma-tised patients and especially for victims who have experienced sexual violence, the patient turned her back on and distanced herself from other people. Cultural and aesthetic values, as these are almost always created or updated in social interaction with others, became increasingly less important. In contrast, through her own ill-ness, her feelings of being under existential threat were again intensified.

Addictive substances in general, and in the case of Frau S. alcohol in particular, are usually used as problem solvers. Similar to medication, for example, against headaches, the consumption of psychoactive substances alleviates symptoms in the short term, but in the long term leads to a deterioration in the patient's condition which becomes chronic. Coping strategies that perhaps existed to a certain degree in the past are pushed increasingly further into the background in favour of the addictive substance. The loss of control—the cardinal symptom of dependency dis-orders—exacerbates this effect and leads to learned helplessness and feelings of guilt and shame in the face of the negative consequences arising from intoxication. During the period when she worked as a building caretaker, the progress of her addiction meant there were phases during which Frau S. was unable to carry out her duties properly, although this was tremendously important to her as she had a very highly developed sense of responsibility. Those around her, the tenants in the coun-cil block in which she worked, increasingly began to make complaints about her and as her excessive alcohol consumption became evident, the patient increasingly found herself on the receiving end of pejorative and addiction-specific stigmatising comments. Due to the depressant effect of alcohol, her sustained consumption led to her developing a manifest depressive disorder.

7.6 The Influences of Culture on This Story

For centuries, Austria has had a strong beer, wine and schnapps culture. It is impos-sible to imagine social and cultural life without alcohol. Austria regularly ranks among the top three nations worldwide for per capita consumption of alcohol. In a country in which alcohol is an innocuous and firm part of many rituals on almost all occasions, the line between what is considered to be socially 'normal' levels of drinking and a pattern of consumption that is considered to be 'abnormal' or 'patho-logical' is a very fine one. A man who can take his drink is still considered to be a 'real man', the threshold for women is significantly lower and society is still quick to ascribe negative attributes, although no longer to the same extent as in the past, to women who consume large quantities of alcohol. This is of particular relevance for the progression of an addiction, as this negative attribution and ultimately the stig-matisation, often results in an addiction continuing to grow in secrecy. Thus, in Austria, approximately 10 years pass from between the time when a patient first manifests alcohol associated problems and when he or she seeks specialist assistance; during this period, the illness progresses and the prognosis for recovery worsens significantly with the continuance of the disease.

7.7   The Influences of Aesthetic Values and the Will to Beauty on This Story

In the case of addictions, and depressive disorders in particular, one of the first steps in treatment involves reactivating experiential capability, i.e. the ability to absorb impressions and to process them emotionally. It is one of the mental characteristics that develops on the basis of a person's individual disposition over the course of their lifetime as a result of their experiences, acquisition of abilities, skills and knowledge. The diverse suggestions and reflections in individual counseling sessions and in the group session aim to strengthen this experiential capability and to bring it into the centre of the patient's consciousness in order to increase their ability to experience pleasure. Pleasure promotes joy, reward, increased well-being and a lust for life. It has nothing to do with severe intoxication and massive alterations of mind. 'Pleasure as the highest form of experiencing beauty should not be confused with fun or quick gratification and absolutely not—as is so often the case today—with consumption at high prices or in large quantities—on the contrary, pleasure stands for the ability to enjoy leisure and relaxation' [2].

The repeated experience of pleasure subsequently raises the level of perceived self-efficacy [3]. Individuals who frequently experience themselves enjoying pleasure, i.e. who are able to put themselves into a sustainable positive mood, possess a more intense conviction that they will be able to successfully overcome difficult situations and challenges with their own resources. In the case of Frau S. this marked the first step in her coming out of her role as a victim and developing an eye for beauty. One of her first accounts of perceiving beauty concerned an experience of nature. She reported something she had experienced that we would like to briefly share:

7.8   Case History (Part III): A Key Experience of Beauty

Her partner died 12 years ago and until then she had only been able to live this relationship furtively and in secret. She began paying regular weekly visits to her partner's grave. These visits were characterised by melancholy, grief and a desire to follow her shortly. Despite the immense suffering these visits triggered on each occasion, she persisted with them, driven on the one hand by a sense of supposed duty, and on the other, by a desire to be near her partner and 'the woman of her life'. One day, the following occurred: as she was standing at the graveside weeping bitterly, a squirrel came and sat on her partner's gravestone where it remained for what subjectively seemed like an eternity and studied her carefully. In the eyes of the beautiful and noble creature she was able to recognise an act of affection for her person—love and respect. She was so deeply touched by what was such a significant experience for her that in contrast to previous visits, where she had only been able to bear staying at the grave for a short time, she remained for a long time. This incident was picked up and reflected upon during therapy. She herself interpreted this encounter as a message and as permission from her deceased partner to live a full and rewarding life. This aesthetic experience characterised by the beauty of the encounter between an animal and a human being marked a milestone in the therapeutic work. For the first time in decades, Frau S. was able to grasp and to experience the beauty of the world in a brief fragment. To not just perceive the power of beauty but to feel it with body and soul and ultimately to utilise the power and energy that reside in beauty.

There is one key requisite for being able to grasp beauty that those who are traumatised and those who are suffering from other forms of mental illness do not possess in adequate measure, the will to beauty [2, 4]. Intrapsychically, this means caring for oneself, wanting something 'constructive' for oneself and to a large extent driving back destructive impulses, having a fundamentally positive attitude towards oneself and others, and ultimately towards the whole world.

Finally, we would like to consider the patient-therapist dyad in the context of Frau S.' treatment and the extension and stabilisation of the process of turning to beauty that was triggered by the initial experience.

7.9 Case History (Part IV): Working Together Towards Beauty

In the 'homeland' of psychoanalysis, the nature of the relationship between patient and therapist is traditionally characterised by distance, in the medical context frequently by a paternalistic attitude in which the therapist knows how it is done and the other person is told how he has to do it. However, to utilise the power of beauty for therapeutic purposes, the therapist is required to adopt a deliberate attitude as a 'friend'. The task is to explore what has been experienced on equal terms—in the case of Frau S. to listen and nudge sensitively when she began to describe similar situations to the encounter with the squirrel. The patient was often overcome with doubt as to whether her view of things was the right one, whether people would consider her to be mad due to her intensive feelings of experiencing beauty in her everyday life. In this situation, the therapist's task is not to confirm the correctness of these views as such, but to work to arrive at a place where what is subjectively felt and experienced is seen as being just as true and valid as if the entire world had unquestionably experienced it in the same way. Self-doubt and the orientation to the norms of others in combination with the taking on board of the values of the collective prevent a patient from opening up and engaging with beauty and rob these experiences of sustainable efficacy.

In addition, the therapist can serve as a model in sensing and experiencing beauty. The patient has the possibility through vicarious observation—even more through vicarious sensing—to experience exposure to beauty without fear and at first at a safe distance. Of course, these experiences are not as intensive and as strong as if the patient were experiencing them directly, but in many cases, they offer the necessary guidance and support.

The final aspect in the patient-therapist dyad in connection with the experience of beauty is the reaction of the therapist to the discovery of beauty in the patient themselves. The patient's intrinsic beauty first has to be discovered and brought out in the therapeutic process. Praise, recognition and conscious appreciation in the countertransference process are suitable instruments to help the patient begin to identify his own beauty. On several occasions during Frau S.' accounts of beauty, the therapist showed how moved he was by the patient's experiences and provided feedback about his enthusiasm for the way she dealt with the situations and their observations. This increasingly reinforced Frau S's affinity to beauty, it became an integral part of her personality and is still a helper in difficult times.

Six months ago, the patient was diagnosed with macular degeneration. The ophthalmologists who are treating Frau S.—a woman with an eye for beauty—have told her that she will soon go completely blind. Of course, she was very upset by the diagnosis and evoked fear regarding her ability to cope with the future, but since then she has begun to prepare accordingly and to train her other senses. Beauty remains and continues to have an effect and as everyone knows, one only sees beautifully with the heart.

7.10 Conclusions

In contrast to traditional forms of therapy, confrontation with the beauty requires much more of an encounter at the eye level. Value discussions with addicts must be carried out very sensitively, as alcohol-dependent persons are very severely affected by guilt and shame at the beginning of therapy. Self-devaluation and mental or sometimes physical self-harm are dysfunctional coping strategies for the preservation of the self. If the therapist begins to offer the beauty too quickly, it is usually not accepted or becomes the object of devaluation. The therapist's task is, therefore, to create situations that make a deep experience of the beautiful more likely and, if that has actually happened, in support to make the beautiful an integral part of one's personality.

Acknowledgements Our thanks go to the patient, who has given open and unconditional information about her life story.

7.11 Guide to Further Sources

Musalek M., (2017) Der Wille zum Schönen I, Parados Verlag, Berlin
Musalek M., (2017) Der Wille zum Schönen II, Parados Verlag, Berlin
www.antonprokschinstitut.at
www.socialaeshetics.sfu.ac.at

References

1. Kendel E. The age of insight. London: Random House; 2012.
2. Musalek M. Social aesthetics and the management of addiction. Curr Opin Psychiatry. 2010;23:530–53.
3. Musalek M, Scheibenbogen O. From categorial to dimensional diagnosis—deficiency-oriented versus person-centered diagnostics. Eur Arch Psychiatry Clin Neurosci. 2008;258(Suppl. 5):18.
4. Musalek M. Human-based medicine theory and practice: from modern to postmodern medicine. In: Warnecke T, editor. The psyche in the modern world. Psychotherapy and society. London: Karnacbooks; 2015. p. 97–115.

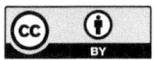

Anorexia as Religion: Ocularcentrism as a Cultural Value and a Compensation Strategy in Persons with Eating Disorders

Giovanni Stanghellini and Milena Mancini

8.1 Introduction

This chapter builds on the philosopher Charland's concept of feeding and eating disorders (FED) as *passions*—long-standing tendencies that represent a rupture in the fleeting and transitory character of emotional life [1]. This view paves the way for understanding the being-in-the-world of people with FED as a kind of *religion* [2], driven, mainly, as we will show here, by cultural values such as ocularcentrism. The values and other elements of this religion are evident in the following personal testimony from one of our case studies.

8.2 Anorexia as Religion: A Personal Testimony

I understand, now, that anorexia was my religion. According to its commandments I knew how to regulate my time, how to spend my days and nights, what to aim to, what was right or wrong. It provided me with undoubtable principles according to which I could behave and choose.

All my questions—who am I, who I want to become, whom I should try to look like and all my doubts about dependence and autonomy—turned into just one scruple: being thin and starve myself. Fat equals sin. Fat was wrong, eating was wrong, starving was right and thinness was right. Fat people were bad; exercising was good. Fat was a sign of loss of control, the sign of a moral sin. Fat people were sinners. Now I can confess that I was fascinated by the dead I guess because I was fascinated by the skeleton.

G. Stanghellini (✉)
Department of Psychological, Health and Territorial Sciences, "G. D'Annunzio" University, Chieti Scalo, Italy
e-mail: giostan@libero.it

M. Mancini
"G. d'Annunzio" University, Chieti, Italy
e-mail: mancinimilena@yahoo.it

© The Author(s) 2021
D. Stoyanov et al. (eds.), *International Perspectives in Values-Based Mental Health Practice*, https://doi.org/10.1007/978-3-030-47852-0_8

69

These ethical principles went hand in hand with aesthetic ones: roundness was ugly; sharpness beautiful. My sensibility was affected. I remember that seeing a ball bouncing caused in me a feeling of disgust. I saw the whole world according to this dichotomy: more than a religion it was a heresy, like Manichaeism! (she smiles). Heaviness and lightness; matter and spirit. I read that book: I too wanted to be light as a butterfly! (she refers to Michela Marzano's Volevo Essere una Farfalla [I Wanted to be a Butterfly], [3]). Always in movement, without touching the ground, not even 1 mg of fat!

This religion had also its ontology—although an involuntary ontology: since I could have no wings, bones were to me the essential part of the body, touching my bones was touching my own Self. Bones were the core of being. Having my bones in my hands, meant to have control over my body, over myself, including my instincts and desires. When I became anorexic I finally knew who I was! Yet I did not realise that my 'philosophy', my 'truth', including its aesthetics, ethics and ontology, derived from my uneasiness about my body. The strength of such a philosophy is its absoluteness: being absolute; that is unconnected with personal needs, necessities and desires. Truth comes from above, doesn't it? What kind of truth may come from the flesh? From the flesh come only dirt, shit, hunger and so on.

But my 'truth' came from there; it came from below—from the disgust for my body; from the fragile bond between my Self and my body. Now, I realise that my philosophy stemmed directly from my lack of being, from my disembodiment, from the weak connection between my bodily feelings, myself and my identity.

8.3   Passions and Values as Sources of Stability

Persons with FED, especially in the early and more fluid period of their condition, often report difficulties of the kind so vividly described in this personal testimony, difficulties of feeling their own body in the first-person perspective and of having a stable and continuous sense of themselves as embodied agents. Doubts about one's identity ('*Who am I, who I want to become, whom I should try to look like*') and about moral issues ('*what was right or wrong*') can be seen as consequences of the person's emotional life being a ceaseless ebb and flow of incoherent and sometimes vaguely perceived feelings [3]. Passions represent an abnormal break in their discontinuous bodily and emotional experience, helping them to answer questions like '*how to regulate my time, how to spend my days and nights, what to aim to*'.

A passion can be defined as a persistent, pervasive and egosynthonic emotion that provides a stable normative structure through which a substantial proportion of relations with the environment are evaluated and processed. Thus passions may help to respond to questions like '*what was right or wrong*' providing '*undoubtable principles according to which I could behave and choose*'. Passions offer fixed points of orientation that endure over time suggesting interpretations and explanations, and at the same time moving the person to action in accordance with fixed goals.

Passions not only help to direct and organise feelings and emotions but also *crystallise* in fixed intellectual ideas or *values*. The fixed ideas involved in passions are indeed just that, values—what a person deems of fundamental importance in her or his life—or are strongly connected with and rooted in values [4]. Valuing is a process founded on the emotional dimension of life. Values are attitudes that regulate the felt-meanings of the world and the significant actions of the person, being organised into concepts that do not arise from rational activity but rather within the sphere of feelings.

Values coalesce in explicit or implicit structures that offer a stable and more or less consistent background for actions. This is also the case with the values involved in FEDs, especially explicit values such as *thinness* and *starvation*, which give to FED persons a steady goal by which to orientate their lives. More implicit values, like the cultural value of *ocularcentrism* (see below), make up the pre-intentional background against which one may experience oneself and the world. Such values include *cultural* values in that they imbue the society in which we live. As such, they can be difficult to detect due to their *mimetic* nature—they are as it were hidden in plain sight, and, yet, reproduced in FED individuals as a direct reflection of the social order to which they belong. We return below to a more detailed account of one of these cultural values—ocularcentrism—and of its role in driving the 'religion' of anorexia.

First, however, there is an even more significant mimetic cultural value than these, to which we would draw attention, namely the search for *identity* and the kind of practice needed to achieve it [5]. People with FED cannot take personal identity for granted. It is for them a task to be achieved. This is because, alienated as they are from their body and emotions, they lack a solid and permanent ground on which to establish their identity. Again, this is graphically described in the above testimony, in terms of the subject's bones: '*since I could have no wings, bones were to me the essential part of the body, touching my bones was touching my own Self. Bones were the core of being. Having my bones in my hands, meant to have control over my body, over myself, including my instincts and desires.*'

8.4 Pro-Anna Websites

Pro-Anna websites and blogs provide further evidence of the religion-like nature of FED. We will illustrate these briefly before returning to the role of the particular sense modality (namely sight) through which we normally experience ourselves and the world, and its role in shaping the values from which the lack of identity of people with FED stems.

Consider this example from: *theproanalifestyleforever.wordpress.com.*

8.4.1 Ana's Rules

1. *If you aren't thin you aren't attractive.*
2. *Being thin is more important than being healthy.*
3. *You must buy clothes, style your hair, take laxatives, starve yourself and do anything to make yourself look thinner.*
4. *Thou shall not eat without feeling guilty.*

5. *Thou shall not eat fattening food without punishing oneself afterwards.*
6. *Thou shall count calories and restrict intake accordingly.*
7. *What the scale says is the most important thing.*
8. *Losing weight is good/gaining weight is bad.*
9. *You can never be too thin.*
10. *Being thin and not eating are signs of true will power and success.*
11. *Ana is a lifestyle not a diet.*

8.4.2   Pro-Ana as a Religion of Thinness and Starvation

Pro-Ana websites and blogs are very good sources for understanding what is valued by anorexia and bulimia patients. *Ana's Rules* make explicit the values of thinness (or as it is sometimes called, *thinspiration*) and starvation (#1, 2 and 3) and their connection with moral themes like guilt and incontinence (#4, 5). These are imperatives whose purpose is to discipline eating behaviour and prescribe a certain appearance. They are mainly related to food intake (#3, 4, 5, 6, 8 and 10) and thinness (#1, 2, 3, 5, 9 and 10). #5 brings together the anti-values of fat and of eating fattening food with punishment, thus with the theme of guilt. Guilt is also present in #4 in connection with food intake. #10 clearly connects thinness and starvation with the values of will power and success. #6 and #7 are about the value of starvation connecting it to what we call digitisation, i.e. counting calories and measuring one's body.

Many of the thinness items are combined with other themes: #1 with attractiveness/look/appearance, #2 health/wellbeing, #3 starvation/purging and #10 power and success. Rule #11 makes clear that this credo is not merely about food and dieting, but prescribes a thorough lifestyle, that is a philosophy of life and a world-view. *Ana's Rules* then are indeed the imperatives of a kind of *religion* - the same religion expressed in our personal testimony above. These imperatives are not merely about food as a partial aspect of life, but about the worth of life and the way to make one's life *meaningful*. They are experienced as the table of commandments by its believers. Also, these rules belong to an overall structure that has the same arrangement of all religions having its own values, goals, creed and practices. Its goal is authenticity and achieving a place in the world, and more generally the Good Life.

The world, one's identity and one's place in the world are chaos without *Ana*. *Ana* is the saviour, a goddess to worship in order to be saved from anarchy and confusion. Food has a moral value: it is a sin and a temptation. Fatness has a moral value too as indicative of laziness, lack of self-care and self-control. Thinness is more valuable than anything else including health because it means self-achievement and self-realisation. Strict rules are needed not to do wrong and to be led astray. Starvation is the unique salvation practice.

8.4.3   Cultural Values: Ocularcentrism

Many of *Ana's rules* bring together values of thinness with appearance (#3). This connection with the dominant medium or sense modality (namely sight) through which we experience ourselves and the world takes us to a key cultural value underpinning the 'religion' of anorexia, *ocularcentrism*. This as we put it above is a 'mimetic' value, i.e. one that is so widely shared by the majority of people in Western civilisation as to be invisible. Yet, its influence is everywhere. Indeed, our culture is permeated by visually imbued social and cultural practices [6].

This is evident in particular in what may be called the 'ocular permeation' of language and the hegemony of visual metaphors. We speak of insight, far-sighted or short-sighted attitudes, we say that one may overlook things and one's reasoning may be more or less perspicuous. Light as opposed to darkness and vision as opposed to blindness play a fundamental role in religious thinking and experience. Wisdom is connected with being clear-sighted—although with some and relevant exceptions: Homer, Oedipus and Tiresias in Greek culture, blind prophets and poets from antiquity to modern times. Western culture is often accused of ocularcentrism—the prevalence of vision over other senses, such as touch and hearing. The hierarchical ordering of the senses and the predominance of sight is claimed not only to affect philosophical theories of perception and knowledge, but also self-experience and self-understanding.

In his masterpiece *The Work of Art in the Age of Mechanical Reproduction* (1936), Walter Benjamin shows how human sense perception is influenced by historical circumstances. Everyone knows that what is valued beautiful or ugly is historically determined—but also the sense modalities (what Benjamin calls the 'medium') can change in the course of human history. The ways human sense perception is organised, the medium in which it is accomplished, is determined not only by nature but by historical circumstances as well. '*During long periods of history, the mode of human sense perception changes with humanity's entire mode of existence*' (p. 216). One relevant change that can be seen in art history is from tactile to visual perception, that is from more to less embodied forms of perception.

Ocularcentrism is the dominant medium implicated in contemporary society. Ocularcentrism is not only the philosophical subtext of the modern and postmodern value-structure. It also permeates our contemporary pop culture and social practices, as argued (among others) by Guy Debord's [7] *The Society of the Spectacle*. Debord calls 'spectacle' the mainly visual representation of our real lives. The society of the spectacle has an alienating power as in it social relations are mediated by the images imposed by media and its implicit or explicit advertisements. Passive identification with the spectacle supplants genuine activity.

8.5   Ocularcentrism and FED

People with FED experience themselves first and foremost through sight, specifically, as we have argued elsewhere [4], through the others' gaze. Another way of expressing this is to say that in people with FED, self- and body-experiences are allocentric, that is, mediated by the other's vantage point. Two factors contribute to this allocentric acquiescence of people with FED to the others' gaze: one is negative, their need for self-definition that is not accomplished by embodied, proximal and self-centred forms of self-perception; the other is positive, the cultural-societal vector of ocularcentrism.

Debord's [7] focus was certainly not on anorexia, but on modern Western society as a whole. Yet his analysis helpfully clarifies how the cultural-societal vector of ocularcentrism may contribute to the allocentric self-perception of people with FED [8]. In our culture, the predominance of sight is claimed to affect the way we experience the world and ourselves. As he puts it 'for one to whom the real world becomes real images, mere images are transformed into real beings' (thesis 18, emphasis added). His explanation of the rise of ocularcentrism continues, since the image's job is to cause a world that is no longer directly perceptible to be seen via different senses, it is inevitable that it should elevate sight to the special place once occupied by touch. In this way, the most abstract of senses, and the most easily deceived, the sense of sight, is also the most readily adapted to present-day society's generalised abstraction.

In the resulting ocularcentric society, the individual is not only a passive receptor of the images coming from the media; rather, *the very relationships between people are mediated by images*. The other is an image for me, and I am an image for the other. Sight, that is the sense that produces images and representations, is the means through which individuals relate to each other. This form of relating through images is the opposite of dialogue. Thus, in this kind of society, images and representations depart from embodied, participated and 'immersed' kinds of vision, being disembodied and passive forms of 'seeing'.

8.6 Conclusions

We have illustrated through personal testimony and evidence from Pro-Ana websites the way in which anorexia may be understood as a kind of religion. In this religion, being fat and eating have an explicit moral value, not simply an aesthetic one. Fatness is seen as indicative of laziness, lack of self-care or lack of self-control, and therefore, contemptible and disgusting. On the other hand, starvation is seen as a salvation practice since it can help regain a sense of self-worth and authenticity. These values in turn we have argued reflect more implicit (or 'mimetic') cultural values illustrated here by ocularcentrism.

Clearly, there is more that needs to be said to fill out this account. First, there is other evidence supporting these observations, for example, the careful qualitative studies of the psychiatrist Jacinta Tan and colleagues in Oxford [9]. Second, a focus on changes in body experience in people with FEDs may be important to establish a differential phenomenology between this condition and other pathologies in which abnormal bodily experiences occur as for instance schizophrenia [10]. Third, a phenomenologically rich account of anorexia and its relation with abnormal bodily experience and the predominance of sense of sight may help translational research to find biological correlates of this disorder [8]. Fourth, a full account would have to encompass the full range and diversity of these and other disorders, and their variation across cultures and different historical periods.

We hope nonetheless that our analysis of anorexia as a religion, and of the origins of this religion in the cultural value of ocularcentrism so dominant in contemporary society, may be helpful not only in illuminating but also in contributing to the treatment of this increasingly important and often devastating form of psychopathological condition. At the very least, clinicians, while projecting treatment plans for people affected by the 'religion of anorexia' and related feeding and eating disorders, should be aware that the unshakable certainty with which the values of thinness and starvation are held by their patients, are not merely negative cognitive distortions. They perform rather the positive role of providing a shelter in which those concerned find relief from their difficulties in attaining a stable sense of self-identity in an age dominated by ocularcentrism.

References

1. Charland LC, Hope T, Stewart A, Tan J. The hypothesis that anorexia nervosa is a passion: clarifications and elaborations. Philos Psychiatr Psychol. 2013;20:375–9.
2. Stanghellini G, Mancini M. The therapeutic interview. Emotions, values, and the life-world. Cambridge: Cambridge University Press; 2017.
3. Marzano M. Volevo essere una farfalla. Milano: Edizioni Mondadori; 2011.
4. Fulford KWM, Stanghellini G. Values and values-based practice. In: Stanghellini G, et al., editors. The Oxford handbook of phenomenological psychopathology. Oxford: Oxford University Press; 2019.
5. Stanghellini G, Mancini M, Castellini G, Ricca V. Eating disorders as disorders of embodiment and identity. Theoretical and empirical perspectives. In: McBride HL, Kwee JL, editors. Embodiment and eating disorders. Theory, research, preventions and treatment. London: Routledge; 2018. p. 127–42.
6. Jay M. Downcast eyes: the denigration of vision in twentieth-century French thought. Berkeley, CA: University of California Press; 1994.
7. Debord G. The society of the spectacle. Paris: Les Éditions Gallimard; 1967. p. 1992.
8. Stanghellini G, Ballerini M, Mancini M. The optical-coenaesthetic disproportion hypothesis of feeding and eating disorders in the light of neuroscience. Front Psychiatry. 2019;10:630.
9. Tan JO, Hope T, Stewart A, Fitzpatrick R. Competence to make treatment decisions in anorexia nervosa: thinking processes and values. Philos Psychiatr Psychol. 2006;13:267–82.
10. Stanghellini G, Ballerini M, Blasi S, Mancini M, Presenza S, Raballo A, et al. The bodily self: a qualitative study of abnormal bodily phenomena in persons with schizophrenia. Compr Psychiatry. 2014;55:1703–11.

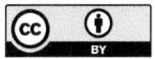

Ethos, Embodiment, Psychosis: Losing One's Home-Identity Stakes

Michèle Gennart

9.1 Introduction

The background to this chapter is provided by phenomenological work on the apprehension of the body by Erwin Straus [1] and on the constitution of identity by Paul Ricœur [2]. This work suggests an understanding of the body as a dimension of the self. The body participates in the self-affection by which the subject's identity is spontaneously constituted, albeit still below any conscious project or act of will. As soon as I am awake, move, and feel the world around me, I also *feel myself* as living this experience. Any bodily experience as it is lived as "mine" supports the feeling of "being oneself" (ipseity). Bringing ourselves into the world and inserting ourselves into an inter-corporeality, our body "anticipates" us in the process of building our sense of subjective identity [3].

According to this approach, our bodily condition is the bearer of an "intersubjective pre-identity," characterized by ethnic particularities, by a "family tune," but also by customs and habits, ways of trading with the world, of being with each other, which outline the main features of the ethos, of the cultural atmosphere, in which we have developed. As much in its appearance as by all the know-how and habits that it carries, our body is thus charged with sketches of identity of which we are not necessarily aware but which support our work of reflection and more deliberate choices and values about what we are and wish to become.

It is therefore through our living body, feeling and moving, that we are primarily present in the surrounding world as well as to ourselves, in what Erwin Straus calls a pre-reflexive pathic communication [1]. Now, different crises can affect this knot through which our body exerts its mediating function between "self" and world. Ruptures of belonging in migration or exile are one form of this rupture. By losing

M. Gennart (✉)
Centre de Recherches Familiales et Systémiques, Neuchâtel, Switzerland
e-mail: gennart@bluewin.ch

© The Author(s) 2021
D. Stoyanov et al. (eds.), *International Perspectives in Values-Based Mental Health Practice*, https://doi.org/10.1007/978-3-030-47852-0_9

the overall familiarity, the tuning, and the "syntony" that was created with the surrounding world and its singular culture, both sensitive and invisible, the subject is exposed to an identity discordance that may require considerable work of re-appropriation of her or him. Not only speaking and understanding the language of the other but also less obvious differences—ways of moving socially, tastes, sounds, landscapes, and atmospheres. All these aspects can be disconcerting and give the migrant subject the feeling of being "maladjusted" and "lost." In psychotic disorders, something of the very knotting of "self to the world" is affected in a more radical way [4]; one's own body seems no longer able to play its full natural or evident mediating function of bringing the subject into the world, and, in the same movement, to collect it "at home."

These considerations are illustrated by the following story in which "Tania Z" (not her real name), a woman of Portuguese descent, feels "betrayed" by her parents in relation to a central cultural value of her native country—namely the safeguarding and trans-generational transmission of the family home. She succumbs to a serious psychic crisis. Showing herself as more loyal than her parents to the values of their native country, but beyond all "reasonableness," she mobilizes a singular way of inhabiting the home in such a way that the latter exercises a function of *self-shelter* analogous to that of the own body. Her story departs from common sense—her family and friends do not understand her at all. Indeed, she puts into words processes that are usually implicit: those that allow the surrounding world to be presented as a *livable, familiar* space, making it possible for the self to exist. Her story thus allows us to understand something of these mysterious conditions of emergence, maintenance, or destruction of the human self [5].

9.2   The Story of Tania Z: Thrown Out of Home

Tania Z, a social worker in her fifties of Portuguese descent, was referred by her general practitioner (GP) for functional symptoms and an anxious state that compromised her ability to work and had led her to become increasingly isolated. The GP insisted that she should undergo a joint psychotherapeutic treatment, which she did not consent to easily. In her view, the problem was not psychological; it had to do with her body and her living space. She accepted nonetheless to meet with us and to give her suffering a narrative configuration.

Her story was that she had developed a severe anxious depression, with melancholic tendencies, when she learned that she was to be forced to leave the family home where she had lived most of her life, first with her parents, then by moving into her own apartment right above them.

Her parents, pressured by the real estate developers who were planning to demolish and rehabilitate the whole neighborhood, had accepted an offer to sell their house. Tania was given no choice in the matter. She was distressed by this situation, which she considered a betrayal by her parents: a betrayal of a central cultural value of their country of origin—namely the transgenerational handover of the family home—and a betrayal of the family spirit itself.

Prior to this, her parents had also chosen to be cremated at their death: this was also against family and cultural traditions. They did not want to burden their children and had organized their funeral themselves. Even then, Tania had felt abandoned: "It was terrifying for me. Even in death, they will abandon me. They did not even consider that I would end up alone in a grave!"

The "ultimate home"—the one that could have been shared by the family across time and generations—was therefore wiped out even before the current home was lost. This first decision taken by Tania's parents had already come as a blow to the family affiliation. The second, the sale of the house, definitely severed the integrity of the transgenerational connection. Tania thought she played an important and appreciated role for her parents by staying close to them; she would stop by on her way home from work, make sure they did not need anything, and advise them when they needed help. And then, they go and decide to move into a small apartment on their own, shattering the mission to which she had devoted herself years ago. The same goes for another implicit mission she had taken on: taking care of the house once the parents could no longer manage it. It was as if the fundamental beliefs that held her world together were being torn apart one after the other.

She appeared inhabited by a terrible indignation toward her parents and was ready to break off contact with them. However, the most intense suffering for her seemed to lie in the loss of the house, which she experienced as an actual ripping apart of her own being. "The day I will close the door of the house," she would say, "I will die. Or I will survive, but my spirit will no longer be." Losing her house therefore exposed her to the threat of losing her life or her spirit—the two possible forms of destruction of the self.

After a few months of acute apprehension, she managed to move, but her new living space was not well adapted to her. It had, for example, big windows that upset her: "I feel projected into an outside that doesn't belong to me. It makes no sense to me." She could not help hanging around the family house, picking herbs from the garden, with nostalgia, incomprehension, and heartbreak. Then, one day she found that there were other people occupying the house as it awaited demolition; she was distraught—"it is like a violation"—and had to hold herself back from violent aggression toward the intruders.

The next dreaded deadline was the demolition of the house—which she was not sure she would survive: "I don't know if I will be able to assume the physical destruction of the house." Through these unusual terms, Tania speaks of the surprising alliance by which our own self is linked to that of a place. She has become the guardian of the house that protected her, and its destruction feels like her own. "When I think about it," she says, "it terrorizes me. 'One day will be the last day'. It's so surreal that I am unable to put it into something real, concrete. It is definite, there is no turning back."

Tania thus describes with sharp clarity her diffracted experience of reality. On one hand, she maintains an access, which is intact, to objective reality, where things and people remain partes extra partes. Yet at the same time, she is experiencing a "surreal" dimension, which she cannot reconcile with concrete reality, and which seems to touch the very conditions of emergence and disaster of that reality for us as human beings. This second dimension refers to the affective or pathic juncture that determines if we have (or have not) a tie to the world that we can (or cannot) be in, or find our place in it. This very alliance is shattered for Tania Z. who, with her house, loses her home and her presence in the world.

She is one with the house, linked by mutual intimacy and protection. The destruction of this anchor leaves her exposed to a preoccupying strangeness, a wandering, and a lack of meaning. Her new apartment feels like a "warehouse" where her things are laid down; "I feel lost in this place. It doesn't suit me. What do I do now? That's where I'm at; it's totally surreal. There is no sense to it, it is attached to nothing. I am floating. I stay with my friend a bit, I stay here a bit. But when I'm here, I'm not. I don't recognize my things. There are no roots. I miss the house. I obsess about returning there. I don't have a home anymore."

The crisis that first affected her living space is reflected directly in her own body space. She floats, feels like a robot. She is worried about a series of neurovegetative symptoms—loss of appetite, vertigo, and tremors—which make her think she has a potentially fatal disease that has not yet been diagnosed. She pressed her GP to arrange various examinations to confirm her sense of imminent destruction of the self. She has lost her love of life, has lost weight, feels numb, old, and without bearings.

9.3   Values Arising

Tania Z did not present florid psychotic symptoms (such as delusions or hallucinations) but nevertheless presents the structure of melancholic experience as described by phenomenological psychiatrists such as Tellenbach [6], with alteration of the basic continuity of the self. Her clinical situation thus sheds particular light on the special role of places, especially the home, with regard to human health and illness. The home concerns, at the same time, one's own body, its potential as oneself and its relation to past and future generations.

Tania's experience, like that of many other patients, gives us, first of all, an insight into the strong link between one's own body and the enclosing home's space. This could be the space in a room or any corner of the world that feels like home. Duplicating the body in a certain way, as a second envelope of the self, as a world's skin around the physical skin, the "home" is an eminent form of space that allows us to gather ourselves together and to become open to other people.

"The non-I that protects I" as Bachelard [7, p. 5] puts it, the house constitutes a transitional space between the "I" and the "other," a space to which we connect ourselves, under the protection of which we can relax and have the confidence to go and explore the world, where we allow ourselves to encounter others. And like the transitional phenomenon defined by Winnicot [8], the home or the "special place" contributes to what "contains" us; it supports our—humanly fallible—experience of continuity and integrity. As Bachelard [7, p. 7] comments, "In the life of a man, the house thrusts aside contingencies, its councils of continuity are unceasing. Without it, man would be a dispersed being. It maintains him through the storms of the heavens and through those of life. It is body and soul. It is the human being's first world." The stability of a home is constitutive of what I would happily call our "psychosomatic foundations."

Tania's story also highlights the essentially *intersubjective* nature of the home. The so-called familiar space is first and foremost the space where our family lives, the space that our "loved ones" have made safe and secure for us. The newborn's welcome into the world is mediated through safe and secure places that provide, in cultural form, an analogue of the protection provided by the physical body. Our connection with the physical space that becomes our own is also mediated through our relations with others. The loss of familiar places, by exile, destruction or, as here, by forced sale, represents both a betrayal of our affiliations and a challenge to maintain our identity.

Psychosis, or as in Tania Z's story being in a state of psychotic vulnerability, by affecting one's security and sense of being oneself, leads to an increased risk of the person feeling "lost in the world," and maybe an increased need to be comforted by secure environments that protect the uncertain boundaries of the self. Tania feels abandoned, cast into the world alone by parents who agree to abandon the family home to housing developers. She lives in her body, in her psychosomatic consistency and identity, the loss and subsequent destruction of her "family home"— under its double intersubjective and spatial aspect.

9.4   Cultural Influences

In the situation described, two cultural models collide: Tania's participative model where the house is part of the family, defining the identity and purposes of its inhabitants, and, on the other hand, the utilitarian model, where the house, a physical object without any essential connection to people, is a disposable financial asset.

Tania's positioning is in line with her culture of Portuguese origin where it would indeed be expected that the family home is passed from one generation to the next, that the children take care of aging parents and that all rest at their death in the same grave. His migrant parents have somehow abandoned the norms and values of the native culture in the native country. And this mutation of the reference values, which appears to her through a series of parents' uncommented decisions, deeply upsets her. As Alfred Kraus, quoted by Tellenbach [5], writes, "social changes in the sense of breaking with the norm or of a contradiction with the norm can engender (...) dangerous general conditions for persons with a melancholy structure."

Among her relatives, Tania finds herself alone in witnessing the essential link that can arise between a material space and a living person—a link that perhaps constitutes what we would call the "soul" of a place. She struggles to be heard, but has nonetheless something to teach us about the significance of the house in relation to our "earthly" human condition. As Ricoeur [2, p. 150] puts it: "In virtue of the mediating function of the body as one's own in the structure of being in the world, the feature of selfhood belonging to corporeality is extended to that of the world as it is inhabited corporeally." Our active body, that is to say our condition as beings who move and feel, is our first way to "be ourselves," to assert out identity. But our embodied identity is never "pure," it is affected by "otherness," by our surroundings, by a world in which our identity is always a little mingled and entwined. To recapitulate Ricoeur's way of putting it, this aspect of the self-identity of the body extends to the physical, inhabited world. The place we inhabit as our "home" (corner, house, and region) typically relates to this aspect of world marked by the "self." Equally, the space perceived as uninhabitable is a space of floating and wandering, where the subject no longer finds a place to "be." Tania speaks to us with rare insight of the link between the possibility of being oneself and *finding shelter* in the world.

This shelter, which involves the practice of building, is one of the most basic foundations of culture. "All really inhabited space, says Bachelard [7, p. 5], bears the essence of the notion of home." As Tania's story makes us aware, society has a responsibility to look after inhabited spaces, not just as material objects, but as places where people move in and establish themselves. The loss and destruction of their home, for the most vulnerable, risk destroying their sense of personal identity.

9.5   Conclusions

Losing her sense of family belonging, Tania desperately attaches herself to the walls of her house - which seem to her more reliable, which can't betray. Like Winnicot's "transitional space," her "home" corner has become like a last bulwark: the ultimate "other" that surrounds and offers shelter and protection. Tania tells us about the essential link that can form between a material space and a bodily person. Opened by all our senses to the otherness of a world, we have to find protection in our exposition to space. This protection engages the practice of *inhabiting* it. The contribution of the habitat to our identity, to our sense of continuity and integrity, goes mostly unnoticed. Certain critical events are nevertheless able to remind us of our vulnerable "terrestrial" condition.

Altering the safety, the "naturality" of being-oneself, psychosis, and psychotic vulnerability are associated with increased risk for the person feeling lost in the world. These may also imply increased need to support the uncertain boundaries of self through the mediation of protective environments. Tania Z's story thus graphically reminds us that we should take care to recognize the primordial role of shared spaces and, from the intersubjective point of view, of this fundamental quality of hospitality offered to the "lost" human.

Acknowledgements   Thanks to the two colleagues who translated this text:

- Cristiana FORTINI, psychologist in charge of service, lecturer, Department of Addictions Medicine, Department of Psychiatry, Lausanne, Switzerland.
- Daniella ARDEL EPINEY, psychologist, Cantonal Service of Youth. Monthey—Switzerland.

9.6   Guide to Further Sources

For a values-based account of the importance of home to well being see:

- K. W. M. (Bill) Fulford and Kathleen T. Galvin (2018) *Values-based Practice: at Home with Our Values* Chapter 23, pp. 230–240, in Kathleen T. Galvin (Ed) Routledge Handbook of Well-Being. London: Routledge.

  For a further phenomenological account see:

- G. Stanghellini (2004) *Deanimated bodies and disembodied spirits. Essays on the psychopathology of common sense.* Oxford: Oxford University Press.

References

1. Straus E. The primary world of senses: a vindication of sensory experience. New York: Free Press of Glencoe; 1935/1963.
2. Ricoeur P. Oneself as another. Transl. by K. Blamey. Chicago: The University of Chicago Press; 1990/1992.
3. Gennart M. Corporéité et présence Jalons pour une approche du corps dans la psychose. Argenteuil: Le Cercle Herméneutique; 2011.
4. Fuchs T, Schlimme JE. Embodiment and psychopathology: a phenomenological perspective. Curr Opin Psychiatry. 2009;22(6):570–5.
5. Gennart M, Vannotti M. Espaces familiers et identité; quand l'espace propre est hanté... Thérapie Familiale. 2014;4:439–50.
6. Tellenbach H. Melancholy: history of the problem, endogeneity, typology, pathogenesis, clinical considerations. Transl. by Erling Eng. Pittsburgh: Duquesne University Press; 1961/1980.
7. Bachelard G. The poetics of space. Transl. by M. Jolias. Boston: Beacon Press; 1957/1994.
8. Winnicott DW. Transitional objects and transitional phenomena; a study of the first not-me possession. Int J Psychoanal. 1953;34:89–97.

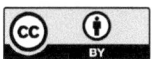

African Personhood, Humanism, and Critical Sankofaism: The Case of Male Suicide in Ghana

Camillia Kong

10.1 Introduction

Suicide in certain African contexts, such as in Ghana, is socially proscribed and subject to widespread moral condemnation. Not only is it illegal to attempt or commit suicide in Ghana—making one vulnerable to criminal prosecution if unsuccessful—but non-fatal suicide attempts are highly stigmatised to the point that individuals (and sometimes their family) are treated as social outcasts. A child will not be named after those who attempt or commit suicide for fears of contagion; sometimes they are refused a proper burial or the dead body may be whipped prior to removal [1]. As a social injury and violation of the common good, moral responsibility falls squarely on the shoulders of individuals and/or family members. These cultural norms are evident in the following narratives:

> *They beat me up mercilessly, hitting me with all kinds of objects—stones, sticks, using their hands. I was weak and tired...[I]t worried me a lot, the way I was disgraced, the fact that I had been a responsible worker before, with a bank … in fact I was traumatized very much. At a point I hid myself and was unable to even step out of the house* [2, p. 276].
>
> *I was told I was not a part of the family again. During family discussions I was disallowed to make contributions. Also even communal labor was very disturbing as people continued to avoid my company and make mockery of me when I attended it; hurling all kinds of insults at me. At a point I thought I should even try hard and end it all. You see you can really feel very bad after the action* [2, p. 277].
>
> *In fact my experience after my suicide attempt was worse than what I was going through initially. It was like everybody turned against me. I thought after the attempt people will be caring and supportive. But they were rather judgmental, they insulted and even my friends did not welcome me into their fold. Each time I visited them in a group I felt abandoned because it was like no one wanted to associate himself with a person who wanted to kill himself* [2, p. 277].

C. Kong (✉)
Institute for Crime and Justice Policy Research, School of Law, Birkbeck College, University of London, London, UK
e-mail: camillia.kong@bbk.ac.uk

© The Author(s) 2021
D. Stoyanov et al. (eds.), *International Perspectives in Values-Based Mental Health Practice*, https://doi.org/10.1007/978-3-030-47852-0_10

Shame associated with falling short of societal expectations around financial secu-rity and masculinity can also motivate suicide attempts:

> *I took a loan from Barclays [Bank] and one other from Ghanafin, a private financial institu-tion that deals with loans … So, Barclays takes from my salary and Ghanafin too … so I went to the bank on Monday thinking I will get something small to take and they said my account has been closed!…I blame myself for all these…I feel ending my life will resolve all these … my creditors will soon start chasing me … the shame and all that …*Man, 34 [3, p. 239]

The phenomenology around male suicide in Ghana reveals a complex, potentially contradictory web of communitarian values that are thought to be central to African personhood—or what it means to be identified and recognised as a person with a certain moral status. Crucially, African personhood is a *socially attained* status that reflects the extent to which one is embedded within communal values. By implica-tion, individuals who violate social norms central to group cohesion and well-being—such as proscriptions against suicide—warrant moral condemnation and blame. Such individuals relinquish (or possibly never attained) the social status of personhood; equally, however, strong gender norms implicitly sanction suicide over shame.

This contradiction could lead to charges of incoherence against the so-called 'traditional' African communitarian values around personhood. However, this chap-ter points to important internal resources within African thinking which encourages critical reflection of values that disregard the humanity of individuals. The Akan[1] tradition of *critical sankofaism* can help illustrate how African cultural values often contain important internal normative resources capable of responding to problem-atic views of shame and male gender norms which make suicide appear as the only option.

10.2   Suicide and Social Values around Gender

In Ghana, suicide is an act of *musuo*—extraordinary, uncommon, and indelible evil 'which brings suffering… to the whole community, not just to the doer alone'; as such, it is a complete abhorrence to the community [4]. As illustrated above, survi-vors are subject to intense moral condemnation, labelled sinner transgressor, outcast antisocial, or criminal, and viewed as deserving social sanction and abuse. Actions that are *musuo* reveal a flawed moral character in Akan moral thought and practice; individuals who attempt or commit suicide are therefore thought to reveal a

---

[1] Akan refers to one of the major ethnic groupings within Ghana and its conceptual schema and moral practices have been systematically theorised in the African philosophical tradition. In this chapter, I use Akan and African interchangeably—this is not to deny the fact of plural and diverse cultures and traditions within Africa. But I follow Gyekye [9] in his assertion that there are similar cultural patterns within Africa, one of which revolves around the communitarian conception of the self and person.

fundamentally evil character which lacks consideration and responsibility to family members and the communal good.

Male suicide is also closely connected to gender norms around avoiding shame. Fears of experiencing dishonour, disgrace, and moral sanction are deeply embedded in Akan moral practice. Various moral maxims describe how disgrace leads to a sense of shame: 'It is unbecoming of the Akan to be in disgrace' (or 'Disgrace does not befit the Akan': *animguase mfata okanniba*) [4, p. 139]. Fear and avoidance of shame function as strong motivation to act in accordance with social-normative expectations. Another maxim states powerfully, 'Given a choice between disgrace and death, one had better choose death' (*aniwu ne owu, na efanim owu*) [4, p. 139].

The shame of failing to meet certain masculine norms has been found to prompt fatal and non-fatal suicidal acts, as clearly illustrated in the man facing financial difficulties [5]. Local sayings promote certain male character traits, such as courage and bravery in adversity: 'a man doesn't cry' (*ɔbarima nsu*); 'a man does not fear death' (*ɔbarima nsuro owuo*); 'it's a real man who takes bitter medicine' (*ɔbarima na ɔnom aduro a ɛyɛ nnwono*) [5, p. 658]. These societal expectations of mental invincibility and physical strength in the face of suffering 'coincide with a general cultural prohibition against men's public expression of such emotions as fear, anxiety, pain or sadness, which are interpreted as forms of weakness', making it 'unmasculine for a man to express or admit feelings of weakness and emotional dependency' [6, p. 475].

Social expectations further uphold masculine ideals of sexual potency, procreation, and providing economically and materially for one's family; achievement of these ideals constitute successful male identity in society. By contrast, those in role reversals—where women function as economic providers—are described as 'useless man' (*ɔbarima hunu*) and subject to social stigma [5]. Virility and sexual prowess are likewise important. The ultimate test of masculinity is to have one's own biological children; impotency and childlessness are met with ridicule accordingly. Failure to achieve valued masculine identities and socially expected roles is a cause for low self-esteem, a sense of personal failure, defeat, and entrapment [5]. Shame around loss of social status generates feelings of defectiveness and helplessness, leading to fatal or non-fatal suicidal behaviour.

Rather ironically, the motivation behind male suicide reveals a strong identification with societal norms and expectations associated with what it means to be a valued male person in the community, as well as the internalisation of the blame directed towards individuals who fail to fulfil those norms. The depth to which these are internalised can paradoxically undermine the resiliency that is socially expected of male individuals. Obstacles and frustrations in fulfilling social responsibilities (procreation, economic provision, etc.) cause substantial anxiety and the perceived—and sometimes real—loss of dignity. A man's exaggerated sense of personal responsibility and self-blame for his own failure accurately reflects social norms where shame and disgrace are tantamount to the loss of personhood. In short, 'local axioms […] seem to provide tacit approval for men to use suicide for addressing shame' [5, p. 663]. Suicide appears to be a fully coherent response, confirmed even by commonplace proverbs.

10.3   Communitarianism of African Personhood

The priority of the community over the individual is frequently cited as a distinctive feature of African personhood, particularly in comparison to Western individualism. Menkiti describes that 'persons become persons only after a process of incorporation. Without incorporation into this or that community, individuals are considered to be mere danglers to whom the description 'person' does not fully apply' [7, p. 172]. Menkiti's formulation lends itself to a strong constitutive reading of communitarianism, whereby 'the individual self is defined by, integrated into, and constituted in the community by the organic processes of acculturalisation, socialisation, moral education, and ritual integration' [8, p. 1010]. This strong reading contains two notable features: first, personhood is a *normative social* concept in the sense that the achievement of moral personhood comes only with the ability to fulfil one's communally-determined duties and responsibilities [8]. This normative conception of personhood presumes that developing persons are inculcated within a society that prioritises certain values surrounding one's pre-eminent responsibility to one's family and community, which become manifest in moral character and behaviour aligned with such commitments. Second, personhood is a *socially attained* status rather than a presumption of human species membership: the achievement of personhood is proportionate to one's participation in communal life and the extent to which the different obligations of one's social role are fulfilled [7].

The attainment of personhood clearly depends on the integration of communal values so that one acts within the constraints and possibilities of what is socially acceptable, making norms of personhood and sociocultural context mutual reinforcing. An individual's understanding of self, responsibilities, and actions must embed the values and interests of one's community. Recognition of a person can then be contingent on conformity with and the achievement of socially determined benchmarks of success. Conversely, 'the decline in the values of a person [...] may also indicate a decline in the values or culture of the community of which the person is part' [8, p. 1008]. All persons therefore share responsibility in contributing to the welfare of the community. The moral status of personhood is earned when social norms are properly internalised and social obligations are fulfilled as an upstanding member of the community [9]. Whether individuals observe or disregard their duties to the social community can mean the attainment, diminishment, or even loss of one's status of personhood. Thus, the communal context *shapes* individual selves while also *evaluating* who deserves the status of personhood based on their compliance to socially expected norms.

On this account, failures to carry out socially expected obligations and roles are viewed as instances of personal irresponsibility, callousness, or generally vicious character. The Akan belief that habitual actions influence the development of one's moral orientation overall means that 'one is [...] responsible for the sort of person one is [and] the state of his or her character' [9, p. 150]. Falling short of the criteria of personhood is therefore morally blameworthy because such actions disclose the wrong normative orientation towards oneself and one's community.

Yet the case of male suicide lays bare the incoherence at the heart of this strongly communitarian conception of personhood: what drives the behaviour of the individuals in the case studies above is not a rejection of social responsibility or disregard for the community, but rather an intense sense of personal responsibility towards fulfilling socially informed norms and roles, particularly associated with gender. For example, the failure to realise male norms related to economic security engenders the self-blame pervading in the man's narrative above, making suicide preferable to social ostracisation. If anything, such examples demonstrate how the *overidentification with* and *internalisation of* socially constituted duties and norms can lead to the very circumstances, motivations, and behaviours that impede the achievement of normative personhood. The worry, then, is that values of African personhood seem to imply 'a cramped and shackled self, responding robotically to the ways and demands of the communal structure', thereby potentially perpetuating and worsening the underlying issues associated with male suicide [9, pp. 55–6]. Moreover, a constitutive account of personhood would have to admit that the failure of individuals to act in a manner aligned with personhood lies partly with the community's values, practices, and incorporation rituals.

This suggests that reflective mechanisms need to be in place to encourage the critical examination of African traditions, particularly in the examination of potentially destructive but socially affirmed norms related to mental health, gender, and personhood. But rather than abandon the communitarian values of African personhood altogether, we must tease out ways in which its humanistic core can temper and limit the demands of the community. Important internal resources are present within Akan moral thinking which would help challenge some of the more pernicious implications of strongly communitarian African values.

10.4   Critical Sankofaism

The case of male suicide may tempt one to reject the communitarian basis of personhood altogether and presume that critical analytical resources need to be imported from Western frameworks. African practices and conceptual schemas are often *reduced* to a static, unreflective tradition while those from the West are seen as *removed from* tradition. Yet this disregards the fact that Akan thinking contains crucial critical resources that belie this mischaracterisation of African social practices and traditions as stagnant and unthinking. The Adinkra symbol of *sankofa* is particularly fruitful in this context: visually depicted as a mythical bird flying forward while looking back, sankofa communicates the philosophy of retrieving lost or forgotten gems from the past as one moves forward; it involves reclaiming parts of African practice, history, and standpoints that have been hidden or distorted [10].

At times the pursuit of sankofa has been interpreted as endorsing the blind revival of African cultural values, leading to the uncritical adoption of the past or certain traditions simply by virtue of it symbolising the renaissance of an African tradition and putative subversion of the Western colonial legacy. This *naïve sankofaism* presumes that African values and ways of life are normatively valuable in a wholesale sense and are capable of being revived in a pristine, authentic, and precolonial form. Yet as Gyekye explains, just as the sankofa bird will spit out rotten seed going forward, so too should approaches to traditional cultural values be critically reflective in ways that consider their functionality and appropriateness to fundamental human needs in contemporary life, captured in the Akan proverb that 'A person cutting a path does not know that the past that he has cleared behind him is crooked' [9, p. 262]. *Critical sankofa* is therefore a process of reclaiming cultural values through the critical evaluation which leads to the reflective endorsement or rejection of past practices or traditions. It demands being conversant with cultural forms to grasp the deeper meanings and possibilities immanent from that tradition; equally it requires a way of working dialectically between one's experiences and needs in the present and the critical interpretation and retrieval of worthwhile values and wisdom from the past. In other words, critical sankofa involves the reflective sifting through, refining and pruning of, different aspects of the cultural past, to determine whether it warrants a place in the current scheme of things. Those values that ultimately deserve reclamation and revival will promote attitudes, practices, and behavioural patterns that are conducive to the attainment of basic human needs—thus functioning as a potential framework for development [9].

Critical sankofa therefore provides an important normative framework *internal* to African cultural schemas, enabling the critical evaluation of problematic dimensions of shame, disgrace, and gender norms within African communitarianism that are manifest in the phenomena of male suicide in Ghana. The core ideals of African communitarianism rest on socioethical values of solidarity, interdependence, mutual aid and obligation, yet, as Gyekye states, '[t]he communitarian social arrangement, as established and practiced in African cultures, has, however, spawned some features that have thrown the worthwhileness and continuity of the arrangement in its old form into question' [9, p. 252]. Problematic masculine ideals and communitarian social arrangements coalesce to some degree, as male norms are closely connected to one's ability to fulfill one's responsibility to meet the needs of group members. Such responsibility is difficult to bear unless one possesses economic wealth and influence [5, 9], meaning values associated with male economic power—and shame when one falls short—intermingle with the communitarian sense of self and one's sense of belonging in deep ways. Yet through the lens of critical sankofa it becomes clear that sociocultural values of what 'being a man' amounts to—reinforced tacitly in local idioms around the preferability of death to shame—corrupt rather than capture the humanism at the core of African communitarian values. Patriarchal expectations associated with economic viability, sexual prowess, and male potency distort the ways in which the needs of the community are to be fulfilled (i.e. support for the needs of those less fortunate, the promotion of familial ties, etc.), and indeed, *devalue* the human being who is subject to such expectations.

To see this, one has to understand the humanism that is the basis of African communitarian personhood. The highest worth of and consideration owed to a human being is expressed in the Akan proverb, 'It is the human being that counts; I call upon gold, it answers not; I call upon cloth, it answers not; it is the human being that counts' [9, p. 258]. To value a person as a human being involves expressing virtues of compassion, generosity, and a sense of moral duty to assist others to benefit their interests and welfare. It is to 'acknowledge that her worth as a human being is equal to our own and that there are some basic values, ideals, and sentiments (such as hopes and fears) that we all share by virtue of our common membership in the human species' [9, p. 259]. The community must therefore uphold and embody certain humanist and egalitarian norms of moral regard, care, and concern for others, which function as the normative framework that enables individuals to actualise the potentiality of attaining the status of personhood. As Nyerere describes, 'In traditional African society [...] we took care of the community, and the community took care of us ... Nobody starved, either of food or of human dignity' [8, p. 1008]. Individuals are presumed to have certain psychological characteristics, such as the ability to make deliberative, freely willed choices, and can be held responsible for fulfilling obligations towards others and one's community as such. Each individual likewise possesses intrinsic worth such that one should 'care for her well-being or needs just as she cares for the needs of others' so that 'altruistic concerns cannot obliterate responsibilities to the self' [9, p. 69].

Thus, from the perspective of critical sankofa there is a clear disconnect between the sociocultural norms around masculinity which engender shame when one falls short as opposed to the core virtues expressed in valuing human beings and developing and meeting basic human needs. Returning to the opening narratives, the man who had survived a suicide attempt anticipated and hoped for care and support but was met instead with bitter condemnation and isolation by both his family and community. Meeting the challenge of male suicide in Ghana will therefore involve counteracting and critically challenging harmful dimensions of sociocultural norms around gender and promoting understanding of those who attempt suicide—recognising how social ostracisation devalues the intrinsic value and needs of human beings, as well as distorts the tradition of mutual aid, compassion, and empathy embedded in the humanistic core of African communitarianism.

10.5 Conclusion

Critical sankofa is an important process which evaluates and retrieves what is worthwhile about the humanism that grounds African community and personhood. The critical reflexivity of critical sankofa challenges pernicious distortions of African values in the context of suicide, as well as more generally the exoticisation and static characterisation of African traditions and values. Critical sankofa also has important implications beyond this context: although discussed as an internal African resource, this approach has clear similarities to Western hermeneutical frameworks that situate current practices within a historical, interpretative tradition. The hermeneutical process involves working dialectically between the acknowledgement and critical evaluation of traditions and cultural practices through the prism of contemporary questions and needs. Western discourses that medicalise suicide can ignore how such behaviours represent a 'life crisis situation' where individuals and their environment interact in dynamic ways, and as such, critical scrutiny of Western sociocultural values and norms around gender are put to one side. A hermeneutical approach modelling a similar process to that of critical sankofa could promote greater reflection on the distorted values, practices, and traditions that can devalue human beings and motivate suicide within Western cultures.

Acknowledgements Thanks to Caesar Atuire, Martin Ajei, Katrin Flikschuh, and others for discussion and feedback on an earlier draft presented at the *Persons—African Perspectives* conference at Universität Bonn, May 2018.

Guide to Further Sources

Gadamer, H.G., Weinsheimer, J. and Marshall, D.G., 2004. *Truth and Method*. Bloomsbury Publishing USA.

Osafọ J, Akotia CS, Hjelmeland H, Knizek BL. From condemnation to understanding: Views on suicidal behavior in Ghana in transition. Death studies. 2017 Sep 14;41(8):532–41.

Presbey GM. Maasai concepts of personhood: the roles of recognition, community, and individuality. International Studies in Philosophy. 2002 May 1;34(2):57–82.

Supremo Mensa. Africa critically needs what we term, "Sankofa"—Prof. Gyekye [Internet]. Supremovisions. 2016 [cited 10 December 2019]. Available from: https://supremovisions.wordpress.com/2016/12/04/africa-critically-needs-what-we-term-sankofa-prof-gyekye/

Wiredu K. The moral foundations of an African culture. In Kwasi Wiredu and Kwame Gyekye. Eds. *Person and community*. Washington, DC; 1992.

References

1. Akotia CS, Knizek BL, Kinyanda E, Hjelmeland H. "I have sinned": understanding the role of religion in the experiences of suicide attempters in Ghana. Ment Health Relig Cult. 2014;17(5):437–48.
2. Osafo J, Akotia CS, Andoh-Arthur J, Quarshie EN. Attempted suicide in Ghana: motivation, stigma, and coping. Death Stud. 2015;39(5):274–80.
3. Akotia CS, Knizek BL, Hjelmeland H, Kinyanda E, Osafo J. Reasons for attempting suicide: an exploratory study in Ghana. Transcult Psychiatry. 2019;56(1):233–49.
4. Gyekye K. An essay on African philosophical thought: the Akan conceptual scheme. Philadelphia: Temple University Press; 1995.
5. Andoh-Arthur J, Knizek BL, Osafo J, Hjelmeland H. Suicide among men in Ghana: the burden of masculinity. Death Stud. 2018;42(10):658–66.
6. Adinkrah M. Better dead than dishonored: masculinity and male suicidal behavior in contemporary Ghana. Soc Sci Med. 2012;74(4):474–81.
7. Menkiti IA. Person and community in African traditional thought. In: Wright RA, editor. African philosophy: an introduction. 3rd ed. New York: University Press of America; 1984. p. 171–82.

8. Ikuenobe P. Relational autonomy, personhood, and African traditions. Philos East West. 2015;65(4):1005–29.
9. Gyekye K. Tradition and modernity: philosophical reflections on the African experience. Oxford: Oxford University Press; 1997.
10. Temple CN. The emergence of Sankofa practice in the United States: a modern history. J Black Stud. 2010;41(1):127–50.

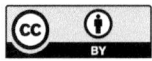

Temitope Ademosu, Tutiette Thomas, and Sola Adebiyi

'Tala kati na yo, nzela ya bonsomi',—'be the change you want to see in the world'

11.1 Introduction

Service users from the African diaspora consistently receive poorer mental health outcomes in the UK. A deeper delve into culture, migration history, religion, acculturative stress and trauma is required to understand how mental illness is conceptualised and responded to by many African diaspora individuals. This deep dive is often ignored or dismissed in the West, resulting in individuals from the diaspora receiving treatment that falls short of their needs.

This chapter explores through a detailed transgenerational case study, of Masimbo, who migrated with his family from Zimbabwe to the UK, to highlight the conceptualisation and journey of mental illness within an African cultural perspective. Comments are provided from all three of us as authors, respectively, a service user and former carer (Tutiette Thomas), an African healer and storyteller (Sola Adebiyi), and a systemic psychotherapist (Temitope Ademosu). The thread that binds us is our lived experiences as members of the African diaspora straddling two cultures and our passion for respecting both Western and African philosophies,

T. Ademosu (✉)
Kings Global Health Institute, University of East London, London, UK

T. Thomas
South London and Maudsley NHS Foundation Trust, London Borough of Southwark, London, UK

S. Adebiyi
Narrative Mindfulness Ltd, London, UK

© The Author(s) 2021
D. Stoyanov et al. (eds.), *International Perspectives in Values-Based Mental Health Practice*, https://doi.org/10.1007/978-3-030-47852-0_11

promoting an approach in which mental illness and the nuances that culture brings is appreciated and worked with.

11.2   Narrative History: *Masimbo*

The background to Masimbo's story is the Rhodesian Bush War that broke out in the 1960s as many majority black citizens fought against the injustices of a powerful white minority rule in Zimbabwe. In its aftermath, the Gukurahundi took place, a civil conflict that lasted 4 years, resulting in nearly 20,000 war-related deaths, many of them Ndebele civilians. This legacy of European colonialism resulted in many Zimbabweans, both Ndebele and Shona, becoming displaced nationally and internationally (Fig. 1.1).

Emmerson (Masimbo's father), of Ndebele ancestry, had spent years developing his lucrative farm just outside Harare (previously Salisbury), Zimbabwe, to sustain his family. Married to his second wife Grace, who raised his five sons, Emmerson lived comfortably in his homeland. A well-known and respected member of his community, Emmerson was a vocal citizen who remained active in politics speaking out against injustices.

It was a bright, stuffy morning when Masimbo, aged 14, his father Emmerson and their family fled from Harare. The war was intensifying and showed no signs of ending. 13 h and 8000 miles later Masimbo and his family arrived in Cardiff airport on a dark, damp morning in 1983. Masimbo and his twin, Dakarai, soon settled into a local school. As the only black boys in the school there were several challenges both boys had to navigate alone. Their father, Emmerson, spent long hours working during the day as a bus driver and his evenings as a domestic cleaner. Their

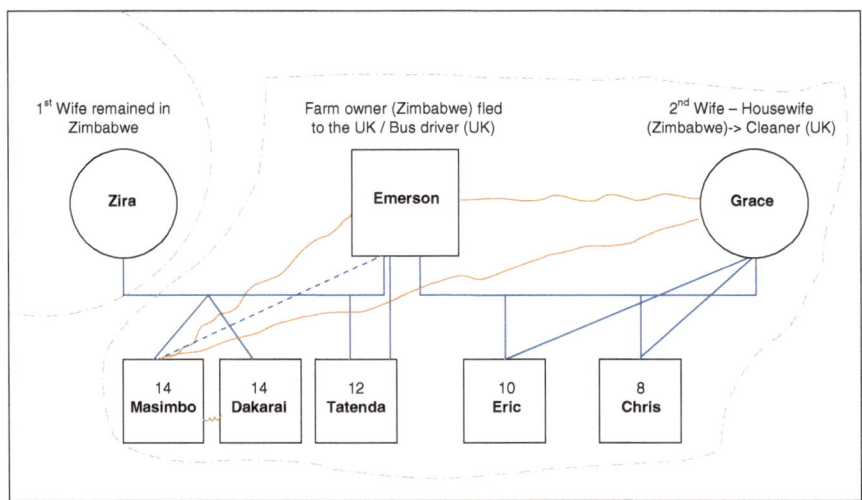

Fig. 1.1 Masimbo's family genogram

stepmother, Grace, showered love and attention on her two biological children only, causing many tensions to arise in the family home. Incidents of conflict around relationships and finances were common.

After 3 years living in Wales, Masimbo and his family moved to Liverpool, a city in the North of the UK. Here Masimbo, by now a musically talented boy, aged 17, struggled in school both academically and socially with his peers. As a result of his quiet, shy personality he was often isolated among his peers. In contrast, his twin brother, Dakarai, was an out-going, lively bright teenager who excelled academically and was extremely popular in school. Academic success was the family currency in Masimbo's family. Emmerson wanted his sons to reclaim in the UK the life and the status they had once enjoyed in Zimbabwe, and he believed education to be the key to survival. Anything short of this was failure. Masimbo was constantly reminded of his shortcoming in this regard.

Despite these difficulties, Masimbo enrolled in university and developed a close friendship group. Girls, social drugs and alcohol were a common feature amongst many students at university and Masimbo used drugs and alcohol recreatively and enjoyed spending many hours mastering Tai chi and his guitar. Again, though, beyond his immediate group of friends, Masimbo's shy temperament led to him once again becoming isolated and feeling lonely as he was unable to connect with his peers. Emmerson, still a bus driver and domestic cleaner glowed with pride when he spoke of Dakarai who continued to be academically successfully and remained the thread and hope to keeping his dream and aspirations alive of reclaiming all he had lost in Zimbabwe. Aged 21, Masimbo now felt he had settled in life. He had a satisfying relationship with his girlfriend, Claire, whom he now lived with, and was well developed in Tai chi. His relationship with his father remained fractious.

It was Dakarai that rung him one evening and broke the news that his girlfriend Claire had cheated on him. This news made Masimbo feel like the scared, vulnerable boy who started life in Wales many years ago. Friends and family saw a steep decline in Masimbo's behaviour as he continued to withdraw into himself. He self-medicated with cannabis, isolated himself from his few friends, and eventually ended all activities with Tai chi. Masimbo then spiralled out of control.

Recognising his decline, concerned friends and family were moved to support Masimbo. Emmerson, worried about his son immediately met with his Pastor at Church to discuss about healing for Masimbo. They strongly believed that evil spirits had entered Masimbo causing him to have this 'spirit of madness'. The Pastor offered an array of treatments for Masimbo that included a consultation, followed by prayer, fasting and deliverance for divine healing.

In 2001 Masimbo had his first mental health breakdown, a psychotic episode that resulted in his arrest and subsequent section (involuntary detention) on a mental health ward. Family, friends and Church members swarmed the ward to visit Masimbo and offer prayers, Holy oil, and a Bible to continue his process of healing. Masimbo struggled for years in and out of the wards as he often refused to take the medications prescribed for him due to their unpleasant side effects. His behaviour remained unchanged. With little improvement and no clear diagnosis being assigned to his son, Emmerson believed his own actions had aggrieved the ancestral spirits resulting in them withdrawing their protection from Masimbo. There was only one solution for this supernatural cause—and it could not be found in the hospital. Emmerson tapped into his transnational network and sought support from African traditional medicine, Hun'aga from Zimbabwe, to identify the underlying cause for Masimbo's illness.

When Masimbo and Emmerson discussed this traditional approach with his clinical team, it was frowned upon. Both father and son were encouraged to continue working with his care team to support Masimbo with medication and therapy. Dismayed, Emmerson agreed to the clinical plan, but continued his pursuit of Hun'aga privately, with renewed fervour.

11.2.1 Values Arising in the Story: What Matters or What Is Important to Those Concerned

Sola: I spent some time with Masimbo's parents. They often stated that perhaps leaving their home was not such a good idea. His father in particular reflected that he knew people 'back home who would have known what to do'. When questioned further, he would smile cryptically and say, 'in our village there are people who have medicines for all illnesses'. It was important for Emmerson to 'tap into' his traditional resources 'back home'.

This was also an important value for Masimbo who would often announce 'my dad did not even want me to get better because he didn't even take me back home!'

Temitope: Sola's point reminds me of my childhood. It was with love that my mother would reach into the 'special cupboard' full of unnamed jars of powders, creams and soaps, with a wide array of colours. She would rub something on a bruised limb, a runny stomach or any ailment.

There are several values that grab me as I read this case study. Emmerson, migrating from Zimbabwe to the UK, lost his livelihood, status and identity in the process. It was important for him to reclaim this to make the migratory journey worth it. In turn, this sudden migration also had a strong impact on everyone in the family. His sons Masimbo and Dakarai as young boys fled from a white minority rule system in Zimbabwe to join a white majority rule in the UK. They both had to balance values as Black boys in white majority settings. Grace left the comforts of her life in Zimbabwe to work, care and support the family in the UK. Although silenced in this case study, I wonder what was important to her. Emmerson's connection with his network 'back home' and seeking healing through religion and culture appear to be Emmerson's act of love and care to his son.

Tutiette: *Ubuntu ngumtu ngabanye abantu*—'A person is a person through other people'.

As a service user and former carer from the African diaspora, I strongly identify with Masimbo's narrative. Although I am a second-generation UK citizen, I connect with Masimbo also having lived with the legacies of the trauma of broken attachments. Masimbo and his family faced a range of acculturative stressors when migrating from Zimbabwe to escape violence, this included as key values, legacies of the trauma of broken attachments through migration, and disruption of his support network that may contribute to the progression of his psychotic symptoms. In seeking to restore his son's mental health through syncretic practices, Emmerson demonstrates African/Abantu discussion of the Cartesian dualism 'Mind-Body problem' (as in the above aphorism).

11.2.2 The Influences of Culture on the Story

Sola: Masimbo was a young man who inherited a dichotomy of cultural influences. On one hand sat an African 'Christian' perspective that viewed mental illness as the result of demonic possession. Interestingly, this perspective also viewed traditional African practices as 'witchcraft and lead by the devil'. However, on the other hand sat an innate connection and draw to healing that drew on traditional medicine and its ability to heal.

Including the *treasure chest of wisdom* from humanity is crucial. The paradox proved confusing for Masimbo. Added to this mix was the Western medication which is implicitly and quietly the route that many 'civilised people' use to address mental illness. I wonder if, without the constraints and stigma towards African-led practices, Masimbo and his family would have had an array of options available to them, particularly ones they knew well.

Temitope: Emmerson, Masimbo and his siblings were born in Zimbabwe with a strong history of colonialism. Growing up in this era as middle-class Black Zimbabweans meant that families felt the visceral pain of livelihoods flushed away, lost opportunities and cheated dreams when they were displaced. The history of Zimbabwean migration to the UK is long-standing. In consequence, Emmerson held simultaneous attachments to both the UK and Zimbabwe as a result of straddling two worlds. It is important to note that despite 20 years in the UK, in various crises, it was still to Zimbabwe that Emmerson 'returned home'.

Emmerson's aetiology of mental illness was strongly linked to spiritual factors. It was important from this perspective for treatment to go beyond the physical manifestations of the problem to include underlying spiritual issues. These explanatory models of mental illness are often not acknowledged or valued by practitioners in the West. This case study, however, highlights how powerful these models are as Emmerson returns to these beliefs to seek help. The cultural and spiritual needs of Masimbo need to be addressed to cater for his physical and mental health needs.

Tutiette: For Masimbo and Emmerson, as service user and carer respectively, the Zimbabwean epistemology, called upon to resolve distress, faced epistemological injustice. Yet, much of the psychiatry and psychology workforce are trained in 'cultural sensitivity' with the aim of providing culturally competent services. If this approach was successfully implemented across the UK, Masimbo, his family and friends would have facilitated Ndebele rites of passage, including access to the psychotropic compounds of the Ndebele.

Acculturative stress and the psychological impact of adaptation to a new culture, along with trauma are factors that may have contributed to the development of

Masimbo's crisis. The need to understand the history of this culture, and to respect the responses to it into which the African diaspora taps, is crucial.

11.3   Storytelling as Healing in African Culture and Beyond

With Masimbo's story in mind, it is worthwhile reminding ourselves that although many African conceptions of the universe and our place in it are different from their European counterparts, there are also parallels. These parallels become clear when we consider the role of mythopoetic stories within each tradition. In Western Christianity for example, the story of humanity's first millennium on earth has a mystical narrative, with divine beings, miraculous happenings and 'holy' visitations. The stories of Jacob, Elijah, David and others have resonance with the stories of a magical universe, not unlike that which African spiritual traditions such as that of the Yoruba, consider as their reality.

The mythopoetic universe of the Yoruba furthermore involves a range of archetypes that in the West might be called Jungian. There is though an important difference. The archetypes of the Yoruba are not 'unconscious' but very much at the forefront of the conscious minds of practitioners. These Yoruba archetypes are known as Orisa (pronounced Oree Sha), and each has a divine essential power similar to that of ancient Greek Gods. Actually, since many African peoples claim that their traditions are the descendants of those of Kemet (Ancient Egypt), and since according to Herodotus (the ancient Greek 'father of modern history'), the ancient Greeks were students of Kemetic masters, this similarity has a logical resonance.

One result of this difference is that storytelling in the Yoruba tradition is *not* just entertainment. To people who live in such a liminal world, their understanding of the happenings of life is actually defined by spiritual narratives. Understood in this way, their practices of choosing specific stories and poems of ancestors through divination, and mining the power of these for healing, communion and for divine solutions to mundane problems, all make complete sense. This is possible, because from such an ontological perspective, there are no mundane solutions. Everything that occurs has a spiritual precedent and the stories provide 'magical keys' to unlock the treasure trove of divine providence, bringing it to bear on specific issues. Again, this is not so very different from European traditions. As Acts 17:28 in the Christian Bible expounds 'in him we live and move and have our being', so too does the Yoruba traditionalist live, move and have their being in the mythopoetic universe of their ancestors.

All this is of course not applicable to the Yoruba alone. I (Sola) once listened to a Zulu shaman, Credo Mutwa, explain how he was taught to calm his troubled mind and also to visualise solutions to problems, through touching the eagle totem in his grandfather's house and listening to stories about it. I have experienced the power of this approach myself when, a few years ago, I was stuck in a depressive and resourceless state from which I could see no way out. I went to see a Babalawo or Yoruba Shaman. He did a divination and told me that he was guided to tell me a specific story as the 'medicine for my woes'. The story he told was of Ogun, the Orisa of iron, and how he began civilisation. This in shortened form is the story he told me.

In the beginning of time when the Orisa came from Orun (heaven) to Ile (earth), Ile was covered by a vast impenetrable forest. All of the Orisa tried with their various mighty powers to pass through: Sango burnt trees with massive lightning bolts, Oya uprooted them with hurricanes, and Yemoya caused tsunami force tidal waves to smash them down. However their success was very limited and despite their combined might, they were unable to win through. Eventually, Ogun stepped up and using his magic sword parted the trees. The Orisa were able to pass through and civilisation began.

Having told me this story, the Babalawo asked me to visualise the forest as the deep unknown area of my unconscious mind and to recognise Ogun's sword as the will focussed on impressing the subconscious mind with its intention. I did this repeatedly also understanding that 'civilisation' was the metaphorical solution to my specific problem and that by making offerings including meditation, I would be able to intuit the antidote to the stuck place in which I found myself. Importantly, and this is crucial, I was told that through participation in tailored rituals (story enactments, songs, dances and offerings) I would also be supported by the divine power of Ogun, The Opener of The Way. I found this to be a uniquely practical and personal way to harness the omnipotence of the 'Divine' to the service of human beings.

11.4 Conclusions

We have shown through the story of Masimbo and his family the importance of adopting an approach to mental health care that has the flexibility to combine Western and African traditions of thought and practice. Displaced from his ancestral Zimbabwe to the UK as a young boy, Masimbo, who is rather shy and lacking in confidence, falls into a depression that proves resistant to treatment. His father, Emmerson, is ready to (as he still puts it even after over 20 years) 'take Masimbo home' to consult with a traditional healer. Consistently with his Yorubo culture, he blames himself for his son's problems believing he had alienated their ancestral spirits. But the Western mental health professionals caring for Masimbo frown on this idea. They remain in the UK, and Masimbo remains depressed. Just what the outcome of Masimbo's story would have been had a more joined up approach been offered we can only speculate. But Sola's experience as a storyteller, on which the last part of our discussion draws, suggests that it may well have had been more positive not only for Masimbo but for family, and notably his father, Emmerson.

There is a growing recognition of the need within contemporary person-centred medicine to take the spiritual needs of service users as seriously as their mental and bodily needs [1]. Masimbo's story reinforces the message of this chapter, namely of the potential contribution of mythopoetry as a resource for meeting the spiritual needs of people of the African Diaspora. Again, our view, as we have repeatedly emphasised, is not that African approaches should displace those of Western medicine. To the contrary, everything we have said in this chapter is to the effect that African mythopoetry should be made available for people of the Diaspora but always alongside other forms and conventions of healing including those of Western psychiatry. Neither is a panacea. If this is true for people of the Diaspora, furthermore, the similarities we have indicated in the origins and manifestations of these apparently very different traditions, suggest that there may be a role for storytelling in the African mythopoetic tradition in meeting the spiritual needs not just of people of the Diaspora but of many others as well.

11.5 Guide to Further Sources

For more on spirituality in Western psychiatry see the website of the Royal College of Psychiatrists Spirituality and Psychiatry Special Interest Group at: www.rcpsych. ac.uk/college/sig/spirit

Reference

1. Coyte ME, Gilbert P, Nicholls V, editors. Spirituality, values and mental health: jewels for the journey. London: Jessica Kingsley Publishers; 2007.

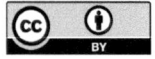

Inside and Out: How Western Patriarchal Cultural Contexts Shape Women's Relationships with Their Bodies

Hillary Lianna McBride and Janelle Lynne Kwee

12.1 Introduction

A woman's relationship with her body is experienced from the inside as it is felt, known, and lived personally through her first-person perspective. At the same time, a woman's relationship with her body is shaped by broader sociocultural influences around her, which are evident in the context of personal relationships, organizations, and media. All of these influences express cultural values about women's bodies. These broader influences can simultaneously feel both invisible and ubiquitous, and they play a significant role in a woman's experience of her physicality: whether she feels she can move freely through the world, enjoy her sexuality, feed herself, go places and know she is safe, dance and play with abandon, and see herself as a holistic agentic being rather than as a sexualized object. How she experiences and expresses her physicality also tells a story about her relationship to her social context, and her phenomenological experiences of being a woman.

Disordered eating appears to be a symptom of these ubiquitous yet sometimes invisible patriarchal cultural values about women's bodies. Girls and women receive 90–95% of eating disorder diagnoses [1] and risk of developing an eating disorder increases with time spent in Westernized cultures [2], which perpetuate a thin ideal female body type, an ideal which is largely unattainable. Narratives of femininity in patriarchal cultures foster the objectification of women and girls and are linked to

H. L. McBride
University of British Columbia, Vancouver, BC, Canada
e-mail: hilarymcbride@gmail.com

J. L. Kwee (✉)
Master of Arts in Counselling Psychology Program, Faculty of Humanities and Social Sciences, Trinity Western University, Langley, BC, Canada
e-mail: Janelle.Kwee@twu.ca

© The Author(s) 2021
D. Stoyanov et al. (eds.), *International Perspectives in Values-Based Mental Health Practice*, https://doi.org/10.1007/978-3-030-47852-0_12

internalized objectification, body shame, low self-esteem, lack of internal awareness, and disordered eating [3].

Below, we present a case history of a woman we will call 'Annie' to illustrate the
influences of a Western patriarchal cultural context on her relationship with her
body, specifically her development of Anorexia Nervosa, and her experience with
medical and psychological treatment within the same Western patriarchal context.

12.2   The Story of Annie

*Annie[1] first came into my (HM) therapy office when she was 28. She was seeking
weekly psychotherapy after having recently been dismissed from an eating disorder
treatment facility for being non-compliant with the treatment provider's interventions. Her physician had labelled her Anorexia Nervosa as 'treatment resistant', she
was considered to be chronically ill, was unable to sustain employment, and was
referred to the treatment facility for more intensive medical monitoring and group
and individual therapy. When she communicated to the treatment providers that she
did not want to participate in one of the group therapy activities involving mechanical eating, she was given a 'warning' about her involvement in the program. When
she shared with her psychiatrist that she did not want to continue on the medication
he had prescribed to her, as it was making her feel too sleepy to participate in individual therapy, she was told she was 'non-compliant' and was being ejected from
the program.*

*During the initial assessment phase of therapy, Annie indicated that her disor-
dered eating behaviour began when she was a child. When she was young, she was
sexually abused by an older male in her extended family. She remembered that after
the abuse occurred she felt dirty and wanted to punish herself by not eating, thinking of herself as not worthy of being fed. On one occasion she attempted to tell her
parents about the abuse but her concerns were invalidated and dismissed, and she
remembered being scolded for making up a lie about this family member. The eating
disorder behaviour increased in frequency and intensity in her late teens when she
began having regular nightmares about the abuse from her childhood. She shared
that she was both restricting her caloric intake as a way of punishing herself, and
over-exercising to the point of fatigue, hoping that that would make it easier for her
to fall asleep and stay asleep at night.*

*Although she initially sought psychotherapy with me to continue treatment for
the eating disorder, she first wanted to address her experience at the treatment facility. How she was managed at the treatment facility left her feeling like she did as a
child when she told her parents about the abuse: punished and shamed for speaking
up about what did not work for her. After this experience in the treatment facility, it
was particularly important to support Annie to have a different experience of treatment in which she would be given a voice about deciding what happened in therapy,
and when. Although the therapist is traditionally viewed as the expert, guiding*

---

[1] Annie is a pseudonym. Story used with the individual's consent.

treatment based on the therapist's assessment of the clinical issues, for the purpose of our work together Annie was seen as the expert of her lived experience and needed to be actively involved in her own healing. This meant that she was given options about what the possible courses of treatment could look like, and was considered a collaborator in treatment planning. Whenever Annie asserted herself in session, or advocated for something (i.e. asking for a particular kind of therapy in one session, asking for a specific concern to be addressed, or saying 'no' to the therapists' requests to engage with particular topics or styles of therapy until more time had passed) this behaviour was celebrated and meta processed as an essential part of the therapeutic process.

Annie stated that it was the experience of being celebrated for having and using her voice that allowed her to feel emotionally safe enough to begin working on the eating disorder behaviour and the trauma that lay beneath it. This allowed her to begin to explore how she had learned to punish her body (through eating disorder behaviour and occasional self-harm) because she had learned from her cultural context and interpersonal experiences that her body was bad, and that this was the reason she was hurt by others. Through this she came to understand how her body was not the problem, but that the Western patriarchal narrative about, and treatment of, the female body was the problem.

As Annie began to think critically about the social context within which her experience of her body was shaped—such as the sexualized violence against girls and women, the sexual objectification of women's bodies, and the silencing of girls' and women's ability to advocate for their own bodies—she began to develop a new relationship with her body: one of trust, kindness, compassion, and nurturance. She began to practice intuitive eating (listening to her satiety cues instead of following a rigid meal plan) and exercise gently to care for herself and build strength, instead of punish or control her body. Although Annie had previously been labelled as treatment resistant, when her resistance was not pathologized but was encouraged as a healthy response to problematic sociocultural context, she began to heal and her eating disorder symptoms slowly began to subside, and were replaced with healthy behaviours. After 18 months of therapy (initially every week, then ever 2 weeks), Annie did not meet diagnostic criteria for Anorexia Nervosa, her weight was stable, and she was able to resume regular employment.

12.3   The Values in Annie's Story

In encountering Annie's story, it is apparent that conflicting values are present in her experience. Through early experiences of sexual abuse, Annie internalized the value that her body was 'bad' and engaged in disordered eating and excessive exercise as a form of self-punishment. When Annie reached out for support from her parents, she was silenced and even punished for speaking up, further perpetuating her harmful attitudes and behaviours towards her own body. At the same time, one can detect an inextinguishable sense of agency in Annie's story, a form of resistance to the external pressures to be silenced, shamed, and punished. From this sense of agency arises evidence of another value emerging from within her as the desire to find and express her voice in and through her body. Exemplifying this, Annie actively resisted pressures to conform to the status quo when participating in the treatment programme for eating disorders.

The idea of 'resistance' from a treatment facility is framed pathologically. From a feminist perspective, however, Annie's resistance can be understood as a way of rising up to the silencing and oppressive forces of her treatment team. Paradoxically, although the treatment existed to address eating disorder behaviours, the dynamics of power and control over Annie as a patient resembled her experience of learning that her body is for others, is to be controlled, and is bad. In engaging a different form of outpatient therapy following her dismissal from the eating disorders programme, Annie was able to embrace the value of discovering her own voice and agency and the value of connecting to her body.

Several values are apparent in the treatment facility and in the attitude of the treating psychiatrists. These values are also conflicting with each other. On the one hand, we can presume that there is a value for patients of this facility to recover from eating disorders and be healthy. On the other hand, this value is expressed in a way that is shaped by power hierarchies in the broader sociocultural context, resulting in a 'top-down' treatment structure in which the so-called experts maintain power, and the patients are expected to blindly comply with treatment expectations. This value of compliance within an externally imposed power structure dangerously misses the need for women suffering with eating disorders to develop voice and agency in their bodies.

Another value apparent in the treatment facility is the value placed on cognitive-based interventions. This reflects a dualistic view, pervasive in the broader sociocultural context, of mind being separate from body and mind existing to control the body. Consistent with this dualistic view in which the body is seen as object to be controlled, the treatment facility exhibits a value on medication used with the aim of suppressing the embodied agency of the patient. Due to the hierarchical power structure of the treatment facility, the patient's resistance to compliance results in further pathologization of the patient.

12.4 The Cultural Influences

Although women who have struggles in and with their bodies, particularly in cases of severe eating disorders, such as Annie's, are typically pathologized as 'sick', it is apparent that their symptoms reflect values of the sociocultural context. Western patriarchal values about the female body measure its worth by appearance and maintain appearance standards which are largely unattainable. The pervasive dualistic view of women's bodies and minds as separate diminishes opportunities for women to develop interoceptive awareness of somatic cues and affect. Instead of supporting women to listen to and develop an attuned awareness of their physiology, an exclusive focus in treatment on changing cognition about one's body or eating has reinforced a disembodied and fragmented perspective of the self [4]. Ultimately, the cultural influences perpetuate a devaluation and the resulting silencing of women. Within this context, sexual objectification of women and sexualized violence towards women is widespread.

12.5   Implications for Therapy

In my (HM's) work with Annie as her therapist, I aimed to exhibit contrasting values with those evident in the treatment facility from which she was expelled. Rather than adopting a hierarchical 'top-down' approach to treatment based on positioning my expertise *over* Annie as the patient, I embraced the feminist values of mutuality and collaboration in which the patient is an active participant in her own treatment and in which her own voice is valued. Within this context, Annie's resistance to the treatment facility and her own opinions about therapy are neither punished nor merely tolerated; they are celebrated and encouraged.

In this approach, guided as it is by feminist values, the therapist embodies a value of the patient's voice, offering a field of development for the patient's voice and agency. This was crucial for Annie. By adopting a collaborative stance in which power is shared and resistance is sought to be understood rather than shamed, the therapist exemplifies humanistic and compassion-focused work in which the patient's perfectionistic inner critic is given an opportunity to step aside while her inner 'knowing' and self-acceptance are allowed to develop. Finally, in contrast to the dualistic separation of mind over body, the therapist demonstrates a value of body-based work centred around the patient developing trust in and through the body rather than attempting to help the patient control her body.

Unlike more androcentric approaches to psychotherapy, such as the interventions and theoretical frameworks used in the evidence-based treatment unhelpful to Annie, feminist approaches to psychotherapy are particularly useful when considering issues of body, agency, and voice, as it relates to women's experiences of distress and suffering [5]. Feminist approaches to psychotherapy see women's resistance to oppressive and silencing systems as a strength, not a problematic behaviour to be challenged or reformed. Additionally, therapists who work within a feminist perspective consider the sociocultural narratives of gender, the idealization of the disappearance of the female body, and the systemic silencing of women, as contributing to women's distress, in which a normal or healthy response to unhealthy cultural contexts is to struggle [6]. This reframes these experiences of women, like Annie, from a pathology that needs to be corrected, to a kind of cultural truth telling, in which the symptoms act as a canary in the coal mine of the social context.

12.6   Conclusions

The programme that dismissed Annie from treatment was following an evidence-based model. However, her story is a reminder of the importance of clinicians, treatment programmes, and theorists, being able to see the individual (and what has been identified as an individual psychopathology) within a social context which has constructed women's bodies in a particular manner. Instead of women's body-based challenges, and their attempt to discover their own agency in treatment being seen as a form of illness, this must be celebrated in the light of cultural contexts that have overwhelmingly silenced women and their bodily knowings.

Acknowledgements Thank you to the client 'Annie' who allowed the use of her story for this chapter.

12.7   Guide to Further Sources

A more extensive exploration of eating disorders and their treatment through feminist, existential, and body-based approaches is provided in a book edited by the authors of this chapter: H. McBride & J. Kwee (Eds.), Embodiment and Eating Disorders: Theory, Research, Prevention, and Treatment. New York, NY: Routledge.

References

1. Levine MP, Piran N. The role of body image in the prevention of eating disorders. Body Image. 2004;1:57–70. https://doi.org/10.1016/S1740-1445(03)00006-8.
2. Franko DL. Race, ethnicity, and eating disorders: considerations for DSM-V. Int J Eat Disord. 2007;40(Supl):S31–4. https://doi.org/10.1002/eat.20455.
3. McBride H, Kwee J. Understanding disordered eating and (dis)embodiment through a feminist lens. In: McBride H, Kwee J, editors. Embodiment and eating disorders: theory, research, prevention and treatment. New York: Routledge; 2018.
4. Sands SH. Eating disorder treatment as a process of mind–body integration: special challenges for women. Clin Soc Work J. 2016;44(1):27–37. https://doi.org/10.1007/s10615-015-0540-7.
5. Gilligan C, Rogers A, Tolman D. Women, girls, and psychotherapy: reframing resistance. New York: The Harrington Park Press; 1991.
6. Lerner H. Women in therapy. New York: Harper and Row Publishers; 1988.

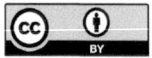

Spiritual, Religious and Ethical Values in a Suicidal Individual

13

Ana Cristina Lopes and Diogo Telles Correia

13.1 Introduction

In a multi-faith and multicultural world, psychiatrists and other mental health professionals are confronted by distressed patients for whom religious beliefs shape psychopathological symptoms and their compliance with treatment. Therefore, religious and spiritual factors should be debated in the context of the patient's psychiatric diagnosis and also taken into account in the process of choosing the appropriate psychiatric treatment.

We present a clinical vignette of a 62-year-old sacristan who was admitted to the Psychiatric Emergency Room for suicidal thoughts in the context of physical sequelae of a cardiac episode. He confessed that, in the process of coping with his illness, he had a distressing experience of guilt and of losing his religious faith and shared the intention to take his own life by hanging himself.

In the discussion that follows we reflect upon the association between spiritual values, religiosity and suicidal ideation, by exploring whether some experiences should be classified as symptoms of a psychiatric disorder or crises within spiritual life. As will be seen cultural values play a key role in this. Themes that emerge include issues related to the boundaries of psychiatric diagnosis, the spiritual dimension of mental health and the values that underlie clinical decision-making regarding a suicidal individual.

A. C. Lopes (✉)
Departamento de Psiquiatria, Centro Hospitalar de Entre o Douro e Vouga,
Santa Maria da Feira, Portugal
e-mail: ana.lopes@chedv.min-saude.pt

D. T. Correia
Clínica Universitária de Psiquiatria e Psicologia, Faculdade de Medicina da Universidade de Lisboa, Lisbon, Portugal

© The Author(s) 2021
D. Stoyanov et al. (eds.), *International Perspectives in Values-Based Mental Health Practice*, https://doi.org/10.1007/978-3-030-47852-0_13

13.2   Narrative Vignette

We present a case of a 62-year-old man who was referred to the Psychiatric Emergency Room by his general practitioner, reporting suicidal thoughts during a routine appointment.

M.S grew up in a traditional family and was living with his wife and daughter in a rural area of the north of Portugal. He used to be socially and political engaged, as well as a practicing catholic, having been appointed to take charge of the church daily care as a sacristan.

In the Psychiatry Emergency Service he was calm and collaborative, talking openly about his health problems. He said that he had suffered from two heart attacks, 2 years ago, and had developed dyspnea on moderate effort and erectile dysfunction, secondary to cardiovascular disease.

To cope with these sequelae, he had been seeking care from multiple cardiologists, with no satisfactory outcome. He came across as very rational, focusing on his somatic complaints and his impaired sexual function, which he could no longer accept.

He found it difficult to express his innermost feelings, but in the course of the interview he described how persistent physical limitation had been humiliating when facing his wife and friends. Believing that he could no longer "play the role of the man of the family", which had come up in recent arguments with his wife, he admitted his intention to take his own life, by hanging himself, once he had taken legal measures relating to his inheritance. "I'm not afraid to die... If I can no longer work... I have no reasons to hang on ... I can't even pick up weights... all I want is to provide a future for my daughter", he claimed. He said he had shared his suicidal thoughts with two friends that told him "to be calm".

Considering his role as a sacristan, we explored his religious commitment and participation, and whether he had used his spirituality to help cope with his illness. In that moment, he tried to avoid the question, claiming that he had continued to be actively involved in all the church activities, but when encouraged to open up and talk about the things he really needed to express, he became more comfortable with sharing his feelings.

He revealed that he had lost his faith and showed signs of spiritual distress. He also shared the belief that his disease was some kind of punishment, since he used to be sexually active and had had an extramarital affair. Such behaviour made him experience feelings of guilt and worthlessness and he confessed that erectile dysfunction had led to reduced self esteem and low confidence.

During the psychopathological assessment he reported no other symptoms compatible with depressive disorder such as depressed mood, loss of interest and pleasure in hanging out with friends, diminished ability to think or concentrate, and loss of appetite. Furthermore, he still looked hopeful, since he carried on making appointments with several cardiologists in order to find a treatment for his medical condition.

13.3   Discussion

Although M.S. revealed some depressive symptoms, his clinical picture is "sub-threshold", that is he does not meet the full clinical criteria for a major depressive episode. Besides, the severity of some of his symptoms (like his feelings of guilt) reflects his use of religion to understand and deal with his disease.

Individuals struggle to make sense of their experiences in the light of their beliefs and religious vocation. How a person copes with an illness, therefore, depends on their beliefs and assumptions about himself or herself and their disease, about their life and what it should look like, their sense of competence and control. Serious illness challenges many assumptions, and the attribution of meaning to the experience of suffering is the crucial element acting as a cathartic agent.

In the case of this man, a practicing catholic and sacristan, an internal struggle is evident, in the conflict between his declared values and his actions, resulting in guilt, anxiety and low self-esteem. In the interview, he also talked about his loss of faith, which reflected his struggle with God, and how this was related to a feeling of loss of contact with this reality and a sense of rejection. It was these that had led to the profound loss he felt in the meaning of his life (an experience shared by many others) and that drove his desperate suicidal intention (contrary to the generally accepted observation that religious commitment may protect against suicide [1]).

13.4   Religion, Values and Mental Health Issues

There are contrasting ways of understanding the influence of M.'s religion on his current problems. On the one hand, the act of adultery within his faith is very distressing because it is considered a mortal sin forbidden by God and it is against one of the Ten Commandments.

From this point of view, it is understandable that M. experienced his disease not only as a loss of dignity or integrity, but also as a punishment for his sin, to the extent that this is congruent with the belief system of the cultural and religious group to which he belongs.

This belief could have a negative effect on mental health, causing feelings of guilt, rumination and angst, and often becoming intricately entangled with depressive symptoms and loss of the meaning of one's own life.

However, these spiritual experiences could happen as non-pathological problems and, as Prusak puts it, "in most spiritual traditions, mild symptoms of depression are often regarded as signs of spiritual development, whereas its clinical symptoms are sometimes associated with the occurrence and solution of a spiritual crisis" [2].

This is evident in particular in what is often called in the mystical tradition he *Dark Night of the Soul.* This expression describes a phase in a person's spiritual life, that is associated with a crisis of faith or spiritual concerns about their relationship with God, and that has intrinsic aspects of spiritual growth. As such it is often distinguished from clinical depression. It is a painful period of set back, disillusionment, spiritual torment and anguish. Those experiencing the Dark Night of the Soul go through a process of attributing meaning to their experience: they consider it as a process of maturation of their spiritual life, as a natural—not pathological—process in their spiritual development [3].

Such is the case of a middle-aged country preacher who finds himself losing his faith, as depicted in Ingmar Bergman's film *"Winter Light"* [4], where God is also the reason for a man's grave confusion. When confronted with his congregation, the character is left in a state of despair over the silence of God, revealing the intention of the director in portraying how a man's psyche may be tricked by shallow faith.

These issues are often undervalued at the time of psychiatric assessment but, in that process, there are problems related to a conflict of values, a conflict that may be aggravated by the empiricist/positivist nature of psychiatric theory and by the prioritization of materialist values over values associated with religious accomplishment [5].

Indeed, psychiatrists are also reported to be less religious than the general population [6] which results in a religious gap between them and general public, but as Proudfoot said "to identify an experience in nonreligious terms when the subject himself describes it in religious terms is to misidentify the experience, or to attend to another experience altogether" [7].

In addition, and since mental health professionals are largely disposed to observing psychopathology in people who express suicidal ideation, the assessment is usually made on the assumption that suicidality is driven by psychiatric disorder, supporting a disease-oriented/medical model [8].

13.5 Suicide and Cultural Values in Portugal

Traditionally, Portugal is one of the countries with the lowest suicide rates in Europe [9]. The standardized mortality rate (SMR) by suicide is 9.8 per 100,000 inhabitants [10], and although this phenomenon may be under-represented, it is officially lower than SMR by suicide in the European Union.

Geographically within our country, northern regions have lower rates of suicide and this traditional north/south divide has strong cultural roots, with the northern region being more catholic overall.

Our country is also among the most religious countries in Western Europe, with more than a third of Portuguese adults (37%) showing high levels of religious commitment [11]. It is recognized that these factors may account for the lower suicide rates in the north of our country, although the urban/rural divide is increasing, which may be related to social and economic factors rather than cultural and religious ones [10].

Indeed, religion and spirituality are often seen as means of protection against depression or means of mitigating its symptoms [12] but this phenomenon is very complex and multifactorial. In the case of M., his traditional values and conservative gender role view make him feel useless and want to die.

13.6 Values, Suicide Risk and Clinical Decision-Making

When it comes to suicidal thoughts, patients suffering from serious mental disorder were assumed to lack decision-making capacity. Given the above, we may consider that involuntary hospitalization is likely to be thought as legally and morally justified, since it allows the patient to recover his capacity for self-determination. The Mental Health Act, implemented in Portugal in 1998, permits the psychiatrists to deprive someone with a serious mental disorder of their liberty, since preventing an individual from committing suicide, and eventually treating the psychiatric disorder that is inducing suicidal thoughts, is likely to bring the patient's actions in line with his or her true values. However, this deprivation of individual liberty and autonomy can be experienced as gravely humiliating, even violent [13]; and if we take into account situations where a person is capable of making treatment decisions—uninfluenced by any mental disorder—we enter into the field of rational suicide [14].

A further consideration is that criteria intended to regulate practice leave scope for discretion, and the values and beliefs of staff may become a determining factor for decisions as long as different models of the clinician-patient relationship warrant different interpretations of the legal criteria for involuntary admission [15]. This presents a challenge for mental health professionals, who have their own world view, and raises complex ethical dilemmas relating to compulsory treatment in suicidal individuals, which by its very nature involves a direct conflict of values between the patient and the psychiatrist.

In the case of M., the psychiatric assessment highlighted the emotional suffering experienced by a male individual, with a chronic disease and his own religious and cultural beliefs, who is at risk of committing suicide, even though his symptoms do not meet criteria for a severe mental illness in current psychiatric nosological systems. This complex clinical presentation raises issues about the limitations of defining the heterogeneous construct of mental disorder and the need for a biopsychosocial-spiritual approach. We should respect and support patients' religious beliefs if these help them to cope better and we should also challenge the beliefs that can adversely affect their mental health. When facing psychiatric symptoms with religious content, we might consider incorporating spiritual matters in psychotherapy, so that the therapist could help patients in the process of discovering their own solutions, promoting mutual respect and tolerance for difference.

Although hospitalization seems to be the safest option when dealing with suicidal patients, psychiatrists risk putting their own professional anxieties above the needs of service users. On the other hand, there is no evidence that hospitalization prevents suicide and suicide risk post-hospitalization, immediately following discharge is 100 times greater than average [16]. Trusting therapeutic alliances are fundamental to reducing suicide risk and promoting recovery and wellness, and modern mental health care highlights a shift from paternalism towards a more human rights focused approach, providing care that is respectful of and responsive to individual preferences, needs and values, ensuring that these guide all clinical decisions.

In the case of M., we suggested that he should start Person-Centred Therapy (Rogerian Therapy), which he accepted, and we encouraged him to meet the hospital chaplain, respecting the value attached to his experience, because he did not feel comfortable in sharing his inner feelings with the priest of his parish.

13.7 Conclusions

Spiritual dimension is important in the lives of our patients, since many of their problems revolve around existential and religious issues, for it reflects the underlying cultural and social values.

In the case of M., a conservative and practicing catholic man, there is an inner conflict between constructs such as guilt, sin and rejection, which play an important part in his religious experience, and the loss of the meaning of one's own life, based on the values and standards of his own cultural framework. This intimate struggle resulted in his intention to kill himself, even though this act is absolutely condemned by his religion.

This case illustrates the association between cultural values, spirituality and suicidal ideation, by exploring whether some experiences should be classified as symptoms of a psychiatric disorder or as crises within one's spiritual life.

13.8 Guide to Further Sources

Durkheim, EC (1912). The elementary forms of the religious life, a study in religious sociology. London: New York: G. Allen & Unwin; Macmillan.

James, William, 1842-1910. (1902). The varieties of religious experience: a study in human nature: being the Gifford Lectures on natural religion delivered at Edinburgh in 1901-1902. New York; London: Longmans, Green.

Van Praag HM. The role of religion in suicide prevention In Oxford Textbook of Suicidology and Suicide Prevention (eds Wasserman D, Wasserman C): 7–12. Oxford University Press, 2009.

Koenig HG; Research on religion, spirituality, and mental health: a review. Can J Psychiatry 2009 May; 54(5):283–91.

Telles Correia D. The concept of validity throughout the history of psychiatry. J Eval Clin Pract (2017) Apr 6.

References

1. Neeleman J, Halpern D, Leon D, Lewis G. Tolerance of suicide, religion and suicide rates: an ecological and individual study in 19 western countries. Psychol Med. 1997;27:1165–71.
2. Prusak J. Differential diagnosis of "religious or spiritual problem"—possibilities and limitations implied by the V-code 62.89 in DSM-V. Psychiatr Pol. 2016;50(1):175–86.
3. Durà-Vilà G, Dein S. The dark night of the soul: spiritual distress and its psychiatric implications. Ment Health Relig Cult. 2009;12:6,543–59.

4. Bergman I. Winter light. Sweden: AB Svensk Filmindustri; 1963.
5. Rashed MA. Religious experience and psychiatry: analysis of the conflict and proposal for a way forward. Philos Psychiatr Psychol. 2010;17(3):185–204.
6. Neeleman J, King MB. Psychiatrists' religious attitudes in relation to their clinical practice: a survey of 231 psychiatrists. Acta Psychiatr Scand. 1993;88:420–4.
7. Proudfoot W. Religious experience. Berkeley: University of California Press; 1985. p. 196.
8. Rich KL, Butts JB. Rational suicide: uncertain moral ground. J Adv Nurs. 2004;46:270–83.
9. Gusmão R, Quintão S. Suicide and death resulting from events of undetermined intent register in Portugal. Revisiting "The truth about suicide", 20 years later. Dir Gen Heal J. 2013;1:80–95.
10. Santana P, Costa C, Cardoso G, Loureiro A, Ferrão J. Suicide in Portugal: spatial determinants in a context of economic crisis. Health Place. 2015;35:85–94.
11. Pew Research Center. Being Christian in Western Europe. 29 May 2018.
12. Blazer DG. Spirituality and depression. In: Peteet JR, Lu FG, Narrow WE, editors. Religious and spiritual issues in psychiatric diagnosis. A research agenda for DSM-V. Arlington, VA: American Psychiatric Association; 2011.
13. Sibitz I, et al. Impact of coercive measures on life stories: qualitative study. Br J Psychiatry. 2011;199(3):239–44.
14. Onkay A. Suicide: rationality and responsibility for life. Can J Psychiatry. 2014;59(3):141–7.
15. Feiring E, Ugstad KN. Interpretations of legal criteria for involuntary psychiatric admission: a qualitative analysis. BMC Health Serv Res. 2014;14:500.
16. Chung D, Ryan C, et al. Suicide rates after discharge from psychiatric facilities: a systematic review and meta-analysis. JAMA Psychiatry. 2017;74(7):694–702.

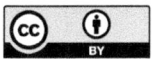

Cultural Values, Religion and Psychosis: Five Short Stories

14

Michael TH Wong, Fiona Wilson, Dennisa Davidson,
Caitlin Hick, and Andrew Howie

14.1 Introduction

Culture and spirituality constrain the way we see our world in ways that sometimes become apparent only when challenged. The issue is more complex still when psychosis and serious mental illness are assessed in the context of spiritual and cultural difference. The following five case narratives—written from different perspectives—illustrate different aspects of these constraints and complexities.

Case Narratives Note: Case narratives one to three are a synthesis and fictional reworking of a number of patient cases and are completely de-identified. Narrative four is based on that of a real person but the name and other identifying details have been changed to protect confidentiality. Narrative five is autobiographical and by a member of the author team.

M. TH. Wong (✉)
Department of Psychiatry, Li Ka Shing Faculty of Medicine, The University of Hong Kong,
Hong Kong, China
e-mail: mthwong@hku.hk

F. Wilson
Manaaki House Community Mental Health Centre, Auckland District Health Board,
Auckland, New Zealand
e-mail: fionawilson@xtra.co.nz

D. Davidson
"Taunaki" Child and Adolescent Mental Health Service, Counties Manukau District Health
Board, Auckland, New Zealand
e-mail: dennisadavidson@yahoo.co.nz

C. Hick
North Tec, Whangarei, New Zealand
e-mail: loulou.14069@gmail.com

A. Howie
Whitiki Maurea Maori Mental Health and Addiction Service, Waitemata District Health
Board, Auckland, New Zealand
e-mail: ajshowie@gmail.com

© The Author(s) 2021
D. Stoyanov et al. (eds.), *International Perspectives in Values-Based Mental
Health Practice*, https://doi.org/10.1007/978-3-030-47852-0_14

14.2 Case Narrative One

"Robert" is a 23-year-old single unemployed New Zealand European male who lives with his parents. His family are committed Church-going Christians of a Pentecostal denomination. Pre-morbidly, Robert was very sociable and academically was a high achiever. While Robert was attending tertiary education, his family became concerned as he had a decline in academic performance, poor self-care and preoccupation with religious beliefs and they contacted mental health services. Robert was hostile and uncooperative with assessment. His parents confirmed that he had reported hearing the voices of God and the Devil for at least a year and explained that was not considered unusual in their Church Community.

Robert was diagnosed with Schizophrenia, paranoid type. He repudiated the diagnosis, continued to be hostile towards mental health services and was non-adherent to prescribed medication. This resulted in a number of admissions to the local mental health unit. Prior to his last admission, Robert had again discontinued his prescribed oral medication, was disorganized and neglected in his presentation and was preoccupied with the belief that he had caused the deaths of a number of people by praying for God to pass judgement on them via an influenza epidemic. He was discharged from hospital on a compulsory treatment order under the Mental Health Act and prescribed depot antipsychotic medication. The treatment resulted in some amelioration of his presentation but he did not return to his pre-morbid level of functioning.

Robert continued to report experiences of hearing the voices of God and the Devil and denied that the prescribed medication had any impact on his experiences. One of the clinical psychologists in the mental health team espoused Christian beliefs and offered to work with Robert; however, Robert declined this. He also declined referral to the mental health chaplain.

On one occasion Robert came to his psychiatry appointment with a collection of his writings. These writings consisted of copied Biblical texts. He said that God had instructed him to read to the psychiatrist. He was focused on a text concerning *"Love your enemies"* and believed that God had told him to change his attitude towards the mental health staff.

14.3 Case Narrative Two

"Aroha" is a 30-year-old New Zealand Māori woman who strongly identifies with her Māori culture. She is unemployed and lives with her male partner in a relationship of several years' duration. She has no children. Aroha is one of a number of siblings, all of whom were exposed to physical, emotional and sexual abuse as children and were removed from their parents' care into state custody. Their foster care was unstable and they experienced multiple caregivers over time. Most of the siblings were separated but Aroha and her twin brother, *"Anaru"*, were placed together. Aroha and Anaru had a very close bond.

In her early twenties, Aroha was diagnosed with Schizoaffective disorder and was treated with anti-psychotic medication. The differential diagnosis was complex Post Traumatic Stress Disorder. She had good engagement with her treating team and had a period of successful psychological treatment. She presented with a marked deterioration in her mental state following Anaru's sudden death in a single vehicle motor crash in another town. She was unable to sleep, distressed and disorganised and had persecutory delusional beliefs that gang members wanted to kill her. She also reported seeing the ghost of her deceased brother, whom she reported was in distress.

Aroha was treated at home with increased support from mental health services and her medication was optimised. In addition, an urgent referral was made to a kaumatua (Māori elder with spiritual authority) under the auspices of mental health services as it is known that Māori may see visions of deceased whānau (family) following their death. The kaumatua advised that Aroha should return to her marae in another town to see the kaumatua there in order to have the appropriate karakia (prayers) and ritual to ensure that her brother's spirit passed peacefully on to the spirit world. (Māori believe that the spirits of the deceased travel to Cape Reinga, northern most part of Aotearoa New Zealand to leave for their ancestral home of Hawaiki). Aroha followed this advice which led to some resolution of her level of distress. She and her partner then moved back to her home town and follow-up was arranged with the appropriate service.

14.4 Case Narrative Three

"John" was a single 25-year-old New Zealand European male living with his parents. He had attained a University degree and was working full time in a responsible position. His family was not religious but as a teenager John had become a committed Christian which was the focus of his life. Also, in his late teenage years, John was diagnosed with Bipolar Affective Disorder. He had three inpatient admissions with mania and psychosis and was treated with Lithium. While adherent to prescribed treatment, he had complete inter-episode recovery with return to full employment.

However, because he had been well for 3 years, he became convinced that he no longer needed pharmacological treatment and slowly discontinued his medication over several months. Unfortunately, this led to a major relapse of mania and psychosis with erratic and disinhibited behaviour at his place of employment and loud, disorganised preaching at his Church. His behaviour was witnessed by many people, and led to hospitalisation and dismissal from his employment.

His mental state had improved such that he was no longer psychotic or manic but he was in danger of becoming depressed as he faced up to the toll that his behaviour, when unwell, had taken on his relationships and employment. He felt that his life was ruined and felt too ashamed to return to his Church. He said that he had no one to talk with except the psychiatrist. He asked the psychiatrist whether they shared any religious beliefs. At that time, the Psychiatrist believed that it was in the best interest of the patient to disclose that they came from a similar religious back-ground without divulging any further information [1]. *John then felt comfortable to talk about his religious beliefs.*

The psychiatrist was familiar with "Spiritually Augmented Cognitive Behaviour Therapy" [2] *which includes encouraging patients to re-engage with their spirituality. With John's permission, the psychiatrist contacted his church minister and a meeting was arranged to discuss how John could re-engage with the church. One of the Peer Support Workers in the mental health team attended the same church as John and undertook to support him with his return to church. A few weeks later, John was happy to report that he had indeed returned to church and was regularly engaged in worship and a small group for prayer and Bible study. He had been uplifted by a Biblical text given to him by a church member: Romans 8:28 "We know that all things work together for good for those who love God, who are called according to his purpose." His mood was euthymic and he was soon able to secure new employment. He was committed to continue taking his prescribed Lithium, seeing that as part of God's plan for his life.*

14.5 Case Narrative Four

The clinician was mid-way in her specialist training when "Richard", a 70 years old widower was admitted to the older-people's inpatient unit following attempting to jump off a highrise building.

Richard had no history of mental illness. Neither was he new to adversity. He had lived through his home being destroyed by a storm and the passing of his wife after a rather brief illness in midlife. He had survived cancer 2 years ago and had moved to a new city to start a new life. Within months after the move, the cancer recurred, leaving him with few options that he chose to decline. He felt an overwhelming sense of futility, loneliness and being let down- Let down by his deceased wife, for whom he had been there till the end, who could not be with him now when his own days were measured. Let down by his children who were too far away in his time of emotional need. Let down by the doctors whom he believed had promised the cancer will not return. Let down by God, whom he had known better in earlier years yet in whom he retained a sense of omnipotence.

He was trialled on a number of medication regimes. Therapists tried hard to engage him. His children came over to visit. The only unwavering response was a stoic withdrawal.

Eventually, after discussing with her supervisor, the trainee psychiatrist gave a copy of the lyrics of the song, 'Precious Lord, take my hand' to the staff to pass on to Richard if he showed interest. Staff laminated it and passed it on to the chaplain who gave it to him. He accepted this and started to come out to participate in the weekly chapel service held in the unit, first sitting at the periphery before slowly engaging more. He went on to engage with other therapies and his family and was discharged much improved. He was reported to continue his spiritual journey post-discharge.

14.6 Case Narrative Five

Case Narrative Five is an autobiographical account of a 17-year-old New Zealand European woman's illness journey. She has called her story "Mental Health with God".

My journey through teenagehood was no walk in the park. I had suffered with Anorexia Nervosa, depression and severe anxiety that had all stemmed from a traumatic childhood. I have believed in God for as long as I can remember, which is kind of strange since none of my family members believe. In fact, my Dad is a proud atheist so when I began to start having serious issues at 14 years of age, I could not relate or talk to my parents about it all.

Without my faith I would have died the first time I tried to take my own life. Some people tell me that God and religion are a crutch just like people use drugs and drink, etc. But I can tell you that it's nothing like that. I found truth about myself out of hard times, knowing that I was loved and cared for, that I was made for a divine purpose and that all of what broke me was not for nothing.

My faith is the backbone of my resilience and the foundation of my present growing self-love. In times where I have been overwhelmed with fear and anxiety, there are verses I can turn to in the Bible that are not just comforting but they ring true in situations from my past as well; and this brings me a lot of resolution.

It's not just a belief, it's a relationship. Unlike coping skills given by my support team, the relationship I have with God helps me on a personal level and it's never something I can overuse. When things are getting difficult again, God is prepared to help me in a way that is intricate and personalised to my exact needs. It doesn't happen like clockwork though and sometimes He comes through for me in the words from other people or even in songs. God doesn't work like an instruction manual either. In all of these battles I have fought, God's love for me is interlaced into everything I have been through.

God working in my life is just having an ever-present father figure or a friend, and I truly feel loved and understood through the things I have learned over the years.

14.7 Values and Cultural Issues Arising

The above five case narratives highlight the various challenges facing the mental health system in New Zealand arising out of the cross-cultural interaction of a number of values between Anglo-European religion, Maori spirituality and secular psychiatry.

First, the underlying historical-political values. Aotearoa New Zealand is a nation shaped by the Treaty of Waitangi signed in 1840 by the British Crown and many of the Māori tribes of Aotearoa New Zealand. The treaty continues as the foundation for Māori in having a partnership with the government for their protection, participation in decisions that impact their well-being and among the articles of the treaty, the rights to cultural practices and freedom of religious beliefs.

Second, the values of immigrants. From the twentieth century onwards, there have been waves of migration to New Zealand from many lands, leading to a rich diversity of cultures, languages and beliefs.

Third, the values of the professionals. In 2018, the RANZCP adopted a Position statement on Psychiatry and Religion/Spirituality [3]. Thus far, there is no specific training for Psychiatrists in this area and a paucity of research in Aotearoa New Zealand. Psychiatrists in New Zealand are Fellows or Affiliates of the Royal Australian and New Zealand College of Psychiatrists (RANZCP), and they are a culturally diverse group.

Fourth, the values of the Māori. Mason Durie's model [4] emphasises that any attempt to separate wairua (spiritual) and whanau (extended family) issues from consideration of well-being will fail for Māori, possibly to an overwhelming degree.

The interaction of these four values is now discussed further through the five case narratives.

The narrative of "Robert" illustrates the challenges of integrating appropriate mental health care and spirituality in a patient who has been diagnosed with a psychotic illness, involving auditory hallucinations and delusions of a religious nature. His lack of insight and persistent hostility towards the treating team poses a major difficulty which the latter tackle by trying to steer a middle course of validating what are appropriate beliefs to the religious persuasion of Robert and continuing treatment with antipsychotic medication to enable him to function adequately in the community. This seems to have worked, and Robert eventually develops a therapeutic relationship with his treating team which supports and helps him stay stable despite remaining symptomatic.

The illness experience of "Aroha" highlights the importance of spiritual and cultural assessment and interventions in a patient who has both a diagnosis of a psychotic illness and an acute spiritual problem. It is recognized that psychiatrists can over-diagnose psychosis in patients who belong to different cultures from their own. In Aotearoa New Zealand, the Treaty of Waitangi documents the partnership between the Government and Māori iwi (tribes) to ensure the protection of their rights. Professor Sir Mason Durie (a Māori Psychiatrist) has developed a Māori model of health, "te whare tapa wha"—a house with four posts, a model that is disseminated widely within Aotearoa New Zealand:

- Taha Tinana (Physical health)
- Taha Hinengaro (Mental health)
- Taha Whānau (Extended Family health)
- Taha Wairua (Spiritual health)

This Māori model of health addresses the enormous impact of colonization on indigenous cultures—spirit-breaking—which has affected multiple generations in areas such as physical and mental health, education, employment and family relationships leading to disconnection from language, culture and land. For "Aroha," this model allows a reconnection with the Māori spiritual understanding of death and the ritual of bereavement, bringing about a resolution of grief and distress and promoting a remission of her psychotic illness.

The psychotic breakdown of "John" and the associated behavioural disturbance not only result in loss of employment and disruption of relationships but also lead to shame, spiritual despair, and self-imposed social isolation. Through the support of his treating team who is sensitive to his spiritual needs, John manages to achieve a good remission, re-engage with his church community and return to the workforce. The narrative of John shows how religion and spirituality are important aspects of patients' illness experience and recovery journey and can have a role in resilience for patients with severe mental illness. While "John" and "Aroha" belong to different ethnic, cultural and religion traditions, they both have benefited from a holistic model of service delivery that covers biological, psychological, cultural and religious/spiritual aspects of care.

"Richard" has given up and as each therapeutic intervention fails, he has become more "set" in his giving up. Spirituality was one of the few interventions that remain. The trainee psychiatrist feels this may be beneficial but struggles with how to approach this. When this is addressed, it seems to awaken in him a renewed sense of meaning and purpose in life and a sense of being cared for by Someone and not being alone. The narrative of Richard represents challenges at end of life and suggests that spirituality may be an appropriate adjunct to offer in therapy [5].

The autobiographical account in Case Narrative Five gives us a glimpse of the traumatic childhood, severe anxiety, eating issues, emotional dysregulation and suicidal ideation of a 17-year-old girl and how her faith has sustained her. Her story of "Mental Health with God" reminds us that spiritual and religious beliefs, and in her case, the Christian Faith remains a source of hope, strength, love, healing and a means to express meaning, significance and sense of well-being for some people [6, 7]. This is despite the fact that the world we live in is increasingly secular and that it is getting difficult all the time for both patients and mental health professionals to speak and discuss spiritual issues with ease and feel safe and comfortable to do so. The latest statistics from New Zealand show that almost half the population see themselves as of "no religion" [8]. It is possible that at times, Christianity may even be perceived as a vestige of colonialism than a personal relationship with God.

14.8   Conclusion

Anglo-European religion, Māori spirituality and secular psychiatry in New Zealand continue to form a complex and dynamic web which is still being woven out with cultural, spiritual and cultural tension.

The particular case of psychosis and serious mental illness discussed here through five case narratives highlights that the experience, expression and perception of psychosis and serious mental illness as well as their diagnosis, treatment, recovery and rehabilitation require a holistic approach that involves not only bio-logical intervention but also psychosocial support and spiritual healing.

Within this clinical framework of values and culture, health and well-being in patients living with psychosis and serious mental illness are not adequately repre-sented only by the control of symptoms or containment of difficult behaviour. Instead, mental health and well-being take on a new perspective of meaning and significance which draws from the cultural heritage and religious tradition of the patients through which fragmented identity is rebuilt, lost roles regained and alien-ated relationships reconnected.

The five short stories narrated here remind us that culture, religion and spiritual-ity continue to play an important role in the practice of psychiatry in our increas-ingly secular contemporary world.

Acknowledgements The idea of this article originates from a symposium the authors orga-nized at the Royal Australian and New Zealand College of Psychiatrists 2018 Congress held on May 17–21 in Auckland, New Zealand. We appreciate the critical and constructive comments from the participants who include patients, carers, hospital chaplains, allied mental health work-ers, nurses, psychologists and psychiatrists from New Zealand, Australia, Asia and the Pacific Islands.

14.9   Guide to Further Sources

Royal Australian and New Zealand College of Psychiatrists. Position Statement PS 96, June 2018. The relevance of religion and spirituality to psychiatric practice. https://www.ranzcp.org/news-policy/policy-and-advocacy/position-statements/the-relevance-of-religion-and-spirituality-to-psyc

WPA Position Statement on Spirituality and Religion in Psychiatry. https://www.seminare-ps.net/positionspapiere/WPA_Statement_Rel_Psychiatry.pdf

Royal College of Psychiatrists. Position Statement PS03/2013, November 2013. Recommendations for psychiatrists on spirituality and religion. https://www.rcpsych.ac.uk/pdf/PS03_2013.pdf

References

1. Florence H. Deciding what belongs: how Psychotherapists in Aotearoa New Zealand attend to Religion and/or Spirituality. PhD Thesis. Auckland University of Technology; 2015.
2. D'Souza R. Spiritually augmented CBT. Australas Psychiatry. 2004;12(2):148–52.
3. https://www.ranzcp.org/news-policy/policy-and-advocacy/position-statements/the-relevance-of-religion-and-spirituality-to-psyc
4. Durie M. Whaiora: Māori health development. Auckland: Oxford University Press; 1998. p. 68–74.
5. Breitbart W, Gibson CA, Poppito SR, Berg AL. Psychotherapeutic interventions at the end of life: a focus on meaning and spirituality. Can J Psychiatry. 2004;49(6):366–72.

6. Wong YJ, Rew L, Slaikeu KD. A systematic review of recent research on adolescent religiosity/spirituality and mental health. Issues Ment Health Nurs. 2006;27(2):161–83.
7. Chang-Ho CJ, Perry T, Clarke-Pine D. Considering personal religiosity in adolescent delinquency: the role of depression, suicidal ideation, and church guideline. J Psychol Christ. 2011;30(1):3–15.
8. http://worldpopulationreview.com/countries/new-zealand-population/

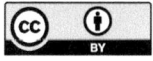

Part III

Practice

Vectors of Best Practice: An Introduction to Part III, Practice

15

Bill Fulford

Where Part II was about theory, Part III is about practice. It shows how a culturally enriched form of values-based practice supports best practice in the design and delivery of mental health services as defined by widely accepted norms of contemporary practice. Parts IV and V are about other aspects of best practice. Part IV, Science, is about best practice in linking science with people; Part V, Training, is about training for best practice. These three Parts together thus cover the elements of values-based practice set out in chapter 1, 'Surprised by Values: An Introduction to Values-Based Practice and the Use of Personal Narratives in this Book' (see Table 1.2).

Returning to this Part, then, contributing chapters illustrate the role of cultural values in relation to the elements of values-based practice most directly concerned with the design and delivery of services. As shown in Table 15.1, these include (1) person-centred care ('person-*values*-centred care', chapter 16, 'Cross-Cultural Factors and Identity in Adolescence'), (2) multidisciplinary teamwork (the '*extended* multidisciplinary team', chapters 17, 'Multidisciplinary Teamwork and the Insanity Defence: A Case of Infanticide in Iraq' and 18, 'Colonial Values and Asylum Care in Brazil: Reclaiming the Streets through Carnival in Rio de Janeiro'), and (3) *shared decision-making* supported by *balanced dissensus* within *frameworks of shared values*', chapters 19, 'Alcohol Use Disorder in a Culture that Normalizes the Consumption of Alcoholic Beverages: The Conflicts for Decision-Making', 20, 'Living at the Edge of Compromise: Balkan Pluralism as a Resource for Balanced Decision-Making', and 21, '"Thinking Too Much": A Clash of Legitimate Values in Clinical Practice Calls for an Indaba Guided by African Values-Based Practice'). Part III concludes with two chapters on a service model of growing

Authors
The editors with input from the contributors to Part III.

B. Fulford (✉)
St Catherine's College, University of Oxford, Oxford, UK

© The Author(s) 2021
D. Stoyanov et al. (eds.), *International Perspectives in Values-Based Mental Health Practice*, https://doi.org/10.1007/978-3-030-47852-0_15

Table 15.1 Annotated table of contents for Part III, Practice

Part III: Practice
• Chapter 15 'Vectors of Best Practice: An Introduction to Part III, Practice'
Cultural values and the person-*values*-centred care of values-based practice
• Chapter 16 'Cross-Cultural Factors and Identity in Adolescence'—Vanya Matanova and Anna Hristova
Cultural values and the *extended* multidisciplinary team of values-based practice
• Chapter 17 'Multidisciplinary Teamwork and the Insanity Defence: a Case of Infanticide in Iraq'—Hasanen Al-Taiar
• Chapter 18 'Colonial Values and Asylum Care in Brazil: Reclaiming the Streets Through Carnival in Rio de Janeiro'—Julia Evangelista and William A Fulford
Shared Decision-making supported by balanced dissensual decision-making within frameworks of shared values
• Chapter 19 'Alcohol Use Disorder in a Culture That Normalizes the Consumption of Alcoholic Beverages: The Conflicts for Decision-Making'—Guilherme Messas and Maria Soares
• Chapter 20 'Living at the Edge of Compromise: Balkan Pluralism as a Resource for Balanced Decision-Making'—D.S. Stoyanov and K.W.M. (Bill) Fulford
• Chapter 21 '"Thinking Too Much": A Clash of Legitimate Values in Clinical Practice Calls for an Indaba Guided by African Values-Based Practice—Werdie van Staden
Cultural values and recovery
• Chapter 22 'Three Points in Time: How Values and Culture Affected My Life, Madness and the People Around Me'—David Crepaz-Keay
• Chapter 23 'Recovery and Cultural Values: On Our Own Terms (A Dialogue)'—Justine Keen and Richard J Shaw

importance in mental health, *recovery practice* (chapters 22, 'Three Points in Time: How Values and Culture Affected My Life, Madness and the People Around Me' and 23, 'Recovery and Cultural Values: On Our Own Terms (A Dialogue)').

15.1 The Bottom Line

The bottom-line message of the Part as a whole is about the potential of cultural values to act as effective vectors for the delivery of best practice. This is well illustrated by the two topics with which this Part opens, person-centred care and multidisciplinary teamwork. Both are widely acknowledged in contemporary health care as aspects of best practice. Yet for both, experience on the ground is that all too often there is a yawning gap between aspiration and practical reality.

There are, no doubt, many reasons for this gap. But that unacknowledged cultural values—specifically, unacknowledged cultural values of service providers—have at least a role to play is evident from observations made in the early days of the development of values-based practice. What these observations showed was that, so long as they remained unacknowledged, and hence hidden, the cultural values of services could act as inadvertent barriers to best practice. Raising awareness of these same cultural values, however, and thus rendering them accessible to the processes of values-based practice, converted them from barriers into effective vectors of best practice.

15.2   Early Observations

We will look briefly at these observations from the early days of values-based practice before returning to how they are filled out by the contributions to this Part. The studies from which they came have been written up in detail elsewhere (see Guide to Further Information at the end of this chapter).

15.2.1   Early Observations Leading to Person-*Values*-Centred Care

We owe the key observations leading to the concept of person-values-centred care to Kim Woodbridge-Dodd (the first author of chapter 44, 'Reflections on the Impact of Mental Health Ward Staff Training in Race Equality and Values-Based Practice'). In preparation for running an early training programme in values-based practice, Kim observed the priorities evinced by team members in one of their case review meetings. Her key finding was that although the service providers in question genuinely believed they were delivering *service user-centred* care, what they were *actually* delivering (as characterised by the topics on which the case review focused) was better characterised as *service provider-centred* care.

Importantly, as the full account of these observations makes clear, those concerned were wholly unaware of, and indeed much taken aback by, the gap thus demonstrated between their beliefs about the kind of service they were delivering and the reality of their practice. This had nothing to do with 'bad faith'. The staff members concerned were genuinely unaware that their priorities in the way they ran their services (as evinced by what they focused on in their case review meeting) were so different from what they believed them to be.

These observations led naturally to the concept of 'person-values-centred care' as it is now used in values-based practice. Person-centred care, this concept spells out, means nothing if the values of the person concerned are left out of account. And the values of the person concerned will inevitably be left out of account if service providers are unaware of (as Kim's group were unaware of) the extent to which their own values as service providers were leading them (all unawares) to make decisions based not on what was important to their service users but on what was important to them.

15.2.2   Early Observations Leading to the Extended Multidisciplinary Team

It was similar observations although in this instance made in the course of empirical social science research that led to the concept in values-based practice of the 'extended multidisciplinary team'. The studies in question were led initially by the British Social Scientist, Anthony Colombo, and then, in a follow-up by a team based in the Mental Health Foundation in London and led by Colin King (the first author of chapter 46, 'Beyond the Colour Bar: Sharing Narratives in Order to Promote a

Clearer Understanding of Mental Health Issues across Cultural and Racial Boundaries').

Both these studies are described in detail in the sources given in the Guide to Further Information at the end of the chapter. The essence of what they showed is, again, as in Kim's study, a failure of self-awareness among staff of their own cultural values. Here, however, the failure of self-awareness was of the extent of the *differences* of cultural values that as different team members with different professional backgrounds they brought to their work. As well-functioning teams, it was natural that they should assume they had shared values. They all believed they were approaching mental health issues with essentially the same biopsychosocial set of priorities. But the priorities revealed by their responses to the case vignette were markedly different. Psychiatrists, for example, focused on biological aspects of mental health (such as diagnosis and medication) while social workers focused on psychosocial aspects (such as stressors and risk management).

As in Kim Woodbridge-Dodds' work, then, there was a gap between belief and reality for staff values. But what is important in this instance was not the gap between belief and reality in staff values as such. It was that the differences in staff values ran *closely parallel with similar differences subsequently demonstrated in the values of service users*. There was in other words a like-for-like matching between staff values within the multidisciplinary team and those of their service users.

It is this like-for-like matching that led to the concept in values-based practice of the 'extended multidisciplinary team'. To that point, multidisciplinary teamwork had been recognised to be important for the range of knowledge and skills that team members from different professions bring to bear in meeting the diverse needs of service users. The like-for-like values matching shown by these studies extended the importance of the multidisciplinary team to include also the range of *different values* that team members bring to bear in meeting the diverse needs of service users.

15.3 With Hindsight: A Confession

With hindsight, the significance of the cultural values revealed by these early observations seems clear: in both cases, the cultural values of service providers were driving their practice; in both cases so long as these cultural values remained unacknowledged, they acted as a barrier to best practice in delivering person-centred care—services were unaware of the extent to which their decisions were being driven not by what was important to their service users but by what was important to them as service providers. In both cases, however, once these same cultural values were made explicit, they were converted into vectors of best practice in person-centred practice.

But it is here that a confession is called for. At the time, the significance of these studies had been understood in terms primarily *not of cultural but of individual values*. These studies, therefor, provide a further and somewhat (with hindsight) startling example of our failure within values-based practice itself, spelled out in chapter 1, 'Surprised by Values: An Introduction to Values-Based Practice and the Use of Personal Narratives in this Book', to attend to cultural values.

As we emphasised in chapter 1,[1] individual values, notably those of the individual patient or service user, are important clinically. For one thing, they are at the heart of contemporary models of shared decision-making. Individual values, furthermore, should not be somehow subordinated to cultural values (recall 'the individual is an n of 1' from chapter 1). But for all that, it was a clear failure of the early days of values-based practice that we failed to appreciate the full significance of these observations for our understanding of the role of cultural values in mental health.

15.4 Values-Based Practice in This Part

The first three chapters in this Part of the book together remedy this failure.

15.4.1 Person-Values-Centred Care

Chapter 16, 'Cross-Cultural Factors and Identity in Adolescence', by Vanya Matanova and Anna Hristova, both of Sophia University, Bulgaria, explores the complex relationships between cultural and individual values in person-centred care. It tells the story of a young woman with self-harming behaviour and the intra-personal and trans-generational conflicts of values that develop when she is brought from her native England to live with her father in Bulgaria. Similar themes are evident in other chapters (for example in chapter 11, 'Madness, Mythopoetry and Medicine' on the African diaspora, see above, Part I). Chapter 16, 'Cross-Cultural Factors and Identity in Adolescence' also illustrates an aspect of the values tool kit: it draws on a culturally attuned form of family therapy to explicate the values issues and thereby develop a strategy for intervention.

15.4.2 The Extended Multidisciplinary Team

Moving now from person-centred care to multidisciplinary teamwork, chapters 17, 'Multidisciplinary Teamwork and the Insanity Defence: A Case of Infanticide in Iraq' and 18, 'Colonial Values and Asylum Care in Brazil: Reclaiming the Streets through Carnival in Rio de Janeiro' pick up similar themes about the extra levels of complexity added by cultural values. Through two very different narratives, these chapters add new dimensions to the significance of multidisciplinary teamwork in mental health. In chapter 17, the forensic psychiatrist, Hasanen Al-Taiar, provides a narrative from Iraq about the role of multidisciplinary teamwork in establishing criminal responsibility for infanticide. In Western countries, such assessments are generally assumed to be matters for expert medical opinion. This story thus extends the role of the multidisciplinary team to a wholly new level of importance. This is

---

[1] See the subheading subsection 4.1.

all the more significant given that in Iraq, in contrast to the legal norms of Western countries, infanticide remains a capital offence.

Chapter 18, 'Colonial Values and Asylum Care in Brazil: Reclaiming the Streets through Carnival in Rio de Janeiro', by Julia Evangelista and Will Fulford, describes a project with which they have been involved in Rio de Janeiro in Brazil, that has the aim of empowering people with mental health issues to, in the words of their title, 'reclaim the streets' through Carnival. Illustrated by the inspiring story of one of their participants, Elizama, they show how the Brazilian concept of Carnival, developed originally as a resistance movement during Brazil's long period of colonisation, has become a potent cultural force in breaking down the stereotypes that drive post-colonial asylum care in that part of South America, thereby empowering people with mental health issues to re-establish their place in society.

15.4.3 Shared Clinical Decision-Making Supported by Dissensual Balancing Within Frameworks of Shared Values

With the next three chapters, we move to the role of cultural values as vectors of best practice in clinical decision-making. Here, the relevant paradigm of good practice is what is widely called 'shared decision-making': clinical decision-making that is shared between the clinician (contributing in particular knowledge and technical skills) and the patient (contributing in particular an understanding of his or her own values).

The story in chapter 1, 'Surprised by Values: An Introduction to Values-Based Practice and the Use of Personal Narratives in this Book' of Mrs Jones and her arthritic knee illustrates shared decision-making in surgery. In Mrs Jones' story, the two sides (the knowledge side and the values side) of shared decision-making were supported respectively by evidence-based practice (represented in this instance by the surgeon, Mr Patel's, knowledge and experience) and by values-based practice (represented in this instance by Mr Patel picking up on what really mattered to Mrs Jones).

But shared decision-making as we went on to indicate, although offering in many situations 'win-win' results for all concerned, and in consequence being widely mandated (see Guide to Further Information), faces many challenges in practice. The challenges moreover, particularly in mental health, often involve cultural values. One example is provided by involuntary psychiatric treatment: this frequently involves a direct conflict between the values of society (to avoid risk of harm) and the values of the individual concerned (to retain individual autonomy). This is where the dissensual decision-making of values-based practice comes into play. Dissensual decision-making allows a balance to be struck within a framework of shared values according to the circumstances presented by the situation in question. This approach has in point of fact been worked out in detail in relation to the conflicts of values presented by involuntary psychiatric treatment [1].

The conflicts between individual and cultural values in shared decision-making are illustrated in chapter 19, 'Alcohol Use Disorder in a Culture that Normalizes the Consumption of Alcoholic Beverages: The Conflicts for Decision-Making' of this Part, in which Brazilian psychiatrists, Guilherme Messas and Maria Soares, examine the challenges of managing alcohol use disorder in a society that normalises (even valorises) alcohol consumption. Messas and Soares' narrative provides a vivid illustration of just how challenging the demands of dissensus may be when it comes to balancing conflicting cultural and individual values in the delivery of person-centred mental health care.

Cultural values, however, as our next two chapters illustrate, provide resources as well as challenges for shared decision-making. Chapter 20, 'Living at the Edge of Compromise: Balkan Pluralism as a Resource for Balanced Decision-Making', by Drozdstoj Stoyanov and Bill Fulford, illustrates through the story of Dr Petrov and his neighbour, the uniquely Balkan capacity for values pluralism. This capacity, gained through generations of having to 'live at the edge of compromise' in order to survive under successive colonising powers, shows that the 'default to monism' identified earlier (in chapter 1, 'Surprised by Values: An Introduction to Values-Based Practice and the Use of Personal Narratives in this Book') as perhaps the key challenge for the essentially pluralistic values-based practice may not after all be inevitable. Balkan pluralism, that is to say, suggests that the default to monism may be a learned rather than innate behaviour; it may be (as Stoyanov and Fulford put it) 'more nurture than nature'.

Chapter 21, '"Thinking Too Much": A Clash of Legitimate Values in Clinical Practice Calls for an Indaba Guided by African Values-Based Practice' illustrates the resources of African philosophy for dissensus. Decision-making in Western cultures relies mainly on consensus (as in evidence-based practice) and dissensus is in consequence a relatively unfamiliar (and hence problematic) concept. But dissensus, as Werdie van Staden shows in chapter 21, is entirely familiar in African cultures. We had intimations of the resources for values-based practice available from African philosophy in Part I, in Camillia Kong's exploration of African Critical Sankofaism (chapter 10, 'African Personhood, Humanism, and Critical Sankofaism: The Case of Male Suicide in Ghana'), and in Tutiette Thomas, Olusola Adebiyi and Temitope Ademosus' account of mythopoetry (chapter 11, 'Madness, Mythopoetry and Medicine'). In chapter 21, van Staden shows how the *indaba*, a distinctively African form of meeting, supports balanced dissensual decision-making in the context of the clinical management of a young man with psychotic experiences. Van Staden and co-author, Samuel Ujewe, explore the use of *indaba* in administrative contexts in a later chapter (chapter 29, 'Policy-Making Indabas to Prevent "Not Listening": An Added Recommendation from the Life Esidimeni Tragedy'). Van Staden has elsewhere developed a general concept of *Batho Pele* as a distinctively African form of values-based practice [2].

15.5 Recovery Practice

Shared decision-making like any other model of care is of course empty if it fails the test of delivering for those with mental health problems. It is with this crucial test that the last two chapters of Part III are concerned. But just what does 'delivering for those with mental health issues' mean? The very concept of 'recovery' in mental health has indeed attracted much debate in recent decades, at least in Western countries.

Chapters 22, 'Three Points in Time: How Values and Culture Affected My Life, Madness and the People Around Me' and 23, 'Recovery and Cultural Values: On Our Own Terms (A Dialogue)', both by those with considerable personal experience of mental health issues, speak to the view of recovery adopted in values-based practice—*recovering a good quality of life as defined by the values of (by what is important to) the individual concerned* [3]. Cultural values as the narratives in these two chapters illustrate may have crucial roles to play in recovery so understood. Chapter 22, by David Crepaz-Keay, is autobiographical. David tells his own story of recovery and how this was influenced (positively or negatively) by the values of the cultures in which at different stages he found himself. Chapter 23, by Justine Keen and Richard Shaw, both members of a group in Bristol working on resources for co-production, is a transcript of an unscripted dialogue between its two authors. They compare notes on what has been important to them over the several years of their respective experiences of coping with mental health issues. The cultures in which they found themselves again emerge as being critically important.

A shared message of these two chapters is that what is important for people with mental health issues (and hence important for recovery), is what is important for any of us, namely the cultural values represented by having friends, a home, and a role in life. Recovery is often equated with recovering independence. But as David Crepaz-Kay has argued in a different context [4], recovery should not be understood as ending with independence if this is defined by individual values such as those of autonomy. Independence so defined is indeed important but only as a step towards achieving the culturally enriched values of *inter*-dependence. There could be no stronger statement of the importance of cultural values as vectors of best practice in mental health.

15.6 Conclusions

This chapter has outlined how the contributions to Part III illustrate the role of cultural values as vectors of best practice in a number of key areas of contemporary person-centred mental health care. So long as they remain implicit and unacknowledged, cultural values (notably the cultural values of service providers) may act as inadvertent barriers to best practice. Made explicit, however, within the framework of a culturally enriched form of values-based practice, cultural values play a number of key roles in delivering best practice:

- They extend the role of the multidisciplinary team in providing person-values-centred care
- They provide novel support resources for dissensus (such as Bulgarian pluralism and the African indaba) in the context of shared clinical decision-making
- They contribute substantively to the quality of life by which the very concept of recovery in contemporary mental health practice is defined

In Part II, we characterised the relationship between theory and practice in terms of a two-way partnership: just as theory informs practice, we said, so practice informs theory. Although not the focus of this Part, its constituent chapters nicely illustrate the many ways in which practice may inform theory. To take but one example from the philosophy of mind, the contributions to this Part, severally and together, provide a rich resource for philosophers interested in personal identity. The Oxford philosopher, Kathleen Wilkes, anticipated this in her seminal book 'Real People: Personal Identity without Thought Experiments' (Oxford, Clarendon Press, 1988). The resources for work on personal identity, moreover, represented by the contributions to this Part, point specifically towards a philosophically neglected but practically relevant aspect of the topic, namely the extent to which cultural values contribute to the formation and maintenance of personal identity over time.

In thus redirecting the focus of theory in this practically relevant way, cultural values show yet again their importance as vectors of best practice in mental health care.

15.7 Guide to Further Information

The observations from which the concept of person-values-centred care is derived are described in [5]. The research underpinning the role of the extended multidisciplinary team in delivering person-values-centred care is reported in [6, 7].

Shared decision-making based on evidence and values is mandated in the UK by professional regulators [8] and in evidence-based guidelines (see, for example, [9]). It has recently been further mandated by a decision of the UK Supreme Court (the Montgomery judgement, [10]).

References

1. Fulford KWM, Dewey S, King M. Values-based involuntary seclusion and treatment: value pluralism and the UK's Mental Health Act 2007. Ch 60. In: Sadler JZ, van Staden W, Fulford KWM, editors. The Oxford handbook of psychiatric ethics. Oxford: Oxford University Press; 2015.
2. van Staden W, Fulford KWM. The Indaba in African values-based practice: respecting diversity of values without ethical relativism or individual liberalism. Ch 28. In: Sadler JZ, van Staden W, Fulford KWM, editors. The Oxford handbook of psychiatric ethics. Oxford: Oxford University Press; 2015.

3. Slade M, Amering M, Farkas M, Hamilton B, O'Hagan M, Panther G, Perkins R, Shepherd G, Tse S, Whitley R. Uses and abuses of recovery: implementing recovery-oriented practices in mental health systems. World Psychiatry. 2014;13:12–20.
4. Crepaz-Keay D, Fulford KWM, van Staden W. Putting both a person and people first: interdependence, values-based practice and African Batho Pele as resources for co-production in mental health. Ch 4. In: Sadler JZ, van Staden W, Fulford KWM, editors. The Oxford handbook of psychiatric ethics. Oxford: Oxford University Press; 2015.
5. Fulford KWM, Woodbridge K. Practicing ethically: values-based practice and ethics—working together to support person-centred and multidisciplinary mental health care. Chapter 5. In: Stickley T, Basset T, editors. Learning about mental health practice. London: Wiley; 2008. p. 79–103.
6. Colombo A, Bendelow G, Fulford KWM, Williams S. Evaluating the influence of implicit models of mental disorder on processes of shared decision making within community-based multi-disciplinary teams. Soc Sci Med. 2003;56:1557–70.
7. King C, Bhui K, Fulford KWM, Vasiliou-Theodore C, Williamson T. Model values? Race, values and models in mental health. London: The Mental Health Foundation; 2009.
8. General Medical Council. Consent: patients and doctors making decisions together. London: General Medical Council; 2008.
9. National Institute for Health and Care Excellence (2015/2017) Suspected cancer: recognition and referral: NICE guideline NG12 (published date: June 2015. Last updated: July 2017) See: https://www.nice.org.uk/guidance/ng12 [and scroll down the page to the statement 'Your Responsibility'].
10. Herring J, Fulford KWM, Dunn D, Handa A. Elbow room for best practice? Montgomery, patients' values, and balanced decision-making in person-centred care. Med Law Rev. 2017;25(4):582–603. https://doi.org/10.1093/medlaw/fwx029. https://academic.oup.com/medlaw/advance-articles. Accessed 19 Jul 2017.

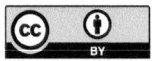

Cross-Cultural Factors and Identity in Adolescence

16

Vanya Matanova and Anna Hristova

16.1 Introduction

In European countries, multiculturalism is a social reality that has widespread official support. Modern societies are characterized by commitments such as respect for others and celebration of the riches of cultural diversity. However, in practice, these commitments run into difficulties especially when they come into conflict with other priority issues.

In this chapter, the story of "B," a young woman with self-harming behavior, and her family, is presented in six episodes that together illustrate the impact of the values conflicts arising from multiculturalism on early child development and on the establishment of identity in adolescence. B's story further illustrates how cross-cultural psychology highlights cultural values as they arise in therapy.

16.1.1 Cross-Cultural Psychology and Family Therapy

Cross-cultural psychology engages with the challenges of multiculturalism by addressing the cultural influences that affect mental processes and behaviors and

V. Matanova (✉)
Sofia University, Sofia, Bulgaria

Bulgarian Association of Clinical and Counseling Psychology and Bulgarian Association of Dyslexia, Sofia, Bulgaria

"Clinical Psychology in Action" Foundation, Sofia, Bulgaria

Institute of Mental Health and Development, Sofia, Bulgaria

A. Hristova
Institute of Mental Health and Development, Sofia, Bulgaria

© The Author(s) 2021
D. Stoyanov et al. (eds.), *International Perspectives in Values-Based Mental Health Practice*, https://doi.org/10.1007/978-3-030-47852-0_16

their impact on individual human behavior in the context of family life, transgenerational relationships, and social experience. It thus supports family therapy and other clinical interventions by helping to make explicit the cultural influences that affect mental processes and behaviors, different cultural patterns, and how they influence human behavior.

In the history of family therapy, tackling cultural differences is an important issue. The roots of this lie in part in the field of anthropology, notably in the work of Gregory Bateson [1] who inspired the first generation of family therapists to use direct observation to describe the patterns and structures underlying family interactions. Against this background, it is natural to ask what we know about Hungarian and British culture, and whether ignorance about significant values and prejudices in them would threaten the counseling and trust relationship in therapy.

In the following narrative, the story of B and her family illustrates the importance of cross-cultural competence in family therapy, involving the ability to understand cultural dynamics within families and across generations and thus react to cultural aspects of a young person's mental health issues in a way that facilitates their development. Further reading on cross-cultural psychology is given in our Guide to Further Sources.

16.2 Narrative Episode I: B Travels from Britain to Bulgaria

B was born from a mixed marriage, her mother being from the UK and her father from Bulgaria, that lasted for just a year (in the UK). After her parents divorce, B.'s mother was awarded custody with her father being granted visiting rights, which he followed strictly over the years.

Twelve years later B's parents agreed that she should move to Bulgaria to live with her father. This was because B's mother could not cope with the self-harming behavior that B had developed. It was a recurrence of this that, 8 months after B's arrival in Bulgaria, led her father to seek psychological support.

Consistently with contemporary multiculturalism, B's father had by this time entered into another mixed marriage. His new wife was Hungarian and they now had a son, age 3. During the first meeting, he shared an additional problem—his present wife, being in Bulgaria for 3 years, had made no attempt to study the local language—she lived in isolation, taking care of their child. Yet another factor that came to light was that B.'s father did business all over the world, travelling frequently and for prolonged periods.

B's father nonetheless declared confidently that there were no difficulties based on cultural differences in his family because everything that went on happened exactly as he said it should, and his wife and others just agreed and complied with his decisions and opinions. This was consistent with his beliefs about family functioning in general, where the man (father and husband) is the leading figure. This authoritarianism was also the basis of his approach to resolving family problems and disagreements.

16.2.1 Values Comment: Cultural Values Hidden in Plain Sight

Note that in B's initial referral, her father was focused solely on her self-harming behavior and made no mention of her new family set up. From a value perspective, the family set up clearly brings the potential for multicultural conflicts straight into focus. B, as a teenager seeking to adapt to a new family, now has to cope with no less than three nationalities and three languages. Yet none of this was mentioned initially by B's father—it was all in effect invisible to him essentially because it reflected local cultural values that being deeply embedded he simply took them for granted as "normal."

We see similar "values hidden in plain sight" later in this part of B's story in her father's confident denial of any difficulties arising from cultural differences. B's father was not being disingenuous. He was simply unaware of any such difficulties because, reflecting traditional Bulgarian values of the "strong father," he had asserted his control as he saw it effectively. We return to this "strong father" cultural value in later parts of B's story.

16.3 Narrative Episode II: Parenting Styles

B's father described her first self-harming injuries in Bulgaria as "scratches" made with a razor blade in the area of her forearm (between the elbow and the wrist) away from the veins, i.e. without being life-threatening.

B had started self-harming 2 years earlier while she was still living with her mother. At this time B was often alone: her mother worked in shifts, also living away to care for a sick grandma and her two dogs. The control she exercised over the B's life was thus weak and chaotic. She tried to compensate for her absence by taking over all the household chores at home, excluding B from them. Thus, overwhelmed by everyday tasks, B's mother hardly ever found time to spend with her daughter.

By contrast, in her new Bulgarian family, B encountered strong authoritarian control exercised by her father, which she described as a "strangle-hold". She was accompanied everywhere, and her requests to be left alone remained unheeded. So, from an overly indulgent parenting style with inconsistent control, B now found herself with an authoritarian father who exercised overly strict control.

The consultations with B's father significantly lowered his parental anxiety about B's self-injury. With greater confidence, he succeeded in letting B have time alone out of their home. To ensure B felt part of the daily life of her new family, he allowed her to make her own choices and included her in certain domestic activities and responsibilities.

16.3.1 Values Comment: Cultural Values and Parenting Styles

In recent years, there has been a visible increase in the prevalence of self-harm in the non-clinical adolescent population in general [2]. Causal factors vary but the style of parenting attributed to B's mother is commonly seen in the families of self-harming teenagers—the child feels rejected by the parent and experiences an ambivalent approach to control, which leads to a chaotic and non-transparent family situation [3].

The inconsistent parenting style adopted by B's mother was driven by internal conflicts of values. On the one side, she was concerned about her own mother and (as became clear later) she was also trying to establish herself in a new career. These were among her values; they were things that mattered or were important to her. But also important to her, on the other hand, was her daughter, B. Hence, caught in a conflict of values, she responded in an inconsistent way that left B feeling neglected and insignificant—as she put it: *"the very last in line, even after the dogs."*

After moving to Bulgaria B found herself subject to the very different values of her father as reflected in his authoritarian style of parenting. As described further below, his values reflect traditional Bulgarian cultural values reinforced by his own family background. But the effect was the opposite of what he had intended in that B's self-harming behavior reappeared. In therapy, helping him to understand the origins of his values, and their unintended consequences on B, allowed him to draw back and let B escape what she experienced as his "strangle-hold".

16.4   Narrative Episode III: B in Bulgaria

The radical change that took place in B's life at this stage of her development was a serious challenge. Her father was trying to understand that B was going through a difficult period but he could not accept the way she had chosen to cope with her experiences. At one point, frustrated by his absolute inability to understand the reasons behind B's behavior, he said: 'This isn't what we do!' By 'we', he referred to himself and his kin; so, without realizing it, he had sent a message to his daughter, which, in the process of identification, could be perceived as: "You're not like us."

16.4.1 Values Comment: The Good Bulgarian Father

This may seem a harsh message. But during the sessions with B's father, it became clear that he represented that aspect of traditional Bulgarian culture where the children are a core priority and value for the parents for the rest of their lives, and the family operates with clearly defined family roles.

This type of family culture necessarily implies clear value expectations: it involves setting aside personal time, interests, ambitions, and right to personal life and liberty. In traditional Bulgarian culture, these expectations are directed primarily toward the mother. In B's previous family, however, they were not directed to her biological mother. B's father claimed that her mother, "while chasing her career dreams, did not devote enough time to their child." He found it unacceptable for a mother to have priorities other than her children and perceived her ambitions and professional commitment as "a desire to compete with him." All this not only contributed to their separation but his reproaches and accusations toward B's mother continued after their separation.

Because of his business, B's father often had formal and informal contacts with people from different cultures, requiring flexibility and a respectful attitude towards diversity. There had thus been significant opportunities for his ideas and concepts about good motherhood to evolve over time. However, his ideal of 'the good mother' remained essentially unchanged.

Believing he was doing the best for his child, B's father tried to convey his idea of 'the good mother' to her by never missing an opportunity to express in front of her his dissatisfaction with her biological mother.

16.4.2 Values Comment: The Good Bulgarian Mother

The explanation for B's father's rather extreme model of the "good mother" lies beyond the framework of his traditional culture and is to be found rather in the dynamics of his own parental family.

His parents were divorced. His mother was granted full custody of their children, and the image of their father was manipulatively demonized. As a result, he and his brothers had no contact with their father for the rest of his life. His mother devoted herself completely to her function as a parent: she deprived herself of her own life, interests, and career; she sacrificed all her time for her family and home and dedicated herself to the role of "mother-heroine," which filled her son (B's father) with loyalty, uncritical trust, and admiration.

16.5   Narrative Episode IV: B Stays with Her Grandmother

During the first session of therapy, B had already left her father's home and moved to her paternal grandmother's house. B had declared her desire to make this move in order to master the local language. Her father had agreed with this, because he found it acceptable for a grandmother to raise her granddaughter—this corresponded with their traditional stereotypes and beliefs. However, he was confused: initially, he was confident that language adaptation was the real reason for B wanting to leave his home, but subsequently he started experiencing some hesitation and anxiety.

In the event B's stay with her grandmother did not go smoothly. A series of transgenerational conflicts followed over issues such as daily chores, going out, and even the way B dressed. Her father was constantly involved as an arbitrator, which was exhausting for him—he had already started a new job and had no opportunity to answer their constant phone calls or to meet and talk to both of them, together or in private. At this stage, B decided to move back in with her father.

16.5.1 Values Comment: Cultural Values Across the Generations

Important to the cultural context of B's story is the strictly hierarchical structure of a traditional Bulgarian family. This is partly a matter of age, partly of gender. In this hierarchical model, the world of men and the world of women are clearly distinguished. The male is dominant (the proper, the good, the right), and the female is the weak (the wrong, the left). The man represents the family before the authorities and in the community; the woman gives birth and cares for the children and the sick. After marriage, the woman enters the new family, loses her name, and takes her husband's [4].

This speaks to the question why B's father failed to mention the different nationalities of his family members in the initial referral (noted above). The problems arising from the multicultural interactions in his family were invisible to him. Being a responsible leader of his family, he did not allow other members to take part in the family sessions. It also explains the transgenerational conflicts between B and her grandmother. B's father had experienced an upbringing that strongly reflected his Bulgarian norms of family life. B, however, did not share these norms.

16.6 Narrative Episode V: Developing Awareness of Values

B's father now realized for the first time that his immense confidence in his mother—in his mind the exemplar "good mother"—had misled him. He understood that B's decision to move back in with him was inspired by his mother—he called this "a coalition behind my back." A "secret coalition" in the family means continuous behavior of two of its members from different hierarchical levels (in this case, grandmother and granddaughter), with the purpose of mutual support, although one of the members (the grandmother in this instance) always demonstrates a certain negative emotional attitude towards the other.

This coalition prompted B's father to put up boundaries for the first time between his mother and his family—he stopped sharing with her his emotional disappointments and anxieties and started seeking support from his Hungarian wife. With the increasing role of B in the family, B's father gained confidence and was inclined to give her a degree of autonomy.

16.6.1 Values Comment: Balancing Values

Up to this point as we have seen, B's father idolized his own mother. Now he faced the reality that she was not perfect. This more balanced understanding, as one of the keys to values-based practice (see introductory chapter), allowed him to begin to move forward in therapy.

16.7 Narrative Episode VI: Crisis as a Starting Point

Realizing the problem of adaptation, B's father made a solo decision and without any prior discussion, sent his second wife to a Bulgarian language course and registered their young son in a local Bulgarian pre-school.

As to B, when she arrived In Bulgaria, she was enrolled in a private English school attended by local children as well as by children of a different background. The latter, however, belonged to a particular ethnicity and formed a single 'in crowd' group. B did not identify with any of the various school communities and failed to develop close friendships. She tried only once to make friends with one of her classmates. They did not get in touch at school but she received invitations to religious gatherings of a community to which her classmate belonged. B's father felt particularly anxious about this friendship and kept himself closely informed of any details about their meetings outside school. B never managed to fit into her peer group. For a short time she joined a Facebook group of English people living in Bulgaria.

Disappointment and difficulties in B's adaptation to Bulgaria, as well as nostalgia about her English friends, ended in B wanting to return to Britain. Her mother was supportive, but her father was against another change. After talking with him about this, B's psycho-emotional state deteriorated.

16.7.1 Values Comment: Crisis as Both a Values Challenge and a Values Opportunity

The strict hierarchy in B's new family was now in crisis. With her father, who as we have seen was a dominating authority, now traveling frequently and being absent from home for extended periods, and with his Hungarian wife (her surrogate mother) adapting more slowly than B to cultural transitions and thus unable to perform her parental role adequately, B faced additional instabilities.

These instabilities, arising as in this story from conflicting cultural values, have the consequence that intra-family tensions between a parent and a teenager can be significantly aggravated. Clearly, there was more work to do. But with the relevant values now finally becoming visible to those concerned, the cultural context of family functioning became an effective starting point for family therapy [5].

16.8   Conclusions

"Identity vs. diffusion" according to Erikson [6] is the time when adolescents actively try to synthesize their experience and to form a stable sense of personal identity. Identity development is formed not only from the psychosocial point of view, but also from the ethnic point of view. Root's model [7] is one of the first to go beyond the paradigm of identity deficit when considering the development of personality in individuals of mixed origin. Adolescents of mixed ethnicity have more than one choice for healthy identification. Root believes that internal conflicts related to the identification of mixed-ethnicity adolescents are due to political, social, or family processes.

The importance of these insights is evident in the story of B and her family. Reading the story as we have set it out here through a values lens informs effective family therapy interventions in the context of the challenges of contemporary multiculturalism.

16.9   Guide to Further Sources

For further information on cross-cultural psychology please see:

1. Henriksen Jr., R. C., & Paladino, D. A. (2009). Identity development in a multiple heritage world.
2. La Roche, M. J., & Maxie, A. (2003). Ten considerations in addressing cultural differences in psychotherapy. *Professional Psychology: Research and Practice*, *34* (2), 180.
3. Romero, D. (1985). Cross-cultural counseling: Brief reactions for the practitioner. *The Counseling Psychologist*, *13* (4), 665–671.
4. Sue, D. W., Sue, D., Neville, H. A., & Smith, L. (2019). *Counseling the culturally diverse: Theory and practice*. John Wiley & Sons.

References

1. Bateson G. Steps to an ecology of mind: collected essays in anthropology. Psychiatr Evol Epistemol. 1972;381.
2. Lloyd-Richardson EE, Perrine N, Dierker L, Kelley ML. Characteristics and functions of non-suicidal self-injury in a community sample of adolescents. Psychol Med. 2007;37(8):1183–92.
3. Burešová I, Bartošová K, Čerňák M. Connection between parenting styles and self-harm in adolescence. Procedia Soc Behav Sci. 2015;171:1106–13.
4. Gavrilova B. "Bŭlgarskoto patriarhalno semeĭstvo: Vlast, zakon, ĭerarkhiya", dots. Anna Luleva, dots. Aneliya Kasabova, gl. as. Mariya Markova, Institut za etnologiyaifolkloristika s etnografskimuzeĭ pri BAN, dots.TanyaBoneva, SU, dots.MariyaKitanovaotInstituta za bylgarskiezik, radioentsiklopediya; 2015.

5. Repetto E. Cross-cultural counseling: problems and prospects. Orientación y Sociedad. 2002;3:29–35.
6. Erikson EH, editor. Youth: change and challenge. New York: Basic books; 1963.
7. Root MPP. Resolving 'other' status: identity development of biracial individuals. Women Ther. 1990;9:185–205.

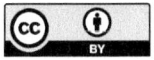

Multidisciplinary Teamwork and the Insanity Defence: A Case of Infanticide in Iraq

17

Hasanen Al-Taiar

17.1 Introduction

Capital punishment still exists in many countries and mainly in the Middle East where Islam is the main formal religion for most states.

Here, the author describes the case of a young woman from Iraq who was arrested by Police on suspicion of murdering her 1-year-old son. Due to concerns about her mental state, it was decided that she would appear before a specialist panel of experienced mental health professionals in the main psychiatric hospital in Baghdad, Iraq. This panel was comprised of consultant psychiatrists, psychologists and nurses whose specialism is in dealing with forensic psychiatric cases. The author has sought consent from the patient who was willing for her case to be discussed for clinical and academic purposes.

17.2 Narrative

The author visited Al-Rashad psychiatric Hospital in Baghdad in April 2018 and he was impressed by the work of the forensic psychiatry committee that determines the criminal responsibility of a large number of cases from all over Iraq. One case that drew a lot of attention was that of a young woman (23) who allegedly killed her 1 year-old infant by dropping the mattresses and blankets over him. The professional committee consisted of specialist psychiatrists (three to four) in addition to psychiatric nurses and psychologists. It met on two occasions to determine the defendant's criminal responsibility. Potential disposals could be admission to a psychiatric hospital via *a Court order should she be found "not guilty as a result of insanity". Alternatively, she could still face capital punishment if she was found guilty of committing the offence.*

H. Al-Taiar (✉)
Oxford Health NHS Foundation Trust, Littlemore Mental Health Centre, Oxford, UK

© The Author(s) 2021
D. Stoyanov et al. (eds.), *International Perspectives in Values-Based Mental Health Practice*, https://doi.org/10.1007/978-3-030-47852-0_17

This patient appeared twice before the panel and it was agreed that she was having a form of a neurodevelopmental disorder i.e. autism and she was intellectually challenged. In addition, she showed some psychotic symptoms e.g. auditory hallucinations commanding her to kill her son to protect her safety. She married at the age of 22 to a local man in her village. She lived with her husband and mother in law. One day, she was cleaning her bedroom and alleged that she mistakenly dropped the duvets on her 1 year old son who suffocated and died shortly afterwards. She was arrested by Police where concerns were instantly raised about her mental welling hence the referral to the criminal panel at Al-Rashad Hospital.

During the two interviews, the lady in question didn't present with obvious signs of a psychotic disorder but was rather showing features of a possible autistic disorder. The panel examined the clinical notes and the criminal case summary (Police and Court documents) over a number of weeks prior to and in between these two interviews.

The conclusion was that this young lady was exhibiting features suggestive of a possible autistic spectrum disorder and a learning disability which would require further assessment. Autism is characterized by qualitative abnormalities in reciprocal social interactions and in patterns of communication, and by restricted, stereotyped, repetitive repertoire of interests and activities [1]. In addition, patients with autistic spectrum disorders have a restricted, repetitive, and stereotyped patterns of behaviours, that could manifest as "compulsive adherence to specific, non-functional routines/encompassing preoccupation with one or more stereotyped and restricted patterns of interest that are abnormal in content or focus; or abnormal in their intensity". This could explain his lack of flexibility around not wearing the used boots. Some patients with autism will exhibit Stereotypy or self-stimulatory behaviour which refers to repetitive body movements or repetitive movement of objects. This behaviour is common in many individuals with developmental disabilities; however, it appears to be more common in autism. Many autistic people have intense and highly-focused interests, often from a fairly young age. These can change over time or be lifelong. Although repetitive behaviour varies from person to person, the reasons behind it may be the same e.g. an attempt to gain sensory input, e.g. rocking may be a way to stimulate the balance system. In the same way, using the phone could provide sensory/auditory stimulation. Such repetitive behaviours can occur to deal with stress and anxiety and to block out uncertainty. Such patients can be supported via modifying their environments, increasing structure or managing their anxieties.

The panel concluded that the patient's behaviour was not calculated to cause annoyance and inconvenience, but rather a symptomatic feature of her possible autistic disorder to the extent that it displays a compulsive adherence to specific, non-functional routines, abnormal in content, focus, and intensity.

In a country like Iraq where Islam is the main formal religion which the majority of population practice, capital punishment is still seen as one of the most ethically challenging prospects. Iraq witnessed many military conflicts over the last four decades and these have eroded the infrastructure of the Iraq economy in addition to the loss of many people (civilians and military). Obviously the criminal responsibility panel has a huge responsibility as it determines life pathways for most offenders who come in contact with it. Its decision could mean that the suspect would face a punitive outcome e.g. custody, execution or a less adversarial outcome such as psychiatric treatment (initially in hospital). Where mental illness is still seen as a stigma in many areas of Iraq especially rural and less urbanized ones, it would undoubtedly be more favourable in the families of their affected ones.

17.3   Cultural Context

Ancient Iraq (Mesopotamia) witnessed the first mention of the Insanity Defence—in the Hammurabi's code that dates back to around 1772 BC [2]. Today, with Islam as the main formal religion (and practiced by the majority of the population), capital punishment is still seen as one of the most ethically challenging prospects.

Iraq witnessed many military conflicts over the last four decades, and these have eroded the infrastructure of the Iraq economy in addition to the loss of many people (civilians and military). Obviously, the criminal responsibility panel has a huge responsibility as it determines life pathways for most offenders who come in contact with it. Its decision could mean that the suspect would face a punitive outcome, e.g. custody, execution or a less adversarial outcome such as psychiatric treatment (initially in hospital). Where mental illness is still seen as a stigma in many areas of Iraq especially rural and less urbanized ones, it would undoubtedly be more favourable in the families of their affected ones.

17.4   The Criminal Responsibility Panel
as a Multidisciplinary Team

The Criminal Responsibility Panel is a specialist team of professionals employed by the Ministry of Health, and they have a close link with the judicial system in which all cases of suspected psychiatric morbidity would be referred to them by the Police or Court. The remit of this panel is to establish the presence or absence of a mental disorder and then recommending any suitable disposals in line with the severity of the offence and the mental disorder.

The panel is set up to meet in the hospital once weekly for a full day when they assess all remanded detainees who are escorted by Police or prison staff.

The panel is chaired by a senior consultant psychiatrist who is assisted by 2–3 other specialists, trainee psychiatrists, in addition to other disciplines such as psychology and nursing.

Obviously, each case is assessed individually and professionals discuss them in huge detail to ascertain criminal responsibility. Two elements are examined here, actus reus (criminal act) and mens rea (criminal intent) [3].

The panel demonstrates a very good model of multidisciplinary team (MDT) work in such a politically sensitive matter. Professionals themselves might find it a challenging task to separate their own personal lives from undertaking their duty especially in the current political uncertainty. Over the last four decades, Iraqis have witnessed a number of military conflicts where millions of souls have been lost to violence. A culture of violence started to prevail among Iraqis in 1980, and an instinct for aggression began to rise in the collective subconscious of the people.

The panel takes in consideration whether the patient was actually mentally ill or simply making up "malingering" or faking symptoms of mental illness for purposes of secondary gain, i.e. avoiding criminal proceedings and consequences such as capital punishment.

Dissociative disorders are also prevalent in countries like Iraq, and they often present with psychosomatic symptoms such as tiredness and generalized pains.

More knowledge about specific disorders and their management, e.g. culture-bound syndromes which are psychiatric conditions, assumed to be specific to a particular culture, that has become the focus of an on-going debate in psychiatry and the social sciences, on the question of the primacy of either universal biopsychological or specific ethnic–cultural factors determining psychopathology.

The fall of the Baath leadership and change of power in 2003 brought with its further complications. Corruption has eroded the infrastructure of Iraq including political, industrial and cultural aspects. The psychological effect of this change resembled the exchange of roles between a master and slave. This reality is explained by the following theory: A society that has two large sects, where one acquires power with the help of external force and the other is subjected to political, economic and psychological frustration, creates sectarian strife. Such medico-legal panels have remained away from political pressures although in would argue that corruption has even invaded the health system. Health professionals especially doctors have been targeted by successive waves of abductions and murders which jeopardized the Iraqi medical community to a large extent. Many doctors have fled the country, relocated work and accommodation, or hired bodyguards for protection.

17.5 Conclusions

The case illustrates a good example of multidisciplinary and inter-agency work and collaboration. It focuses on a number of cultural issues such as stigma and mental illness especially in women. Many families keep their daughters' mental illnesses in a very discreet manner for fear of stigma. Many psychiatric patients experience stigma and discrimination from the society and sometimes from families, friends and employers. It is evident that discrimination and stigma have a detrimental influence on patients' lives. Such discriminatory experiences can also worsen patients' mental health problems and hinder their access to treatment recovery. Social isolation, poor housing, unemployment and poverty are all linked to mental ill health. Stigma and discrimination can trap people in a cycle of illness.

Acknowledgements The author would like to thank all staff members who assisted his visit to Al-Rashad Hospital, especially Dr. Ali Al-Amery (forensic department lead) and members of the criminal responsibility panel.

17.6   Guide to Further Sources

http://applications.emro.who.int/dsaf/EMRPUB_2009_EN_1367.pdf

References

1. World Health Organization. International statistical classification of diseases and related health problem (ICD-10).
2. Downey M, Farhat F, Garofolo A, Jones R. History of forensic psychology; 2008.
3. Bronitt S, McSherry B. Criminal justice and procedure (LAW109). Macquarie University.

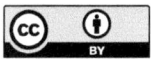

Colonial Values and Asylum Care in Brazil: Reclaiming the Streets Through Carnival in Rio de Janeiro

18

Julia Evangelista and William A. Fulford

18.1 Introduction

Brazil's cultural values are intrinsically linked to its colonial past. The country was transformed almost overnight from a colonial Portuguese outpost to the country's official seat of government when its royal family and entourage of 15,000 courtiers fled Napoleon Bonaparte's forces to arrive *en masse* on 22 January 1808. Rio de Janeiro was anointed its new capital city which was quickly "Europeanised" through a huge programme of infrastructural investment. European cultural values were established as infinitely superior and in direct contrast to any of the myriad of non-European cultural values that had'existed pre-1808. The poor, who were predominantly of native Indian and African descent, were seen as a barrier to this Europeanising project as their behaviour and customs were labelled "mad" and uncivilised [1]. No longer welcomed in the city's modernising centres, they were criminalised and displaced to the outskirts of the city, often finding themselves arbitrarily incarcerated in the newly built networks of prisons and asylums that came to dominate Rio de Janeiro's suburbs. It is in one of these suburban-built asylums, a sprawling 20-acre complex first opened in 1911—the Pedro II Psychiatric Centre, later renamed the Nise da Silveira Institute—where the carnival project, Loucura Suburbana, continues to challenge both the divisive legacy of Brazil's colonial past and stigmas associated with mental illness.

Carnival emerged as a form of resistance against the forces of colonialism in the second half of the nineteenth century, challenging the right for the disenfranchised to occupy the city on their own cultural terms, even if only temporarily and often at

J. Evangelista
Centre for Cultural and Media Policy Studies, The University of Warwick, Coventry, UK

W. A. Fulford (✉)
Faculty of Architecture and the Built Environment, The University of Westminster, London, UK

© The Author(s) 2021
D. Stoyanov et al. (eds.), *International Perspectives in Values-Based Mental Health Practice*, https://doi.org/10.1007/978-3-030-47852-0_18

155

great personal risk. The main language of this occupation was a form of music and dance called "samba" that emerged from Brazil's segregated quilombos,[1] favelas and suburbs, and it is within this context that samba has been described as "resistance in motion" [2]. But today, resistance plays little role in the commercial activities and VIP areas of the main carnival parades. This remains the domain of local "bloc" or neighbourhood carnivals like Loucura Suburbana, who are using "resistance in motion" in their neighbourhood of Engenho de Dentro to provide platforms for diverse and repressed forms of cultural expression.

The project is illustrated here by the story of patient Elisama Ranoud (her real name, used at her request) and psychologist Ariadne Mendes (again her real name and used at her request).[2] Their story shows that it is the project's capacity to enable groups of diverse individuals to express a whole range of differing cultural values in both intimate semi-public and extrovert very-public expressions of solidarity that helps challenge fixed notions of identity and space that become barriers to recovery.

18.2   The Story of "Patient" Elisama and Psychologist, Ariadne

Elisama first came to the Nise da Silveira Institute in 1991 as a young mother seeking help for her 5-year-old son who had been diagnosed with a hyperactive disorder. A community centre had been set up in one of the Institute's abandoned buildings, and on the recommendation of her son's psychologist, she signed him up for some of the free activities they were offering.

Elisama and her son attended these activities alongside a family support group until he turned 18 years old in 2003. But although her son's mental well-being improved significantly over this period, Elisama's own mental health had started to deteriorate. This deterioration was driven in part by her son no longer being so dependent on her, which was obviously a good thing, albeit one that left Elisama with a gap in her own life. This sense of loss was compounded by an unfulfilling and poorly paid job as a cleaner and a broken marriage with a controlling husband and father-in-law she could not escape due to a lack of financial resources. Now 39 years old, her behaviour spiralled out of control and she fell into a deep depression: "*I began to cry all the time and I thought about bad things and didn't even want to leave the house. I had no perspective and I increasingly withdrew myself from the world.*"

Her increasingly dishevelled appearance made her feel like an outcast from society. She was called "mad" by her neighbours and was losing her sense of identity and self-worth. Elisama's son's psychologist had also noticed these changes and recommended she seek out help at an adult support group at the Nise da Silveira Institute that was being supervised by Ariadne. In 2005, Ariadne took direct control

---

[1] Quilombos were settlements located in places hard to access created by fugitive slaves who resisted slavery.

[2] Using their real names when reporting on the Loucura Suburbana project is seen as an important part of the process of reclaiming citizenship and validity as producers of culture.

of this group, and when it was disbanded about a year later she took Elisama on as a patient, in part because she was concerned about her being medicalised by other doctors who did not understand her case history: "*I could understand that Elisama's case wasn't about taking drugs as she had already started improving and doing other recommended activities [being held at the Institute] such as Tai Chi and drawing classes.*"

Meanwhile, in 2000, Ariadne was part of a small group that founded the carnival project Loucura Suburbana, inspired in part by other projects that were bringing people from the local community into the psychiatric centre to attend workshops and classes alongside patients. Loucura Suburbana was designed to take this one step further by not only bringing people from the local community into the psychiatric centre to prepare for the carnival, but also then collectively taking to the streets - patients and non-patients together - to parade through their local neighbourhood.

In 2006, Elisama joined the project. At first, she stayed in the background, using her experience growing up with her aunt and uncle in the culture of the Barracão, the name for the place where the carnival costumes and props are made, which also often serves as a rehearsal and social space for those taking part in the carnival. Elisama worked for 3 years helping organise Loucura Suburbana's Barracão: "*which was nothing like it is today,*" she says proudly, "*it was a mess and there weren't many costumes like there are now.*" It was in the Barracão where Elisama began to define a new role for herself that not only enabled her own recovery but also helped others in the process.

I make hats, I dress everybody, I normally get late because I want to get everybody dressed with makeup…Someone tells me "I want to be a Baiana[3]*" then I go and make them a costume of a Baiana, or I want to be this or that…What matters in these stories is that we do not forget that they touch our soul. There was a man who was hospitalized in an emergency here, but he heard about me and was curious to meet me and asked to see me. So, the doctor who was looking after him came down and told me, "my patient wants to see you because he dreams of wearing a wig." He was bald, so I found a wig and gave it to him. He could not go to the carnival parade, but he left happy dancing with his wig.*

In 2009, the carnival bloc was looking for a new Porta Bandeira, an important symbolic figure in carnival folklore who leads the parade dressed in bright flamboyant clothes and makeup. Buoyed by her increased confidence working in the Barracão, Elisama volunteered. This new very public role represented a step change in her recovery, giving Elisama the chance to present a version of herself to her local neighbourhood that moved beyond the stereotyped image of someone suffering from mental illness in which she felt she had been trapped.

When I went to the streets for the first time, the local people showed prejudice, because I live here. But the way and the moment that door was opened to me and I exited the hospital, many things changed, because now the people themselves take part in the bloc, they accept me and give me compliments and say very good things about the centre. Because when you talk about a psychiatric hospital, people think horrible things, that we will be aggressive

---

[3] A Baiana is a distinctive traditional form of dress typical of women from Bahia in the north east of the country that has strong Afro-Brazilian roots.

towards them, and this is not true. We are people like anybody else. We just need to be looked after... If you give us opportunity, it can take a little while, but we can learn. I learnt to sew, I learnt about informatics...I will never forget the day I went to the Sapucaí[4] with the costumes I always dreamt of...my neighbours saw me and began to see me in a different way because before I was not a Porta Bandeira...you grow as a person. You become a person you did not think you were capable of becoming.

Elisama has continued to play a prominent role both behind the scenes in the Barracão and front of house as the Porta Bandeira. In doing so, she has learnt new skills and met different people that have helped shift her own perceptions about herself and those around her. She has found her identity, or in some cases identities, and an ability, confidence and platform to express these identities both privately and publicly through the various activities of carnival.

This year I am writing...the theme is about prejudice, of race, colour, especially in relation to the condition of the woman, harassment. So, the theme is drag [as in drag queen], about the fight against stigmas. We are what we want to be. I do not want to be a "watermelon[5]" I want to be a drag! Since 2016 I have had this in my mind...a drag is related to my thinking as a woman.

The impact of this renewed confidence has been significant. Although her personal situation—a stressful home and working life—remains largely unchanged, the support mechanisms provided by Loucura Suburbana's activities have given her better tools to cope. "*I feel like I broke barriers. Everybody is capable! I have high self-esteem again! Our self-esteem grows every time the bloc grows, because at the beginning we were nothing.*" Such has been the impact on her health and well-being that Elisama now feels a tremendous sense of loyalty to the Nise da Silveira Institute where the project takes place and the people within it, calling for more projects like Loucura Suburbana that offer creative activities and platforms for cultural expression as alternatives to medication [3].

This sense of project loyalty is one reason why Loucura Suburbana's participants resist the idea of anonymity when talking about the project. As Ariadne explains:

I defend that [not changing names when reporting on the project] because if we want citizenship, I am not talking about clinical cases or giving diagnostics...but we are talking about human lives. Of course, I ask permission where it's required, but in general I use the real names and surnames because these people are citizens, and these are their stories.

When asked if she has ever had anyone refuse permission to use their name, she responds: "*no this has never happened! In fact, it's the opposite. In the carnival bloc the name of each patient appears alongside their role in the carnival. Because everybody has a role. The Porta Bandeira or the Mestre-Sala. They all have a role to play.*"

---

[4] The Sapucai is the principle thoroughfare for the main carnival of Rio de Janeiro that holds 90,000 spectators and is televised internationally.

[5] "Watermelon" is a derogatory caricature of a woman with a curvaceous body-type who is considered by society to have nothing to offer except for how she looks.

18.3   Colonisation, Mental Health and Carnival as Resistance

A defining aspect of colonisation in Brazil has been the imposition of one relatively homogenous set of European cultural values over the myriad of diverse cultural values that either pre-existed or emerged during colonisation. This process of cultural imposition involved a mixture of techniques to ridicule, dehumanise and demonise those that did not fit within the narrow confines of European values and norms of behaviour, which in turn became the foundations for the construction of madness and notions of "normality" versus "deviance" that remain strong in Brazil today. As the country sought to Europeanise, hundreds of thousands of Brazilians were arbitrarily locked up in the network of asylums that were, by no coincidence, built alongside the abolition of slavery in 1888. This is a largely ignored period of Brazilian history, and details are only recently starting to emerge about the horrific conditions and number of unexplained deaths that occurred in many of these asylums. One author has labelled this period the Brazilian Holocaust with more than 60,000 people known to have died in one hospital alone [4].

In time, the Europeanising project extended to carnival, where the "collective" presence of white and black people in a shared space was considered a threat to the morality and social order of the country [1]. As such, people from non-European backgrounds and their associated forms of cultural expression, particularly those rooted in Afro-Brazilian religions and cultures, were banned from taking part. Carnival as resistance in the colonial context in Brazil thus emerges around the second half of the nineteenth century as a direct reaction against this cultural crackdown. By the beginning of the twentieth century, in a series of very public displays of resistance, and despite heavy and often violent responses from the police, the culturally marginalised began to venture collectively into the streets of Rio de Janeiro to express their right to the city and cultural expression through dancing and singing to the sound of drums in deliberate opposition to the polished carnival of the elite, which in general took place in the private spaces of Rio de Janeiro's clubs [5].

However, the colonial legacy in Brazil remains strong. Today, many of its asylums continue to house a disproportionate number of people from non-European backgrounds, and particularly those of African descent, fed by a toxic combination of political powerlessness, economic uncertainty and the constant bombardment of overt and more subliminal messages about cultural inferiority. This toxic combination creates a form of "disrupted self-hood" [6] that exacerbates the likelihood of such populations suffering from mental illness.

Elisama's story shows how suffering from the stigmas of mental illness created the conditions for cultural and social exclusion which only exacerbated her already perilous condition. The Loucura Suburbana carnival project enabled Elisama to resist these forces of exclusion, reasserting her right to occupy the neighbourhood from which she had felt excluded. It also gave her a platform to express her own cultural values while projecting a positive image of herself in both public and more private situations which enabled her to break free from an aspect of her history as someone who suffers from mental illness in which she had felt trapped.

18.4   Conclusions

This chapter began by showing how Brazil's colonial past established European cultural values as infinitely superior to those from other cultural backgrounds. Carnival emerged as a form of resistance against such colonial processes, symbolising a time of year when marginalised communities could gather *en masse* to resist, even if only temporarily, such forms of cultural repression by occupying parts of the city from which they would normally be excluded and playing music and dancing to rhythms that had been rejected as uncivilised.

The story of Elisama and the Loucura Suburbana carnival project show these same forces of resistance at work. A central part of her recovery has been the opportunity to take centre stage during the carnival parades, reclaiming her right to be in a city from which she had felt excluded because of her history of mental illness. In reclaiming the streets as part of a respected carnival parade, Elisama was able to re-build her sense of identity and self-worth beyond the stereotyped image of a mental health patient within which she felt she had become trapped.

The combination of the very public and more private roles behind the scenes in the carnival project have given Elisama the tools to become a producer of culture on her own terms. She is writing her own performances and expressing her own identity, or sometimes identities, all wrapped up in her own sense of important cultural values. This combination has led to huge improvements in Elisama's general sense of mental well-being, even though her own personal circumstances that were major contributing factors in her spiral towards mental illness have remained unchanged.

Acknowledgements The authors would like to thank Psychologist Ariadne Mendes and Porta Bandeira Elisama Ranoud for their time and honesty in answering our questions during these interviews.

18.5   Guide to Further Sources

The authors have a wide variety of photographic and other materials illustrating the Loucura Suburbana—see for example:

- https://www.loucurasuburbana.org
- https://www.bbc.com/news/av/world-latin-america-47419917/the-carnival-parade-shining-a-light-on-mental-health
- https://vimeo.com/40817909
- https://www.youtube.com/watch?v=G-Nizn1wDJ4
- https://www.youtube.com/watch?v=uQh1ixxSkFQ
- https://www.youtube.com/watch?v=bVZ8n2ksbvo
- https://www.youtube.com/watch?v=LtBRBWpttOs

References

1. Cunha MCP. Ecos da Folia: Uma historia social do Carnaval carioca entre 1880 e 1920. São Paulo: Companhia das Letras. p. 2001.
2. Browning B. Samba: resistance in motion. Indianapolis: Indiana University Press; 1993.
3. Evangelista J, Fulford W. Performing urbanity through carnival on the streets of Rio de Janeiro: practical approaches for reducing stigmatization of the "mad" in cities. In: Okpaku S, editor. Innovations in gloabl mental health. Cham: Springer Nature; 2019. p. 1–21.
4. Arbex D. Holocausto Brasileiro: Vida, Genocidio e 60 mil mortes no maior hospicio do Brasil. Lisboa: Guerra e Paz Editores; 2004.
5. Coutinho EG. Os Cronistas De Momo: Imprensa e Carnival na Primeira Republica. Rio de Janeiro: Editora UFRJ; 2006.
6. Selligman R. Possessing spirits and healing selves: embodiment and transformations in an Afro-Brazilian religion. New York: Palgrave Macmillan; 2015.

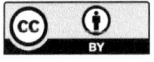

Alcohol Use Disorder in a Culture That Normalizes the Consumption of Alcoholic Beverages: The Conflicts for Decision-Making

19

Guilherme (G) Messas and Maria Julia (MJFR) Soares

19.1 Introduction

Disorders associated with the use of alcohol always reflect the cultural values of the societies in which they occur. This applies equally to Brazil, a country whose culture minimizes the risks of consumption. Current representations of alcohol in the media and in music lead to the invisibility of the social risks of alcohol and hinder the effectiveness of the laws that regulate its sale and use. For example, many young people initiate the use of alcohol with the consent of their parents, although the country's law prohibits minors under the age of 18 from drinking alcohol. Thus, consumption begins to be normalized within family relationships.

Given this cultural liberality in relation to the use of alcohol, what dilemmas arise for the therapeutic management of patients with harmful use of alcohol? Here, we briefly address two questions: What are the values that permeate the treatment of individuals who seek a healthier relationship with alcohol consumption? How does culture permeate therapeutic choices?

The following narrative tells the story of a Brazilian we will call Bruno, who values family, health, and work. After a hospitalization for complications due to the use of alcohol, he tries to stay healthy, but cannot maintain abstinence. Together with his wife, he goes to see the psychiatrist.

G. (G) Messas (✉)
Department of Mental Health, Santa Casa de Sao Paulo School of Medical Sciences, São Paulo, Brazil

Postgraduate Program on Phenomenological Psychopathology, Santa Casa de São Paulo School of Medical Sciences, São Paulo, Brazil
e-mail: guilherme.messas@fcmsantacasasp.edu.br

M. J. (MJFR) Soares
Postgraduate Program on Phenomenological Psychopathology, Santa Casa de São Paulo School of Medical Sciences, São Paulo, Brazil

Hospital do Servidor Público Estadual de São Paulo, São Paulo, Brazil
e-mail: majufrs@gmail.com

19.2 Narrative: *The story of Dra Sousa and Her Patient, Bruno*

Bruno (fictitious name) patient who receives treatment for Alcohol Use Disorder. He sought medical care for the first time with symptoms of Alcohol Abstinence Syndrome, tremors, psychomotor agitation and altered level of consciousness. In addition to this diagnosis, alcoholic hepatitis was also found. He was hospitalized and remained in a psychiatric ward for 10 days; after clinical stabilization, he continued treatment in the hepatology and psychiatric outpatient clinics of the service that assisted him during hospitalization. In a regular and punctual manner, the patient always went to the medical consultations, accompanied by his wife, Lucia (fictitious name).

At that time, Bruno was very frightened by the impact of alcohol consumption on his health and decided to stop drinking. He does not remember when he first drank; he tells us that since he was a child when his father came home, he offered wine to his three children. He tells, lightly, at once, that his mother was irritated by his father's habit. In response, he made the children drunk. Bruno doesn't know how old he was at the time, but he believes that this story occurred when he was around 7 years old. Neither Bruno and Lucia understand Bruno's father to be an alcoholic, because he did not cause "embarrassment", but they list some of his maternal uncles who are alcoholics, one of whom died of liver cirrhosis.

As an adult, Bruno started to drink after working hours, always in the same place, Lucia's brother's car jet wash, close to his house, with the same people that he calls "drinking buddies". He consumed beer, accompanied by cachaça (brazilian spirit). He often stopped at the car jet wash after work and drank heavily, When he arrived at home he used to be already drunk. As he usually drove back home he put himself and other in risk. Normally he went to work the next day with a hangover. He tells us that he did not consider it right to go to work after consuming alcoholic beverages, and that is why he only drank after work. Even among heavy drinkers in Brazil, drinking and working are assumed as a serious misbehavior.

After the hospital admission and the return to routine, Bruno could not maintain the abstinence achieved with the doctor. And, in a follow up consultation, he said that he had drunk six cans of beer at home at night, only once. "Sorry", he said, "I would no longer consume alcohol". Thus, he remained abstinent for 2 months. However, within a couple of months, he had started drinking alcohol again, about three to four cans of beer, at his house, during the night, daily.

Bruno says he is still very concerned about his health. He comes to appointments monthly, takes the physical examinations and tests requested, and takes all medications prescribed regularly. Lucia's presence and care are also important, helping him with the dates of his return and organizing the medicines. Bruno believes that his wife is the person he can trust the most.

Bruno tells us that, in his opinion, his current use of alcohol is not as harmful as before. He stopped going to the car jet washer and meeting with his "drinking buddies". Currently, he only uses beer at home at night and does not mix beer with any other drink or with cachaça, as he did before. He believes that beer is lighter than other drinks, because when he drinks beer, he believes, he never gets drunk, and everybody drinks beer. Bruno also emphasizes in the consultation that he no longer goes to work with a hangover, he believes, in this way, there is no impact of the drink on his work or his life. And he always thinks that the day will come when he is able to stop drinking forever, but he does not want to make that decision now.

Lucia does not hide her concerns about Bruno. She says that her husband minimizes his alcohol consumption, and that although the changes reported by him are true, she is afraid that he will increase the amount of alcohol he takes, returning to previous levels. Lucia does not believe there is anything more that can be done for Bruno to help him to decide to stop using alcohol, she said: "I try to talk to him, he never listen, he always do, what he wants to do, so he drinks anyway". She believes that it would not be helpful to readmit him, because she does not believe that he will remain abstinent after discharge. And she requests that the medical follow-up, with the medications and returns, remain frequent, because she is always concern about bruno's health, warning that the so that her husband is close to the care he needs for his health—and if he needs further hospitalization, he will already be linked to the institution, and to the physician who has helped him.

Dra. Sousa (fictitious name), after the hospitalization, started to see Bruno. She receives him in a welcoming way, listening to his complaints, his symptoms, his relationship with alcohol, with his medication, and with his wife. She then sees Lucia, asking her to describe her complaints about Bruno's behavior and her concerns. After understanding what is important for each of them in relation to Bruno's treatment, Dra. Sousa explains the available treatment options.

Dr Sousa bases her advice on available evidence-based medicine guidelines. She proposes pharmacological treatment with topiramate, recommended in the treatment of Alcohol Use Disorder, to reduce the urge to use alcohol, and naltrexone, which reduces the pleasure sensation generated by alcohol. Two other therapeutic strategies proposed for the patient were refused: Bruno chose not to start using disulfiram, a substance that induces discomfort when the patient uses alcohol, he explain that he does not intend to feel any harm if he decides to drink, and refuse to do Group Therapy, offered by their service. Bruno explains that he does not want to use disulfiram at that time because he had decided not to abstain. As to Group Therapy he believed that he would not benefit currently from therapy of any kind, because he did not feel comfortable talking about his problems with people he does not trust, and did not believe that therapy could help him stop drinking.

19.3 Values Arising and Clinical Care

Dra. Sousa began the approach to this case by identifying the fundamental values of the patient, which could support the establishment of treatment: the presence of Bruno's family, of his wife, Lucia, his concern for his health care and well-being, and his wish to perform well at work. These factors had all been important in helping Bruno to reduce his alcohol intake. Also important were his wife's, Lucia's, care and supportive concern. It is usual in Brazil that wives support their husbands in alcoholism, supporting them in their appointments, helping with the administration of medications, and supporting the changes that the treatment imposes, like Lucia did with Bruno. This support is maintained even when there is a case of marital violence against women. Alcoholism plays an important role in gender-based violence in Brazil, and despite the existence of a specific criminal law to combat violence against women (Lei Maria da Penha), this is still a widespread practice in Brazil [1]. The change in mood provoked by the state of drunkenness is understood by some men—especially in the lower classes—as a supplement of courage to offend and attack their wives. Surprisingly, the offended women often take on the role of caregivers of the husband after being persecuted. The main reason for this is the interpretation that her man is a good man, only alcohol drives him mad, and it is her responsibility to keep the man away from this source of risk.

It was also essential to identify the values that were in conflict with these supportive values. Dr. Sousa's view, based on scientific evidence, was that the best course for Bruno would be complete abstinence. However, Bruno expressed no desire for this option. In the same way, Lucia, his wife, however, much she wished for Bruno's abstinence, did not believe that he would be willing to take this course at that time. In short, the couple's shared wish was that Bruno's health should continue to be cared for, even though he was still using alcohol.

Dra Sousa thus aimed to secure a clinically effective approach to case management by taking into account her patient's values even though these conflicted with her evidence-based view that he should become abstinent. As described above in the case history, she prescribed naltrexone to reduce Bruno's desire for alcohol (by reducing the pleasure he experienced while drinking), together with topiramate, an anticonvulsant, to control his compulsion to drink. This approach thus drew on Dr. Sousa's knowledge of the relevant evidence-based medical information to propose an approach to treatment that respected the patient's value of reducing alcohol use. Similarly, she understood her patient's refusal of group psychotherapy and the use of disulfiram as an expression of the value Bruno placed on continuing to drink.

This reflects a person-centered approach to treatment in that all decisions were made in partnership between Dr. Sousa, Bruno, and his wife, Lucia. Consistent with her values as a clinician, however, Dr. Sousa continued to emphasize the harmful effects on health of alcohol use, always included Lucia in consultations, and remained alert to the possible adverse effects of continued alcohol use on Bruno's work.

19.4   The Influences of Culture on This Story

Like Bruno, most Brazilians who drink begin to use alcohol before the age of 18, the age at which the use of alcoholic beverages becomes legal. There is a culture that beer is a lighter beverage, not bringing the same risks as other alcoholic beverages, such as cachaça, the typical Brazilian spirit. Beer is often considered a nonalcoholic beverage, as in publicity regulation [2]. Beer is the most consumed alcoholic beverage in the country [3]. It is also commonly the case that alcohol is consumed after work, at home, even if in front of minors, contrary to the Brazilian law. It is also common for people to go back to the same establishments to consume alcohol, often in environments not suitable for alcohol consumption, as in Bruno's case when he went back time and again to his 'drinking buddies' in his brother-in-law's jet wash. When people go to the jet wash, they usually go by car; if they drink, they could be a risk to themselves and other people.

It is believed that alcoholics are only those individuals who abuse alcohol (which means for many brazillians causing embarrassment to others), while daily over-consumption is not widely recognized as a harmful habit. Bruno's family, for example, when he was a child, did not see their father's behavior (giving wine to his children) as harmful to their health. Alcohol consumption is trivialized by common expressions such as cervejinha (little beer), vinhozinho (little wine), and barzinhos (little bar). In the same way, excessive drunkenness is even actively cultivated, often as a sign of virility.

Alcohol consumption is embedded in the daily life of Brazilians, expressed in popular music of all different musical styles: for example, in the brega "... and to kill sadness only at a bar table, I will take them all, I will get drunk..."; in the samba "... I drink yes, I am living, there are people who do not drunk and are dying..."; and in the sertanejo "... drowning in alcohol, sound of the car in the stem...". On television, in advertisements known as "Skol (beer brand), the beer that goes down round" or "Brahma (beer brand), the number 1".

In addition, the main laws that regulate the use of alcohol in Brazil are ineffective, such as the law that criminalizes the sale of alcohol to minors under 18 years of age, or permissive, such as the determination that a beverage is only considered an alcoholic beverage for advertising purposes if it has more than 13 GL of alcohol [2]. In conclusion, Brazilian society is very poorly protected and enlightened about the harm related to the use of alcohol in the country [4]. For this reason, a recent initiative has been launched, introducing Value-Based-Practice as a tool for alcohol regulation in Brazil [5].

19.5 Conclusions

Substance misuse emerges from different psychopathological experiences involving personal and cultural values, which highlights the need to consider the different values when determining treatment [6]. VBP is a tool for assessing personal and cultural values and increases the effectiveness of management when it involves complex and conflicting values [7].

In the previous pages, we showed an example of how alcoholism is interpreted in Brazil, by a case of a patient, Bruno, his wife, Lucia, and the clinician, Dr. Souza. We could see how the pattern of use of Bruno jeopardizes him, his relevant others, as well as population in general. His behavior regarding alcohol shows us that, for Brazilian culture, especially in men, the most important topic defining alcoholism is any compromise to the professional role. Other natural consequences of alcohol misuse of, as inflicting harm on others, as, for instance, intramarital violence, drinking and driving, or drinking in front of minors, are not ranked among "alcohol problems".

Intramarital violence related to alcohol is a frequent theme in Brazilian culture. Usually, offended wives are implicated in the treatment of their male aggressors at least at the beginning of the husband's alcoholism. As we could see in this case, Lucia was fundamental for the continuity of Bruno's treatment. Her role was to simultaneously accept the patient's desire—a desire not to be abstinent—and to point out the issue to be addressed by the clinician, for example, to tell the clinician that he could be drinking more than he suggested. Thus, Lucia plays the role of bringing back the truth to the treatment and helps in the clinical process. This attribute of telling another narrative (distinct from the patient's narrative) to the clinician and, as a consequence, helping the clinician to be aware of what is happening in a treatment is usually a female role in Brazil.

The narrative exemplifies the application of an approach based on the basic principles of VBP [7]. First, the decisions were shared between the patient, the main stakeholder, and the medical professional who assists them. Bruno, part of the Brazilian culture, exhibited a behavior that minimized alcohol consumption, not considering the usual hangover as a problem related to alcohol and stating that if he does not have clear problems working with alcohol, he sees no reason to suspend the use of beer, the main drink consumed in the country. Thus, Dr. Souza, despite understanding that abstinence could be the best option for the patient to avoid new liver complications, decided, together with the patient and the stakeholder, to implement harm reduction [3]. In more severe cases of alcoholism in Brazil, the decision-making process on the problem related to alcohol includes several stakeholders, in order to reach a consensus on the treatment of the patient. The Brazilian culture adopts the idea that the misuse of severe alcohol is not exclusively an issue of the individual and, as a consequence, cannot be addressed by an isolated individualist perspective. A clear evidence of this perception is the great increase in the number of lay and religious Therapeutic Communities (TCs) in contemporary Brazil. In these, abstinence is the main target of care, based on a whole reorganization of community life [8].

The medications prescribed to Bruno were chosen based both on patient values and on scientific evidence, an important principle of VBP, and both naltrexone and topiramate are recommended by the American Psychiatric Association for the treatment of alcohol use disorders [9, 10]. The treatment in this case serves exclusively as a tool for a harm reduction strategy as desired by the patient. It is, however, only a pharmacological harm reduction, since the patient does not accept a broader harm reduction, in which more restrictions would be included. The preference for narrow harm reduction strategies, usually pharmacological, is also a characteristic of Brazilian culture.

The patient's adherence to treatment was important, and the decision to base the choices on values resulted in a decrease in the impact of alcohol use, both in the difficulties previously seen in the social environment, as well as in better family and work relationships, and in the health care of Bruno, who now had direct contact with the health service and is aware of the risks he runs when he consumes alcohol.

Acknowledgements   We wish to thank Bill Fulford for previous reading of this material. We also thank the Hospital do Servidor Público de Estadual de São Paulo for supporting this initiative.

19.6   Guide to Further Sources

- Woodbridge-Dodd K, Fulford KWM. Valores de Quem?. Tradução, adaptação e revisão técnica: Arthur Maciel Nunes Gonçalves The Sainsbury Centre for Mental Health 2004 (Brazilian Edition of british guide Whose Values?)
- The Brazilian VBP network. https://valuesbasedpractice.org/what-do-we-do/networks/brazilian-vbp-network/
- The Committee of Alcohol Regulation (CRA) is a civil society initiative, led by Guilherme Messas, which brings together many stakeholders in the field of substance misuse. The aim of the Project is to offer and implement succesful regulatory measures for reducing the burden of alcohol use in Brazil. CRA uses value-based strategies for the development of its policies. See http://fcmsantacasasp.edu.br/cra/
- The VBP network for Co-production in Addiction. https://valuesbasedpractice.org/co-production-in-addiction-services/

References

1. Zaleski M, Pinsky I, Laranjeira R, Ramisetty-Mikler S, Caetano R. Intimate partner violence and alcohol consumption. Rev Saude Publica. 2010;44(1):53–9. https://doi.org/10.1590/S0034-89102010000100006.
2. Brasil. Lei n°. 9294, de 15 de julho de 1996. Coleção de Leis do Brasil. Diário Oficial da União 16 Jul 1996;1:13074.
3. World Health Organization. Global status report on alcohol and health—2014. Geneva: World Health Organization; 2014.
4. Messas GP, Silveira S, Maximiano V. A Hora e a Vez de uma Política do Álcool para o Brasil Orientada pela Saúde Pública (The time and place of a public health oriented alcohol policy for Brazil). RDM. 2019;2: RR-2.1-15.
5. Comitê para Regulação do Álcool (CRA) [Committee for Alcohol Regulation]. http://fcmsantacasasp.edu.br/cra/. Accessed 5 Dec 2019.
6. Messas GP, Fukuda L, Pienkos E. A phenomenological contribution to substance misuse treatment: principles for person-centered care. Psychopathology. 2019;52(2):1–9. https://doi.org/10.1159/000501509.
7. Fulford KWM. Bringing together values-based and evidence-based medicine: UK Department of Health Initiatives in the "Personalization" of Care. J Eval Clin Pract. 2010;17(2):341–3. https://doi.org/10.1111/j.1365-2753.2010.01578.x.

8. Macedo JP, Abreu MM, Fontenele MG, Dimenstein M. The regionalization of mental health and new challenges of the psychiatric reform in Brazil. Saúde Soc. 2017;26(1):155–7.
9. Fulford KWM. Values-based practice: a new partner to evidence-based practice and a first for psychiatry? Mens Sana Monogr. 2008;6(1):10–21.
10. Reus VI, et al. The American Psychiatric Association practice guideline for the pharmacological treatment of patients with alcohol use disorder. Am J Psychiatry. 2018;175(1):86–90.

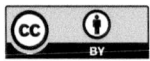

Living at the Edge of Compromise: Balkan Pluralism as a Resource for Balanced Decision-Making

Drozdstoy Stoyanov and Bill Fulford

20.1 Introduction

A culture's distinctive values are often a product of its history. Totalitarian, democratic, individual, and communitarian values, not to mention a whole raft of religious and spiritual values, all offer cases in point. This much is familiar. Less well recognized is the extent to which a culture's history may drive its characteristic ways of *processing* or *working with* values.

It is this processing aspect of cultural values that is illustrated in this chapter by a story from the Balkan region of Eastern Europe, the story of Dr. Petrov and his neighbor Ivailo. The Balkan history of repeated colonization has given its people a particular capacity for balancing different and at times conflicting sets of values. Balkan people survived colonization by learning to live 'at the edge of compromise' between their own values and the values of their colonizers.

Here, Dr. Petrov's uniquely Balkan capacity for living at the edge of compromise allows him to balance the conflicting values involved in supporting his neighbor, Ivailo, through a difficult period.

20.2 Narrative: The Story of Dr Petrov and His Neighbor, Ivailo

Ivailo (not his real name) was a 48 year old Bulgarian working as a psychiatric hospital attendant (orderly) and in the evenings on a part-time basis as a taxi driver. He had suffered several clinical episodes over the past 10 years diagnosed as psychotic mania with associated history of alcohol abuse.

D. Stoyanov
Medical University Plovdiv, Plovdiv, Bulgaria

B. Fulford (✉)
St Catherine's College, University of Oxford, Oxford, UK

© The Author(s) 2021   171
D. Stoyanov et al. (eds.), *International Perspectives in Values-Based Mental Health Practice*, https://doi.org/10.1007/978-3-030-47852-0_20

His mother left Bulgaria in the early 1990s and went to live in New Zealand. His father although remaining in Bulgaria had been a major source of various traumatic experiences throughout Ivailo's life. His father was constantly abusive, with both verbal and physical aggressive behavior, and entering into frequent conflicts about property and relationships. He repeatedly threatened to disinherit Ivailo and leave him and his family practically homeless.

Ivailo lived in the same house with his father, wife and two adolescent children until July 2011 when his father died from a rapidly progressive cancer. His wife had been unsupportive throughout and now set out to antagonize Ivailo's two sons against him. In September 2011 Ivailo stopped taking his medication and gradually returned to abusing alcohol.

A couple of months later during a brief period of sick leave he turned up at the home of a psychiatrist, Dr Petrov (again, not his real name), who was living nearby, asking for a loan. Dr Petrov was not Ivailo's physician but recognized that his behavior was unusual: he was struck by his somewhat awkward and untidy appearance and unusual behaviour. After talking with his (Ivailo's) wife however he came to the view that Ivailo's presentation was understandable given his complicated family situation and low income.

He thus decided to help Ivailo with a loan while encouraging him to take care and to consult his own doctor. Ivailo came back 3 weeks later asking for a further loan but now in a more obviously disturbed state. On this occasion Dr Petrov refused the loan but again urged Ivailo as a friend to see his doctor.

Ivailo however did not seek medical help and over the following 18 months his condition deteriorated to the point that his behavior became destructive and dangerous. Following a further period of sick leave he was finally admitted as a patient to the hospital where he had previously worked as an attendant.

From this point Ivailo's situation gradually improved. Over 3 months of inpatient treatment he restarted his medication and stopped drinking. Within a few months of discharge he was well enough to return to his job as an attendant in the same acute psychiatric ward on which he had been a patient. Ivailo's family problems continued. But he now felt more prepared to cope with them while holding down his job.

One of the first things Ivailo did after being discharged from hospital was to return Dr Petrov's loan.

20.3   What Values and Whose?

Reading this story, the reader may reasonably want more information particularly about Ivailo. Was his 'relapse' perhaps a pathological grief reaction to the death of his abusive Father, for example, and what were his actual symptoms? Without such information, we are left speculating about his values, about what mattered or was important to him. We are in the dark similarly about Ivailo's wife. What values were driving her antagonism, for example? What about Ivailo's father? Why did his mother leave so early in his life and move to the other side of the world? Then again, the institutions involved would have had their own priorities. That Ivailo was allowed to return to work in the same hospital suggests a very supportive employment policy.

As to Dr. Petrov, though, it is clear from the information provided that in deciding how to help Ivailo, he was faced with a number of conflicting values. On the one hand, there were considerations of prudence. Giving Ivailo a loan might seem (Dr Petrov's wife thought it was) financially risky. Not only that but from a professional perspective, it might be seen as breeching professional boundaries. True, Dr. Petrov was not actually Ivailo's doctor. But he was putting his professional reputation on the line. One of Dr. Petrov's senior colleagues commented 'you did something quite stupid giving him money and not helping the police to catch him'.

Dr. Petrov was well aware of these negative considerations. On the other hand, however, and on the positive side, he saw Ivailo as someone in trouble. As a neighbor, he simply wanted to help Ivailo in the difficult situation in which he knew him to be. Although not exactly friends, they had been acquaintances for many years. Dr. Petrov also knew Ivailo through his work at the hospital. In this context, he had had experience of him when well as a hard working and conscientious character.

Dr. Petrov balanced these conflicting values differently on the two occasions when Ivailo asked him for a loan. On the first occasion, he said 'yes' though encouraging Ivailo to seek medical help. On the second occasion, only 3 weeks later, he refused the loan. In the interim, Ivailo had not sought medical help and he was now in 'a more obviously disturbed state'. Note therefore that the same two sets of values were in play on both occasions but balanced differently according to the particular circumstances presented.

Balancing values in this way is what is called in values-based practice dissensual decision-making. As indicated in chapter 1, 'Surprised by Values: An Introduction to Values-Based Practice and the Use of Personal Narratives in this Book' of this book dissensus is difficult. One of the aims of training in values-based practice is to develop the skills that support dissensual decision-making. Dr. Petrov's instinctive use of dissensual decision-making was supported by his Balkan cultural heritage of living under colonization at the edge of compromise.

20.4 The Influences of Culture

Bulgaria's history is a history of serial colonial domination running from the Ottoman period (1396–1878) through to its recent period as a satellite of the Soviet Union.

Throughout the Ottoman occupation, Bulgarians adopted many survival strategies. The indigenous Christian population for example were obliged to build their churches so that they appeared lower than Muslim mosques. The Twentieth Century saw the adoption of a number of similar compromises. Between 1934 and 1944, for example, the Saxe-Coburg-Gotha governing dynasty, backed by a number of pro German politicians, brought Bulgaria into alliance with the Axis and National-Socialist Germany. It was in response to this that King Boris III captured the idea of 'living at the edge of compromise': he advised his diplomats to be *"always with Germany and never against Russia"*. King Boris' son, Simeon II, embodied the same 'edge of compromise' principle by reigning as King from 1943 to 1946 and then going on to become the Prime Minister of a republican Bulgaria from 2001 to 2005.

A further example of the Bulgarian capacity for compromise is provided by the way her period as a satellite of the Soviet Union came to an end (in 1989). The demise of the Soviet empire in most Eastern and Central communist countries was by popular uprisings of the people against the local regime. In Bulgaria, the regime was deposed from within by a party *coup d'état*.

20.5 Implications for Values-Based Practice

Balkan pluralism as evinced by Dr. Petrov in his relationship with Ivailo offers a direct response to the central challenge for implementing values-based practice noted in our introduction to values-based practice (chapter 1 and in a number of other contributions to this book, the challenge of pluralism.

The elements of values-based practice tend to work together as a whole. The story of Dr. Petrov and Ivailo more fully explicated illustrates many aspects of values-based practice [1]. We summarize these in Table 20.1. In this commentary,

Table 20.1 Some of the areas of values-based practice involved in the story of Dr. Petrov and Ivailo

Elements of values-based practice	Main areas highlighted
Premise	
Mutual respect	
Process elements	
Clinical skills	
1. Awareness	✓
2. Knowledge	
3. Reasoning	
4. Communication	✓
Service model	
5. Person-value-centered care	✓
6. The extended MDT	
VBP and EBP	
7. Two feet principle	
8. Squeaky wheel principle	
9. Science-driven principle	
Decision-making	
10. Partnership based on dissensus	✓✓
Outputs	
Balanced decision making within	✓
Frameworks of shared values	
Value toolbox	

however, we focus on the example it gives us of dissensual decision-making supported in particular by a key aspect of values-based communication skills, a focus on strengths as well as needs and difficulties.

20.5.1 Balkan Pluralism and the Default to Monism

First, then, what has this story to tell us about the challenge of pluralism? Values-based practice, we pointed out in chapter 1, is top-to-bottom—from its theoretical basis in (a particular take on) the logic of values through its reliance on process to its outputs in balanced dissensual decision-making—irreducibly pluralistic in nature. Yet, when it comes to values our default position, as we put it, drawing on the work of the moral and political philosopher Isaiah Berlin [2] is not pluralism but monism.

Good idea, then, values-based practice may be in principle but what chance it has in practice? Like so many other good ideas in principle, it looks set to fail the test of implementation. Values-based practice, it seems, has an inbuilt design flaw. Intrinsically pluralistic, it is ill-fitted to a value environment dominated by monism. We gave a number of examples in chapter 1 of Berlin's default to monism at work, notably, in the case of mental health, with the values-based Guiding Principles supporting implementation of the UK's Mental Health Act 2007.

But Balkan pluralism puts a very different and more optimistic slant on all this. It points to and indeed challenges an unacknowledged premise guiding Berlin's observations and the implications we took from them for the challenges of implementing values-based practice. The unacknowledged premise is that the default to monism is inbuilt in human nature. It is as it were in our value genes. Balkan pluralism points to the possibility that the default to monism may be more 'nurture than nature'. As indicated above, Balkan pluralism is a learned behavior, a survival strategy adopted in response to several hundred years of serial colonization.

20.5.2 Dr Petrov as a Values-Based Practitioner

It will be worth reflecting for a moment on how closely Dr. Petrov adopted, by nature, a values-based dissensual balance in his dealings with Ivailo. Dr. Petrov was caught between the (in this instance) conflicting demands of financial prudence and humanitarian neighborliness. Both values were in play. Both had the status of prima facie principles. They formed part of what amounted to a framework of (implicit) values shared by Dr. Petrov, his colleagues, and family and, given the happy ending of the story, Ivailo himself.

Neither value moreover, neither financial prudence nor humanitarian neighborliness, was somehow to be simply set aside. There was no general rule that placed one against the other in principle. The two values had instead to be balanced one against the other according to the particular circumstances presented by the decision in question. On the first occasion of Ivailo requesting a loan, humanitarian neighborliness won out for Dr. Petrov against financial prudence. Both values, however, consistently with values-based dissensual decision-making, remained in play. One indication of this is that others weighed them differently (Dr Petrov's senior colleague weighed them differently). On the second occasion, the balance, for Dr. Petrov, came out the other way around, with financial prudence outweighing humanitarian neighborliness.

Also important in this story is the attention paid by Dr. Petrov not just to the needs and difficulties experienced by Ivailo but also to his strengths. You will recall from chapter 1, 'Surprised by Values: An Introduction to Values-Based Practice and the Use of Personal Narratives in this Book' that exploring strengths, aspirations, and resources (StAR Values) as well as needs and difficulties is a key aspect of the communication skills for values-based practice. Thus, the familiar (to many medical students, at least in the UK) acronym ICE is used in communication skills training as a reminder to explore a patient's Ideas, Concerns, and Expectations; but this becomes in values-based practice, ICE *StAR*. On coming to his balanced dissensual decision, Dr. Petrov we are told knew Ivailo through his contact with him at the hospital where he was employed, to be 'hard working and conscientious'. This information thus critically shifts our picture of Ivailo. Without it, he is a failed family man and employee on the downward slope toward destitution. With it, with the information about his strengths (his StAR Values), he is a man struggling with a devastating life situation but with the personal resources for recovery. This proved to be so in the event. He recovered and indeed immediately repaid Dr. Petrov's loan.

20.5.3 Implementing Values-Based Practice

Dr. Petrov, it is worth pointing out, was not at the time of his interactions with Ivailo, consciously engaged in a dissensual balancing of values. He had indeed at this stage in his career never heard of values-based practice. This should not come as a surprise. As emphasized in chapter 1, values-based practice is all about recognizing and building on best practice. Indeed, the point of the story of Dr. Petrov and Ivailo is precisely to illustrate the *natural* capacity of Balkan people for value pluralism derived from their cultural history of colonization. Balkan people offer a timely exception to Berlin's default to monism, thus highlighting and challenging Berlin's (and our) hidden premise of values defaulting to monism.

Merely recognizing that the default to monism can be learned and, hence, unlearned, opens up new possibilities for implementation. With its origins in philosophy, it is perhaps natural that implementation strategies for values-based practice have relied perhaps over-heavily on argument. Ideas can after all change the world. As to the arguments of philosophers, Bertrand Russell, writing in the mid-twentieth century, at about the same time and with many of the same concerns as Isaiah Berlin, argued that philosophy could teach us 'how to live without certainty, and yet without being paralysed by hesitation' [3, p. 14]. There could be no more accurate statement of the aims of values-based practice. Yet to date, as we saw in chapter 1, the resources of analytical, ethical, legal, and professional arguments, appealing to 'win-win' and other supposedly motivating outcomes, have all been deployed against the default to monism to only limited effect.

Understood rather as learned behavior, however, the default to monism is opened up to that whole range of additional empirical resources represented by the sciences of change management. There are no doubt those who will object to the idea that good and bad behavior should be 'reduced' from matters of principle to the 'mere' contingencies of an empirical science. Certainly, any form of 'moral determinism' (such as evolutionary ethics) is inconsistent with the theory supporting values-based practice (see Reading Guide to chapter 1). But the example of pluralism in (natural) action represented by Dr. Petrov in his dealings with Ivailo is a salutary pointer to empiricism as a resource for implementation. By the same token, it requires us to take empiricism seriously rather than hiding behind a supposed in-principle analytical high ground.

All of which is not to underestimate the challenges of implementation faced by values-based practice. We lack as yet even an agreed outcome measure (this is discussed further below, in our concluding chapter). As a resource for tackling such challenges, the change management sciences themselves are after all very much sciences at the cutting edge. The challenges of implementation will no doubt thus require, like other sciences at the cutting edge, the full methodological resources of philosophy as well as of empirical science. But the intimations of success provided by the story of Dr. Petrov and Ivailo, seen through the cultural lens of Balkan pluralism, allows us to approach these challenges more optimistic of success.

20.6 Conclusions

Through the story of Dr. Petrov and his neighbor Ivailo, we have illustrated the importance of historically derived Balkan cultural pluralism for values-based practice. Faced with the conflicting demands of financial prudence and humanitarian neighborliness, Dr. Petrov came to what is called in values-based practice a balanced dissensual decision about how to proceed. In this, however, he drew not on training in values-based practice but rather on a Balkan capacity for living 'at the edge of compromise' developed over several centuries of living under one or another colonial power.

As a learned capacity, Balkan pluralism suggests that the default to monism identified by Isaiah Berlin may not after all be an insuperable barrier to implementing the inherently pluralistic processes of values-based practice. The default to monism thus illuminated, appears to be a barrier not of principle but rather of historical contingency. It is a learned behavior and hence one that can be unlearned.

This revised understanding of the default to monism holds out promise for a number of areas of mental health calling for a full partnership between evidence-based practice and values-based practice. It is important for recovery practice. We noted also its potential relevance (read with other contributions to this book) to contemporary concerns about the disproportionate use of involuntary psychiatric treatment among young black men.

Acknowledgements The story of Dr. Petrov and Ivailo was first presented by one of us (DS) at a conference of the International Network for Philosophy and Psychiatry held in 2013 at St Catherine's College, Oxford, on 'Making Change Happen'. This presentation was subsequently published as Fulford and Stoyanv [1].

20.7 Guides to Further Sources

For a more extensive account of the elements of values-based practice illustrated by Dr. Petrov in his dealings with Ivailo and their relevance to mental health, see reference [1].

References

1. Fulford KWM, Stoyanov D. Living at the edge of compromise: Balkan pluralism as a resource for new philosophy of mental health. Chapter 1. In: St. Stoyanov D, editor. Towards a new philosophy of mental health: perspectives from neuroscience and the humanities. Newcastle upon Tyne: Cambridge Scholars Publishing; 2015. p. 2–26.
2. Berlin I. Two concepts of liberty. Oxford: Clarendon Press; 1958.
3. Russell B. The history of western philosophy. London: George Allen and Unwin; 1946.

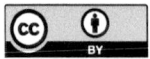

"Thinking Too Much": A Clash of Legitimate Values in Clinical Practice Calls for an Indaba Guided by African Values-Based Practice

21

Werdie Van Staden

21.1 Introduction

The practical concern of this chapter is with legitimate values that are clashing in clinical practice. The chapter illustrates an accountable way of dealing with such clashes as guided by an African version of values-based practice (A-VBP), [1, 2] which averts default responses to these clashes that tend to be destructive and failing both the clinician and the patient. For example, when values clash between a clinician and a patient, A-VBP averts the professionally eroding response by which to do "whatever the patient wants," sometimes advocated in the name of anti-paternalism or respecting personal autonomy [3]. A-VBP averts on the other hand the domination of the clinician's values in, for example "I offer only what is medically best—take it or leave it" [1].

The role of A-VBP in clinical care is illustrated here by the story of Akanya.[1] This concerns two major decision points in his clinical management: when he presented to health services with an acute psychotic episode for the first time and 8 years later when he wanted to discontinue his antipsychotic medication.

21.2 Akanya's Background

Akanya's grew up as a lonely and unusual child in a rural community in South Africa. Whilst his father and most of the community in which he lived were Setswana speaking, his mother's mother tongue was isiZulu and she was considered to be, like

---

[1] Akanya is a pseudonym meaning "to think" in Setswana.

W. Van Staden (✉)
Centre for Ethics and Philosophy of Health Sciences, University of Pretoria, Pretoria, South Africa
e-mail: werdie.vanstaden@up.ac.za

© The Author(s) 2021
D. Stoyanov et al. (eds.), *International Perspectives in Values-Based Mental Health Practice*, https://doi.org/10.1007/978-3-030-47852-0_21

her only child, an outsider. His mother had a rather critical perspective on most people and their actions. She took pride in her neat organised way of doing her daily chores. His father was often alcohol intoxicated, usually over weekends. Both his father and mother lived in a rural community all their lives, were illiterate and made a living through communal subsistence farming.

In contrast with his illiterate parents, Akanya was an avid reader. His favourite books were science fiction, popular psychology and books that espoused Buddhism. His parents and most of his community hardly knew anything about these topics and they considered his conversations as strange. Attempts at befriending him never lasted. His teachers were similarly puzzled, even more so because his marks were inconsistent and incongruent with the extent of his knowledge of and insights into some topics. They thought he underachieved in obtaining merely average marks in spite of various indications that he was actually exceptionally bright. The teachers and community attributed all these oddities to "thinking too much", which they thought was foreboding much trouble to come.

21.3   The First Major Decision Point

The troubles they had anticipated, culminated when Akanya was 19 years of age and in their view, his "thinking too much" got out of hand. A general medical practitioner identified various persecutory delusions, by which he was accusing his parents that they wanted to deliver him to Satan and they had been colluding with the community leaders to have him put away. He also had delusions of though insertion by which his ancestors were putting thoughts into his head—thoughts that were not his and had been taking over control of his life. During the preceding week, he had been verbally abusive towards his parents, and threatened to kill them and the leaders of his community. He also expressed ideas of killing himself rather than giving them the "joy" of doing so.

The practical and ethical difficulty at this time was about invoking the Mental Health Care Act (MHCA) and admitting him to hospital on an involuntary basis. His parents were reluctant that he be taken away to a psychiatric hospital. One of their reasons was that they did not want to do precisely what their son had been accusing them that they would be doing, i.e., colluding to have him incarcerated. His parents had no appreciation of his behaviour being part of a psychiatric disorder and insisted on taking him to a traditional healer instead.

These demands posed several difficulties for the general medical practitioner, Dr Robertson, who was called to see Akanya for the first time. It seemed clear to him that Akanya was suffering a psychotic episode and needed hospitalisation even though he was resisting this. But being of a different culture, Dr Robertston was concerned that by invoking the MHCA for involuntary treatment, he would be alienating the parents and even be accused of being dismissive of and perhaps violating the cultural beliefs and practices of Akanya's parents. The MHCA also required that the parents complete an application form for involuntary treatment and that one resorts to another applicant only in exceptional circumstances. Weighing against these considerations, Dr Robertson was acutely worried about Akanya's volatile mental state and high risks of harm to his parents, community leaders and himself. He remembered being taught as a medical student that homicidal and suicidal behaviours were rather unpredictable in situations like these. Finally, in addition to his concerns for all those involved, Dr Robertson was aware of his own professional and legal obligations to apply the MHCA in this situation.

21.4   Course of Events Before a Second Major Decision Point

After his period of involuntary hospitalisation, Akanya regularly attended as an outpatient at a public mental health facility and the need for a second hospitalisation did not arise. Whilst his acute psychotic symptoms abated on a standard dosage of anti-psychotic medication, his depressed state remained for about 6 years in spite of trials on various antidepressants. He considered his depressed mood as precious to him, saying "feeling depressed is all I have". Excessive feelings of guilt dominated his clinical presentation about failing to live up to his parents' expectations in everyday activities at home, hardly ever venturing outside the house, and not even trying to get a job.

He often had suicidal ideas and his psychiatrist, Dr Mahlangu, reckoned that it would not be surprising to receive a phone call with news of his suicide. Yet, he considered continuous hospitalisation as unsuitable and tried instead to contain the risk of suicide within a therapeutic relationship. Subsequently, Akanya's depressed mood gradually disappeared and his suicide risk decreased but only over a period of about 6 years.

21.5   A Second Major Decision Point

Eight years after the acute psychotic episode, the need for a second major decision arose. Akanya had been seeing Dr Mahlangu every 3 months for monitoring and supportive psychotherapy. A trusting relationship was well-established, which contrasted with Akanya's skepticism and distrust towards people in general. As had been the pattern since adolescence, Akanya resorted to keeping his own company, avoiding social contact as far as possible. He experienced the social world as too daunting, overwhelming, insincere and pretentious. Not being employed, he spent much of each day in his room, often reading and collecting pictures and other items that would aid his memory as he had been trying to counter continually losing precious ideas. He subscribed to an unusual and complex world view, which he valued proudly as unique and shared with no one in particular. For example, his view was that expressing one's thoughts brought them to life in a universe of thoughts. Within this universe, thoughts might influence each other, and some modified thoughts might come back to one, or find entry into the mind of someone else. This universe of thoughts was but one of an infinite number of parallel universes.

*Akanya now wanted to discontinue his use of antipsychotic medication. This was a difficult decision, particularly for Dr Mahlangu who was not keen to do so at all. He believed Akanya was at high risk of relapsing into an acute psychotic episode should antipsychotic medication be discontinued. He based this on his assessment of Akanya's history, his impaired current functioning, and professional literature. On the other hand, Akanya maintained the medication was a means of the psychiatric profession sustaining their hold on patients. Dr Mahlangu was concerned that he would be exposed and criticised professionally, even found negligent, if he did not continue prescribing an antipsychotic medication in this situation as would be professionally expected, based on best practice and evidence based guidance. Confounding the difficulty for the psychiatrist was that he assessed Ankaya's unusual thoughts (as above) to be overvalued ideas but not delusions. He was aware, however, that his colleagues might consider these delusions for which an **increased** dosage of antipsychotic medication would be indicated. When the psychiatrist shared his concerns with Akanya, Akanya took them as evidence for his conclusion about a professional hold on patients.*

21.6 Values and Evaluations of the Stakeholders

There are many potential conflicts of values both within and between the stakeholders in this narrative: the parents, the general medical practitioner (Dr Robertson), the community, Akanya, the psychiatrist (Dr Mahlangu) and the wider society.

The **parents** ascribed to the cultural value of consulting a traditional healer. This value is common to both Tswana and Zulu cultures (his father's and mother's, respectively). Regarding personal values, Akanya's father valued drinking alcohol, whereas his mother valued proudly her neatly organised way of doing her daily chores. She also evaluated critically most people and their actions. Both parents valued negatively their son being taken away to hospital and both were concerned that he would construe their actions as confirming his accusations of collusion. Furthermore, the narrative suggests indirectly through Akanya's take on the expectations of his parents, that his parents held the values that Akanya should participate differently in everyday activities at home, should venture outside more often and should attempt to get a job.

The **general practitioner**, Dr Robertson, evaluated Akanya's clinical presentation as comprising delusions with considerable risk to others and himself. He was particularly concerned that the parents, the community leaders and Akanya should not be harmed or even killed. The general practitioner recognised as important the cultural values of the parents, particularly with his culture being different. He valued negatively the alienation that might result from this difference and that he might be regarded as dismissive of and even violating their cultural values. He also valued compliance with the values of his profession and society (see below) regarding professional and legal obligations. With these values being in part conflicting, he evaluated the situation as difficult and demanding ethically and practically.

The **community** attributed Akanya's situation to "thinking too much," under-pinned by their values that his thinking was excessive. They considered "thinking too much" as foreboding trouble if it got "out of hand," implying that it should not have been allowed to do so. They evaluated Akanya as "strange," an "outsider," and incapable of having lasting friendships, implying values by which he should not have been so. His teachers valued his academic abilities as exceptionally bright. They also held the values that he should have achieved better than average, consistent with the extent of his knowledge and insights.

From early on, **Akanya** valued his reading as a precious activity, especially on topics of science fiction, popular psychology and Buddhism. In his acute psychotic episode, he valued negatively the intentions and actions of his parents and community leaders, as if these were to his extreme detriment (e.g. delivering him to Satan; colluding against him to put him away). He evaluated control of his life as being taken over by his ancestors putting thoughts into his head—thoughts that were intrusive, unwanted and not his. He also ascribed value to committing suicide or to others killing him as holding potential "joy."

After the psychotic episode, Akanya valued his depressed mood as precious. Also, his ideas were precious and for this reason, he had to counter "losing" them by collecting pictures and other items in aiding his memory. He ascribed values of failure and guilt to his not meeting the expectations of his parents about everyday activities at home, venturing outside often enough and trying to get a job.

Akanya valued that he was different and had a "unique" worldview about parallel universes of thoughts. This was in conflict with the values of his community by which he was considered "strange" and an "outsider." He evaluated the social world as being too daunting, overwhelming, insincere and pretentious. Like his mother, he evaluated others skeptically with distrust towards people in general. He valued in a similarly negative way the psychiatric profession as maintaining a hold on patients through medication.

The **psychiatrist**, Dr Mahlangu, valued highly a trusting relationship with Akanya, considering this an achievement given Akanya's tendency to distrust others. He also valued highly the need to prevent Akanya from relapsing and hence was concerned about discontinuing his antipsychotics. In this, he valued following best practice based on best evidence. He also valued meeting professional expectations and standards in the assessment and treatment of Akanya. He recognised that his evaluation of Akanya's thoughts as being overvalued ideas rather than delusions might be at odds with an evaluation by his colleagues and profession. He valued negatively being exposed, criticised or found negligent by going against professional norms and expectations. Compounding these concerns was a recognition that an actual relapse could be evaluated as proof of his failure to prevent it.

In addition to the community values highlighted above, **other societal values** may also be identified. The values by which Akanya was considered abusive and threatening were shared by the wider society beyond that of the local community. Societal values were also captured in the Mental Health Care Act, which included obligatory values that prescribe how Akanya must be managed. Furthermore, some of the values of the general practitioner and the psychiatrist highlighted above were also shared by society generally.

21.7 An Indaba to Process the Conflicting Values at the *First Major Decision Point*

"Indaba" is a word from isiZulu, the meaning of which includes "meeting", "matter" and "story." It captures a process common in sub-Saharan Africa, described inclusively as a meeting to discuss a matter where individuals and communities have a voice in generating a common story to tell about a matter of concern [4–6]. An indaba is an African way of following the communication pointer of values-based practice, whereby communication is meant to be an end in itself rather than the mere means to an end [1].

At the first major decision point described above, an indaba was held among the parents and Dr Robertson preceding the application of the MHCA. Although it would have been ideal, Akanya did not participate in this indaba since his parents and Dr Robertson thought that he was too disruptive and threatening. The indaba generated a shared story framed and driven by the common value, namely, Akanya's best interest. It crucially accounted for the differences and specifically the conflicting values in this story. By adopting an appositional (i.e. on the same side) rather than an oppositional attitude in the indaba, Dr Robertson skilfully led the process by locating the clash as being between legitimate values rather than between people. The values of the parents were deliberately included in the story-making together with his professional values as well as societal values. The key question that drove the indaba was *how may (the story of) their shared decision account for the differences between values without dismissing or changing anyone's values?*

Dr Robertson ensured that the differing values were made explicit in the indaba by providing space for the stakeholders to explain and understand each other's concerns and interests. The parents explained their need for a consultation with a traditional healer and their worry that their son would construe their agreement to hospitalisation as confirming his accusations of collusion. Dr Robertson took these concerns seriously and explicitly said that they need to make a plan by which to incorporate these in their joint decision. In turn, Dr Robertson explained the provisions of the MHCA as an expression of how seriously society viewed this situation involving the need to protect Akanya, the community leaders as well as the parents. He also explained his position by which he was legally and professional compelled to proceed with involuntary admission procedures, but he did so in a way that these societal and professional values were placed next to, rather than displacing, the values of the parents. He explicitly shared his concern that his action to proceed with involuntary hospitalisation would alienate them or be interpreted as him being dismissive of or violating their cultural values.

The indaba accordingly afforded a joint decision by which the prescriptions of societal values encapsulated in the MHCA were followed, because all were law-abiding citizens who had to make decisions within the law. The parental values nonetheless were also part of the decision. It was decided that they would not complete the application forms for involuntary admission but that a community leader would do so instead. This, they felt, absolved them factually from their son's accusation that they would have incarcerated him. A further decision was that consulting a traditional healer would be postponed, being made either in discussions with the treating team during hospitalisation or thereafter.

21.8 An Indaba to Process the Conflicting Values at the *Second* Major Decision Point

Whereas the values of Akanya had to be put on hold temporarily during the acute situation, they featured centrally in the indaba 8 years later at the second major decision point. Dr Mahlangu skilfully made space for them alongside his values, maintaining a being-on-the-same side attitude even though their respective values were clashing. He made it clear that he considered it therapeutically important to account for Akanya's reservations and interpretations about antipsychotic medication in their shared decision. They nonetheless also accounted for the professional values of Dr Mahlangu by which it would be medically best to continue and even increase the dosage of his medication. Akanya clearly understood Dr Mahlangu's concern about the high risk of relapse on cessation of medication and even his concern that his colleagues may disagree with him on his assessment of Akanya's current mental state. Akanya had no doubt that Dr Mahlangu would want him to continue with the medication.

As in the preceding indaba 8 years earlier, the key question that drove this indaba was: *how may (the story of) the decision account for the differences between respective values of Akanya and Dr Mahlangu without dismissing or changing the values of either?* Confronting this question conjointly and creatively, they made a shared decision that was the best in this specific values context even though not medically context even though not medically. They decided to discontinue the antipsychotic medication, while accounting for Dr Mahlangu's concerns by conjointly agreeing a plan to identify early a deterioration of his condition with an advanced agreement to revert to antipsychotic medication earlier rather than later. The outcome to date, 4 years on, has been good as evaluated by both. Being now without antipsychotic medication for this period, Akanya's condition has remained largely unchanged. Dr Mahlangu suspects that the relationship cemented with Akanya through this trying indaba may have helped therapeutically to avert a relapse.

21.9 Conclusions

Indabas as Akanya's story illustrates avoid a battle 'to persuade' without anyone sacrificing their values. Although framed by shared values, consensus on these did not, and could not, account for the legitimate differences of values among the stakeholders. The indabas rather exemplify dissensual decision-making where no one had to change, compromise or sacrifice their values. All stakeholders could preserve what mattered to them in those specific circumstances. Dr Robertson and Dr Mahlangu did not relinquish what would be medically best, nor did they have to persuade Akanya or his parents to change or sacrifice their values as prerequisite to making a decision. The indabas afforded creative decisions that accounted not merely for what would have been best medically, but was instead best for the specific circumstances in which all stakeholders had legitimate values.

Without dissensual decision-making, Dr Robertson could have merely applied the MHCA. He had societal, professional and legal warrant to do so, but that indeed would have displaced the values of Akanya's parents as if not legitimate. Dr Mahlangu could have maintained that he had to do what was medically best, but that would have ruined the therapeutic relationship with Akanya. He could have tried to persuade Akanya to continue taking his antipsychotic, which would have set up both himself and Akanya for potential failure, usually labelled as non-adherence.

Alternatively, Dr Mahlangu could have argued that Akanya was not incapacitated by his mental disorder and he could decide for himself on whether to discontinue his antipsychotic medication. Dr Mahlangu could also have justified this in virtue of Akanya's legal status as being a voluntary mental healthcare user or as if so prescribed by the ethical principle of respect for personal autonomy. Although the merits of these justifications are not disputed here, note that without the dissensual decision-making, Dr Mahlangu's professional contribution would have been eroded and, importantly, also Akanya's participation in setting up sensitive arrangements to prevent a relapse early.

Thus, an indaba in the African version of values-based practice (A-VBP) holds in high regard differences of values. It caters for uncommon ground, even though framed within common ground. Doing so is premised on person-centred and interconnected-people orientations expressed in the African terms of "batho pele" and "ubuntu" [1, 4] reflected upon elsewhere [3, 7, 8].

References

1. Van Staden CW, Fulford KWM. The indaba in African values-based practice: respecting diversity of values without ethical relativism or individual liberalism. In: Sadler JZ, van Staden CW, Fulford KWM, editors. Oxford handbook of psychiatric ethics. Oxford: Oxford University Press; 2015.
2. Fulford KWM, Van Staden CW. Values-based practice: topsy-turvy take home messages from ordinary language philosophy. In: Fulford KWM, Davies M, Graham G, Sadler JZ, Stanghellini G, Gipps R, Thornton T, editors. Oxford handbook of philosophy & psychiatry. Oxford: Oxford University Press; 2013.
3. Crepaz-Keay D, Fulford KWM, Van Staden CW. Putting both a person and people first: interdependence, values-based practice and African Batho Pele as resources for co-production in mental health. In: Sadler JZ, van Staden CW, Fulford KWM, editors. Oxford handbook of psychiatric ethics. Oxford: Oxford University Press; 2015.
4. Van Staden CW. African approaches to an enriched ethics of person-centred health practice. Int J Person-Centered Med. 2011;1:11–7.

5. Van Staden CW. Spiritual and other diversities at the heart of invigorating leadership: a South African spark. Int J Leadership Public Serv. 2010;6:73–7.
6. Van Staden CW. Stuck in the past or heading for flourishing people in diversity. S Afr J Psychiatry. 2010;16:4–6.
7. Kirmayer LJ, Mezzich JE, Van Staden CW. Health experience and values in person-centered assessment and diagnosis. In: Mezzich JE, Botbol M, Christodoulou G, Cloninger CR, Salloum I, editors. Person-centered psychiatry. Heidelberg: Springer; 2016.
8. Christodoulou GN, Van Staden CW, Jousset D, Schwartz M, Mishara A, Mezzich JE. Ethics in person-centred psychiatry. In: Mezzich JE, Botbol M, Christodoulou G, Cloninger CR, Salloum I, editors. Person-centered psychiatry. Heidelberg: Springer; 2016.

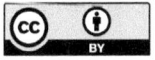

Three Points in Time: How Values and Culture Affected My Life, Madness and the People Around Me

22

David Crepaz-Keay

22.1 Introduction

The experience of hearing and seeing things that others do not, when it brings the observed behaviour of the person experiencing it into conflict with what is expected of them, is commonly regarded as a psychiatric problem. This has, in the western world, historically been regarded as a clinical problem that requires a clinical solution.

In this chapter, I explore three stories taken from my teens and twenties as I was growing up hearing and seeing things in middle class middle England. The impact of these experiences on my life, both in the moment and on its future direction, was affected as much by the culture it took place in as by any clinical conditions or responses.

22.2 Episode One: *Schizophrenia Is Just Like Diabetes…(Circa 1979–1982)*

I started hearing and seeing things in my early teens (in the late 1970s). They were frightening things and my responses ranged from flinching to running away or hiding, depending on the severity. This was initially an infrequent occurrence and though I'm sure it caused my parents concern; it only became an issue when it happened in the presence of people outside the immediate family. As the frequency of "escapes" increased I was taken to see our family doctor, but I did not find him someone I could talk to. After several years and several diagnoses, I found myself with a diagnosis of schizophrenia and on antipsychotic medication.

D. Crepaz-Keay (✉)
Applied Learning, Mental Health Foundation, London, UK

© The Author(s) 2021
D. Stoyanov et al. (eds.), *International Perspectives in Values-Based Mental Health Practice*, https://doi.org/10.1007/978-3-030-47852-0_22

My father had type one diabetes and took daily insulin. On the rare occasions that he experienced a "hypo" his behaviour became extremely unusual and the family had a well-established plan to respond. Our doctor described schizophrenia as "just like diabetes, as long as David takes his medication, he will mostly be fine; it's not 100% effective but it's very dangerous to not treat this illness."

Like many people with the same diagnosis I found that the medication had no effect on what I heard or saw, but it did make running away a lot more difficult. With my escapes less frequent (and when they did happen, a lot slower), my parents were, if not delighted, at least satisfied. I was both increasingly frustrated and less willing/ able to articulate my concerns and this unstable hiatus held for some time.

Nothing really prepared me for the experience of hearing and seeing things; it was the most frightening experience of my life. Although I was reluctant to talk about the experiences themselves, my reactions to the things I could see and hear and my subsequent "fight/flight" (predominantly the latter) responses meant that medical involvement was inevitable. I had always got on well with our family doctor and so when he explained that my experience was an illness like many others, I initially found this reassuring; particularly, the only alternative I could think of was that I was going mad.

Unfortunately, the medication I was prescribed failed to prevent me from hearing and seeing things. It did, however, affect my thinking, feeling, speed and balance. When I explained this, I was given different doses and variants, but they all had the same lack of impact on what I was seeing and hearing and made little difference to the (substantial) negative effects of the drugs.

The impact of these effects was that I responded less rapidly to what I was seeing and hearing. To me, this made the experience more frightening, but to those around me, I seemed calmer and my behaviour less disturbing and unusual. I continued to describe the effects as unhelpful and disruptive, while my parents told the doctor that I appeared to be much better. In short, the perceived impact of my experiences and the efficacy (or otherwise) of treatment was affected by the values of the perceivers.

A summary of the key values is presented in Box 22.1.

Box 22.1 Values in Episode One

The Family Doctor
- His primary relationship was with my family, this had been a long-standing relationship and the larger part of this had centred around managing my father's diabetes.
- His approach to me was based wholly on a simple illness—treatment control—control of symptoms model and I'm sure that he would have seen this as entirely objective in terms of culture and values.
- If forced to consider values and culture, success would be based on achieving a normal healthy nuclear family, by treating illness with the prescribed medicine.

My Family
- My family's values and culture were strongly influenced by a desire for their children to achieve more than they had (they had both been the first in their respective families to have white collar jobs, whereas their parents were blue collar and such things were important to them). At that time, this meant O levels, A levels and a university degree.
- They were also drawn to a medical explanation of my behaviour; it matched their experience of diabetes and removed any sense of responsibility for my condition.
- They would not have challenged a medical opinion and would take the view of a doctor as gospel.

Me
- I very much wanted to be "normal", just like my friends. I definitely did not want to be "mad" or mental".
- I respected medical opinion but was disappointed that I was treated as a family son not as an individual.
- I valued my schoolwork and friends and felt my treatment was impairing both without affecting my hearing and seeing things.

22.2.1 Cultural Influences

In addition to the impact of values, the cultural context was also important. The middle-class middle England culture of social improvement and deference to medical professionals was a strong influence on this stage of my life and development. Clearly, a desire to achieve the best for me was the strongest cultural influence; the goal of me being the first in the family to go to university was shared by all of us; but sometimes, I think social embarrassment was a strong motivator.

22.3 Episode Two: *The Great Escape… (Circa 1985–1987)*

I found myself detained in a secure ward in the psychiatric department of a large hospital just north of Slough. I was told I had been "sectioned"; I had no idea what this meant and just wanted to know when I could leave.

The environment was entirely alien to me and it took a long while to get to grips with it. For the first week or so I just wanted to leave but once I started talking to the other patients everything became a little easier. The medication was still not affecting what I saw or heard but it become clear that this was quite common amongst us.

Staff contact was minimal, and most was with student nurses, porters or cleaners. Qualified nurses stayed in the office or were off ward entirely. The psychiatrist was pleasant but only visited weekly.

I eventually settled into a comfortable inertia which seemed to be regarded as a positive outcome by pretty much everyone. We started to receive regular visits from a remarkable woman who ran the local Mind; she told me to stop wasting my talents, get out and do something more useful with my life.

The key to escape was to be seen as "normal" and the person to convince was my psychiatrist. Fortunately, an enthusiasm for cricket and a sound knowledge of economic policy and practice seemed to be the key skills required for this task.

Life on the ward as a detained patient was unlike anything I had ever experienced. Our movements severely constrained (constraints that were equally applied to patients whether they were subject to detention under the mental health act or not). Restrictions were not limited to our movements; information about treatments (which at that time meant either drugs or electroconvulsive therapy (ECT)) was not freely available. Plain language leaflets about medication, which were published by Mind, were distributed by volunteer visitors but confiscated by staff. Negative comments about treatment regimens were regarded as symptoms of illness or lack of insight. Anyone caught not taking oral medication would be switched to injections. If we refused to comply with injected medication, restraint was used (this was a routine occurrence); if patients repeated this behaviour, we would be subject to seclusion.

Wards were highly hierarchical, with the consultant psychiatrist at the top and clear demarcations at each subsequent clinical level. Although the psychiatrist was clearly the person who made the clinical decisions, including the most important one regarding discharge, they only saw us every other week at best. Nurses were more present, but even they spent most of their time in nursing offices with the doors firmly shut and they took a dim view of any interruptions. Conversations with nursing staff were entirely at times of their choosing and only about symptoms and treatments. Student nurses and domestic staff were around much more of the time and most of our social interactions were either with these staff or with each other as patients.

My main recollection of time on the ward was of boredom. Any contact with the outside world was exciting and the regular visitor from the local Mind association was the one person who remained ambitious for me. My primary goal was to get out of hospital for good. The titular great escape did not involve motorcycles, vaulting horses or any great physical feats; rather, it meant appearing to be "normal" and that this meant not questioning clinical regimes and not causing any kind of disruption (incidentally, the skill of pretending to be normal is very useful in day-to-day life) (Box 22.2).

Box 22.2 Values in Episode Two

Me

- I wanted to be out of this environment, driven by values of independence, distrust of the clinical approach, which I knew was not working, but an understanding of the importance of "playing the game".

Consultant Psychiatrist
- Had a clear idea of what normal was and this seemed to entirely match the values I was brought up with: the manners, knowledge and life experiences (by now, I was at university and had started working for the civil service during my holidays).
- Expected adherence to treatment and a return to conventional behaviour.
- Was clearly used to being at the summit of ward hierarchy and this was universally accepted.

Student Nurses and Non-clinical Staff
- The most compassionate and humane of all I came into contact with during my stay.
- Almost universally seemed to be driven by a desire to make our time there as pleasant as possible.
- Present more often than anyone else and much more likely to engage in conversation that was not about medication or symptoms.

Hospital Visitor
- Driven by a desire to see people reach their potential.
- Directive and assertive in style, she was not afraid to tell people what she thought they should do.
- Her style put off as many people as it appealed to—she had the ambition for me that had been sapped by defensive psychiatric practices and excessive medication.

22.3.1 Cultural Influences

Although it is common to talk of "ward culture," it would probably be more accurate to consider "ward cultures."

There was the day-to-day culture of normal life on the ward. This was generally comfortable if dull. Hierarchies were apparent throughout and were not restricted to the clinical staff side. Even as patients we group ourselves in a number of ways, including diagnosis, medication and duration of detention.

The nursing culture was designed to deliver a quiet and controlled ward and levels of medication, seclusion and restraint were all used to maintain this. Most interaction with nursing staff centred around medication or food. There was little social interaction between staff and patients (apart from with student nurses). Discussion about medication and treatment was actively discouraged and the notion of informed consent was quite absent. Every now and then, we (patients) would get hold of a BNF or perhaps a Mind leaflet on treatment, but these would be confiscated if discovered.

The psychiatric culture was one of the quiet authority and it was clear that the ward (and indeed the department) was his domain. As the psychiatrist was the ultimate judge of "normal," it was extremely helpful for me that we came from similar social backgrounds and in many ways his "normal" was my aspirational "normal".

Pam, the hospital visitor, was entirely counter-cultural in this respect (and most other respects). She believed that people should be in control of their own lives. It is not clear how she achieved this in the then-prevailing culture.

22.4   Episode Three: *Every Cloud… (Circa 1992)*

At the end of a prolonged experience of hearing and seeing a sinister cloud, I found myself running through the Chilterns in only my pyjamas, dressing gown and slippers. It was a stormy night and I was soaked through and over five miles from home. I found a telephone box and called my then girlfriend asking for help.

We had been going out for a couple of months or so and she was aware of my psychiatric history but had no first-hand experience of me hearing and seeing things with this degree of impact. I had met her mother a few times and we got on well.

They both came to collect me, took me home and looked after me until we all agreed it was fine for them to leave me. About a year later we were married and last year we celebrated our 25th wedding anniversary…

Until this point, I had taken an individual approach to what might these days be referred to as my recovery. The goal being to get by on my own and to be able to cope with all that is thrown at me. This was a reasonable response to the illness/deficit model that I had initially been confronted by and the emphasis placed on individual "wellness" (the normality of episode two). The important development in my own values was the understanding that the meaningful and fulfilling life I sought was more about how I related to others than how independent I could be.

I was fortunate to find not just one person who shared and explicitly exhibited these values, but two. Their response to me at my most "mad", and my willingness to seek support from them at that point, was the most significant event in my development from dependence, through independence to interdependence.

The behaviours of all players in this episode took a degree of confidence in each other that defied rational analysis, but which came to define my values from that point on (Box 22.3).

Box 22.3 Values in Episode Three

Me
- My final steps towards interdependence. The first time I *really* trusted a third party as a part of how I might survive and thrive in the context of hearing and seeing things.

My Girlfriend
- Driven by a desire to understand what the right thing to do was and how it might be done.
- Instinctively humane and compassionate.
- Sceptical of a clinical approach to something that defied any explanation.

Her Mother
- Integrity and a desire to do the best for her daughter and, by extension, someone who was important to her.
- Entirely non-judgmental of my "condition".
- Compassionate and supportive.

22.4.1 Cultural Influences

The culture of support and compassion without clinical judgement shone through. It echoes and amplifies the culture and values exhibited by student nurses, cleaners and porters from episode two. These are values which I aspire to and which have influenced the way I work.

22.5 Conclusions

In this chapter, I have explored the impact of cultural values on mental health through a series of episodes from my own experience of "psychosis" over a number of years. Key to these experiences was the extent of the match between my own cultural background and various cultures in which I found myself. Thus, in episode, "schizophrenia is just like diabetes," the culture of my family and the immediate community around me placed my non-conformist experiences firmly in the clinical space as a simple chemical imbalance that could be managed with carefully titrated medication; in episode two, "the great escape," variations in what the prevailing culture considered normal directly affected decisions about how people would be detained and treated; in episode three, "every cloud," the simplest of human values helps mitigate a complicated and distressing problem. None of this is to argue that mental health services could be replaced by simple kindness—just that the values and cultures of different participants and organisations (and in particular the differences between them) have a clear impact on both processes and outcomes in mental health.

A number of important themes emerge from my story: the diversity of individual experiences of madness; the importance of context (including cultural context) on the outcomes (favourable or unfavourable) of these experiences and, perhaps most importantly, the importance of narrative within the "oral tradition of the survivor movement," in allowing one's own story to be told rather than someone else "putting it up on a power point."

Acknowledgements I would like to acknowledge the importance of all those who have enabled me to live a mad life well: the pioneers of the survivor movement who fought for so many then counter-cultural principles which we now take for granted, allies who gave us the space and support to battle effectively, my close friends who value me, and above all Margaret and Lavinia who have given me a mad life worth living and values to aspire to.

22.6   Guide to Further Sources

Although it is somewhat daunting to explore the full range of cultures available, searching for the following terms will broaden most people's cultural horizons: "hearing voices", "white privilege". For those too young to understand ward culture in the 1970s and 1980s the following always remind me where we've come from: "on being sane in insane places" [1] and "one flew over the cuckoo's nest" [2] (please note other cultures are available).

References

1. Rosenhan D. On being sane in insane places. Science. 1973;179:250–25.
2. Kesey K. Penguin Classics edition (2005) One flew over the cuckoo's nest. The Viking Press: New York; 1962; or in the film version, Forman M (Director). One flew over the cuckoo's nest. USA: United Artists; 1975. Widely available including: https://www.youtube.com/watch?v=lcAU0-OfdVs or https://play.google.com/store/movies/details?id=lcAU0-OfdVs or https://itunes.apple.com/gb/movie/one-flew-over-the-cuckoos-nest/id278291787.

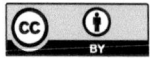

Justine Keen and Richard J. Shaw

23.1 Introduction

The dialogue in this chapter is about recovery in the sense of achieving a good quality of life as defined by what is important to (i.e. the values of) those concerned rather than by professional and service delivery priorities [1, 2]. The speakers, Justine and Richard, recorded their discussion live. They met in an informal environment and shared their experiences entirely unscripted.

At that time, they had no expectation of the dialogue being published beyond being a contribution to the work on co-production of a local group. Yet, the themes that emerge reflect a number of key ways in which cultural values may impact positively or negatively on recovery from severe mental ill health issues. These factors are given below with subheadings. Although not part of the original dialogue, the subheadings were agreed and introduced through a co-writing process in which the speakers themselves had an equal voice with the editors.

The factors identified as influencing recovery—the negative impacts of homelessness, loss of control over one's own life, plain discrimination, and the positive impacts of a home, friends, and a role in life—are not new. Indeed, it is a tragedy of contemporary approaches to mental health that these factors have been well recognised since the path finding work of the sociologists, Ann Rogers, David Pilgrim, and Richard Lacey nearly 30 years ago [3]. Just ask those concerned, their work showed, and it will be clear that what matters to people with severe long-term mental health problems is not more and not less than what matters to us all. As one of the speakers in the dialogue (Justine) put it in an earlier conversation and adapting a recipe for happiness widely attributed to Immanuel Kant: happiness requires 'something to do, somewhere to go, someone to love.'

J. Keen · R. J. Shaw (✉)
Service User, Bristol, UK

© The Author(s) 2021
D. Stoyanov et al. (eds.), *International Perspectives in Values-Based Mental Health Practice*, https://doi.org/10.1007/978-3-030-47852-0_23

23.2   The Dialogue

In the dialogue that follows Richard's words are in black type and Justine's in bold italic.

23.2.1   Street Culture

When I came to Bristol, I had come directly out of the psychiatric unit in Preston who had amazingly worked out that there was nothing wrong with me without even talking to me.

That sounds familiar

So I was "hoofed" out of the psychiatric unit with no medicine, no help, nothing. So my dad gave me a couple of hundred quid and I decided I'd start again in Bristol. That turned out to be a mistake 'cause, er, when you're homeless in Bristol you're not treated very well. I have found it one of the worst places that I have been homeless; I have been homeless before. I was homeless in Blackpool, there are plenty of Bed and Breakfast in Blackpool, and they run 'em properly and so you have nothing to worry about. I was robbed and bullied by the owners of the Bed and Breakfasts who don't treat the homeless nicely even though we are paying them rent.

That seemed to be lost on him (the landlord) so I was illegally evicted by the Police, and I was forced to go and live in a flat with absolutely nothing for 2 months; if it hadn't been for me Mum putting food in a big box and putting it on DHL and sending it me down, I don't know what I would have done.

The owners stole a lot of my property, they stole my wallet, they stole the loan money I'd got from the DWP (Department of Work and Pensions) to buy property, they stole my wallet with that in it, and the Police said "we're not doing anything about it and this is a private matter" and I've said 'you're a Cunt'"—its not a very nice word but that's exactly what he said to me and he didn't do anything about it. So even the Police are not very nice to the mentally ill, and if these public servants can't be how is anybody going to learn?

Yep been there on different variants on a theme…

Yeah, um, I've had a mixed experience with the Police. I have to say that I had one very good experience with a Policeman who got me out of my flat before they had to break the door down.

Right…

He persuaded me to come out of the door, got my keys and locked it, gave me the keys and took me to hospital

Well that's a Policeman doing his job the right way.

Yes, and I've had the reverse experiences where….

Oh aye, they're not very nice to me, they're not very nice to me at all.

No, for instance I've been found drunk and incapable, but because they don't know why I am incapable they just put me in the cells, to sleep it off they think. And I got so lucky one time that I vomited and so they called the police doctor to examine me and he looked at my pupils and he said that there was something wrong, so they sent me to A&E escorted and what they discovered a long time later after blood tests came back that I had actually taken, I didn't know how many because I had no way of counting, that I had taken paracetamol in a very severe overdose, and had I been left to sleep it off overnight I would have been dead in the morning. If I wasn't dead my liver and pancreas would have been shot.

They (the Police) should be ordered by the government to uphold the law and tell the truth, but you try getting them to do that. If they don't want to do that, then they bloody well won't. You can take a horse to water but you

Can't make it drink

Can't make it drink. But as I've said to the police, I'll take you to water, I can't make you drink, but unfortunately on this occasion, we'll drown you in it.

23.2.2 Loss of Autonomy and Control

Yes unfortunately, I have been down the old 'the only answer I've got is kill myself, at least I can control when I…'

Die

When I die, I can be in control of that

Same here—exactly that feeling… I can't control anything else in my life, everyone else is running my life telling me what to do, when to do it, how to do it, if to do it, not to do it.

Its horrible isn't it?

When you are in that bit of your life, all you want to do is to get the hell out of it … you don't care how.

How

My life is different from that now. There are good things in it. Not perfect, it doesn't do…. I don't have many close friends. I have good friends but I don't have anybody I would pick the' phone up to and have a chat. Do you understand what I mean?

I do understand that. I'm very guarded when I am talking to people because I can say things and people can say "that's unbelievable, we don't believe you" I've had that, you know people will say "we don't believe you, you're lying—you're making it up"

I'd believe you every time Richard

I don't make anything up, my Dad was a flaming Magistrate and he didn't raise a fantasist, a liar or a peeing idiot.

No

23.2.3 Unwarranted Assumptions

But some people make these broad assumptions about the mentally ill and then dismiss us out of hand. 'Cause I know more than you because I'm a mental health professional, which is poppycock and balderdash, absolute poppycock and balderdash.

Very good choice of phrases there Richard, and yes there is a large section of society that know next to nothing about mental illness except for maybe mild to moderate depression and anxiety, and that's what they think mental illness is. And they will campaign and place on their Facebook pages. And yes, it's important. I don't for a moment deny that mild to moderate anxiety and depression is extremely debilitating, extremely nasty, and I class those people as having a mental health condition.

They have

...but you take the next step along and start looking at things like whatever psychosis encompasses, whatever OCD, Obsessive Compulsive Disorder, encompasses; that's another serious mental illness.

And these are the ones that are ignored, and I would wish... Mind have tried... they have done a campaign but a lot of it was about mild to moderate anxiety and depression, but there were a couple of 'um short documentaries on their website about people coming into psychosis for the first time.

Mm... it's not nice

23.2.4   The Fear Factor

Like, one of the ones that really struck me for a personal reason was a lad who after his diagnosis no-one would leave their children alone in the room with him.

Yes, I had a friend who is sadly no longer with us ... um 'Andy', we'll call him; that's his name. He suffered from schizophrenia, we used to sit and talk, about our voices, and he'd tell me what they were saying. He had three young boys, and his voices were telling him to kill his children.

Ohhh Oh no

So he had spoken about this up [name of police station] on one of his things and then all hell broke loose.

It would

In the end, he was allowed to keep his children. He wouldn't hurt them; he loved them. It was obvious that he loved them enormously. He's like me, he's like you, he doesn't respond to what the voices say, and he wouldn't do it. He loved his kids.

23.2.5   Self-Managing Our Voices

It's fine to respond to the voices, it's not fine to do what the voices want. It's to attack myself in some way that would prevent me from doing what the voices want.

Well I just argue. You see, I don't think my voices are right in any way shape or form about anything that they say.

Mine are extremely persuasive

Mine are too. Go kill yourself Richard they say.

Yep exactly, mine tell me to kill myself because I'm a paedophile. They tell me that I am a risk to children. That I shouldn't go near children. You know that I'm a bad person…you know all of that.

I know, I know, I live with it, it's a constant battle to keep your bloody pecker up with these lot.

Yes.

23.2.6 To Be Happy

But you see my ultimate goal… my ultimate goal is to achieve happiness in life.

Yeah

I think that's a reasonable objective and goal for everybody to achieve some modicum of happiness in life.

Yes to have during the day on average an hour when are sat there chilled and happy. Then you can deal with the rest of the day.

I do. I live on my own, and I am perfectly happy living on my own. If I want to socialise I can talk to my neighbours and go up the pub.

23.2.7 Pub Culture

Could you say more about your mates at the pub.

Yeah brilliant. I call on my mates up the pub. They all know me, good bunch of lads, they're all working hard. Builders, roofers, and people like that and they've all been really good to me. When I came to Bristol, I was completely on my own, I was so immersed in my psychological distress that I wasn't effectively communicating properly with anybody, and I actually found communicating very difficult because I was in such a state of mental distress, which was only made worse through the treatment of Bed and Breakfast owners, the Police, and NHS, and they really put me through the mill. I really thought "my life is over here."

Er so… I… I… I… had already been through several suicide attempts, the last one, the last time I attempted, I had to go and see a psychiatrist who wasn't very useful. I think he was a CPN. He wasn't very useful. Anyway, they weren't very useful and so I basically knew that my problem was my problem, and the only person that was going to resolve my problem was the person that is aware of my problem…

Which is you….

23.2.8 The Culture of Mental Health Services

Which is me. The people that should help me with the problem weren't listening to my problem. Too busy…

Filling in their forms by any chance?

Yeah. Whitewashing over my problem. Saying it's not a problem, and its all in your head. That's absolute bloody rubbish, and it's a real problem.

Yes, and are you saying, like I am saying, "the voices I am hearing are real"

Well, they are real to me. I hear them, I appreciate nobody else does.

Well I never know, I can't tell… because I don't know if they are hearing them and pretending not to—to be nice to me.

No, nobody can hear inside your head apart from you. I'm telling you that now. Ears are not that clever.

I'm still unsure about mine

23.2.9 Taking Back Autonomy and Control

You see… I hate being told what I'm thinking because I am a believer that nobody knows that apart from the person that is doing the thinking.

That makes sense, that's you.

Nobody can tell me what I am thinking. You can ask me. You can enquire… but if you say "you're thinking this Richard"… No I am not thinking that at all. You are telling me conveniently so when you argue that I am thinking that. You are not listening to me.

Ahhh OK, OK That's making some sense to me. Your culture of how you deal with so-called professionals and your diagnosis is quite different from mine. I sort of (um), cave in to (um) what I've been told about what I have experienced.

It's almost as if sometimes it feels as though certainly with the police they pressurise you. Do this, do that, believe this, believe that.

Yeahh…

23.2.10 And Being Listened to

Y'know Until people are made to listen to mentally ill people and respond appropriately to their needs, we've successfully come up with a way of failing them.

Yeah…

I do feel let down on occasions certainly by the Police and the NHS and I do feel failed. It's almost as if the whole system is rigged against mentally ill people. Sometimes, it does seem to me that you got this inner battle within yourself. You know we are all responsible for ourselves, so we have some…We as mentally ill people have to be careful about our behaviour. What we're saying, where we're going, and make sure that we don't put ourselves in harm's way or danger.

Correct. I rarely go out when it's dark.

I don't at all

Even in the short days when it can go dark at 4:30. If I am out somewhere at that point I am heading home as fast as my little legs will carry me.

23.2.11 Pub Culture Again

I mean going back to my mates in the pub. They're all good lads. They're all grown up, mature, working, and responsible adults. That's fine that pub during the day. But you wouldn't catch me drinking; well, I avoid drinking in there in an evening because you get all the young lads come in.

Uh Huh… and they tease you

Well, no, no they're alright. I get the odd comment, or I might get laughed at…but you know I have learned to accept in life that some people are just ignorant, and they are perfectly happy to stay ignorant.

In fact, if I ever get any aggravation, one of my mates warns them off!

23.2.12 Management Culture and Leadership

I know what I know, and I know enough; but you know nobody knows it all, and I don't think you can have too much knowledge. I think, think you can suffer from not having enough…but there is a lot to learn in this life and anyone who thinks they know it all and stops learning is stupid 'cause you can't know it all. There's an awful lot of things in this life that I don't know.

Life is immense in all its different ways and bits of knowledge. It's how you use what you've got and how you use it to expand in the right direction and in the right way. And for me it's about making the best use of limited resources, 'cause resources are not infinite.

No they're not… no they're not

The mental health services, not only are they poorly resourced, which is the first thing that is wrong, but the second thing is…they have tiers of middle management that I just, maybe naively… y'know I'll take an argument saying I'm wrong… but don't seem to do much other than manage people. Managers for managers? Y'know, why?

Well, I mean a lot of how I understand management is leadership. An important part of management is leadership. There has to be someone at the helm, nailing it, getting it right, leading from the front, setting an example, and everybody to raise their game.

Yes, level up not level down.

Sometimes, in this life, we are expected to dumb down our expectations to fall in line with the shoddy…

What's available

… the shoddy or the piss poor services that as you quite rightly just stated, are massively underfunded. You know, and it seems that we are palmed off with the second rate and shoddy when really that is not in the country's best interests to treat people like that.

No 'cause you treat somebody badly they expect they are bad…and when they expect that they're bad they're going to act bad.

23.3　Conclusions

This dialogue makes uncomfortable reading for many of us. But the issues raised are key to understanding the impact of cultural values both positive and negative on recovery. On the negative side of the balance are prejudice and discrimination from many directions: landlords, the Police, members of the public, and services. This much—forcefully expressed in this dialogue from first-hand experience—is sadly all too familiar. Yet, there is also a positive side: one speaker's help from his family and later through companionship in his local Pub; the other had had on one occasion help from the Police.

It is important to acknowledge the balance here. Yes, despite many campaigns (MIND is mentioned at one point), people with severe long-term mental health conditions experience continuing discrimination. But there is also hope for recovery here. Hope not in expanded services as such (though both speakers emphasise the need for better funding) but in the initiatives of the speakers themselves in taking back control. It is when they regain control of their lives, when they take a stand against being told by professionals what is 'good for them', that they find their turning points towards recovery. What this means, though, is not simply independence but—as David Crepaz-Keay puts it in his story in chapter 22, "Three Points in Time: How Values and Culture Affected my Life, Madness and the People Around Me" "Alcohol Use Disorder in a Culture that Normalizes the Consumption of Alcoholic Beverages: The Conflicts for Decision-Making"—*Inter*-dependence. It is Richard's pub culture that gives him his 'hour of happiness' and it is Justine's lack of just such a group of friends that leaves a continuing gap in her life.

Acknowledgements　We are grateful to the Bristol Co-production group for their continuing support and many kindnesses.

23.4　Guide to Further Sources

There are now extensive recovery resources available—please see Guide to Further Sources supplied by Waldo Roeg in his chapter 32, "Discovering Myself, a Journey of Rdiscovery" "Linking Science with People: An Introduction to Part IV, Science."

For a profile of the Bristol Co-production group, please go to: valuesbasedpractice.org/who are we/organisations (and scroll down to the Group's listing).

The work of the Bristol Co-production group on assessment in mental health is described in:

Fulford, K.W.M., Duhig, L., Hankin, J., Hicks, J., and Keeble, J. (2015) Values-based Assessment in Mental Health: The 3 Keys to a Shared Approach between Service Users and Service Providers. Ch 73, in Sadler, J.Z., van Staden, W., and Fulford, K.W.M., (Eds) *The Oxford Handbook of Psychiatric Ethics.* Oxford: Oxford University Press

For a short film recording the Group's experience of working together, please go to the Bristol Co-production group profile - see website above.

References

1. Allott P. What is mental health, illness and recovery, Ch 1. In: Ryan T, Pritchard J, editors. Good practice in adult mental health, Good practice series 10. London: Jessica Kingsley Publishers; 2004.
2. Slade M, Amering M, Farkas M, Hamilton B, O'Hagan M, Panther G, Perkins R, Shepherd G, Tse S, Whitley R. Uses and abuses of recovery: implementing recovery-oriented practices in mental health systems. World Psychiatry. 2014;13:12–20.
3. Rogers A, Pilgrim D, Lacey R. Experiencing psychiatry: users' views of services. London: The Macmillan Press; 1993.

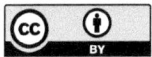

Linking Science with People: An Introduction to Part IV, Science

24

Bill Fulford

That values-based practice links science with people is easily said, but as the chapters in this Part illustrate, it is often far from easy to put into practice. Here as elsewhere in the book, cultural values have a key role to play. Left implicit and unacknowledged, they may act as barriers to the process of linking science with people. Made explicit on the other hand, as part of a culturally enriched form of values-based practice, cultural values become powerful facilitators of the process.

24.1 Three Principles of Values-Based Practice Linking Science with People

The first four chapters in this Part between them explore the three principles of values-based practice defining its partnership with evidence-based practice in linking science with people. As described briefly in our introduction to values-based practice (chapter 1, "Surprised by Values: An Introduction to Values-based Practice and the Use of Personal Narratives in this Book"), and indicated in Table 24.1, the three principles are the Two Feet Principle, the Squeaky Wheel Principle, and the Science Driven Principle.

The editors with input from the contributors to Part IV.

B. Fulford (✉)
St Catherine's College, University of Oxford, Oxford, UK
e-mail: kwmf@kwmfulford.com

209
D. Stoyanov et al. (eds.), *International Perspectives in Values-Based Mental Health Practice*, https://doi.org/10.1007/978-3-030-47852-0_24

Table 24.1 Annotated Table of Contents for Part IV, Science

24.1.1 The Two Feet Principle

The *Two Feet Principle* states that *all decisions are based on the two feet of values and evidence, including decisions about diagnosis.*

It has become a truism in contemporary health care that clinical decisions should be evidence based. The *Two Feet Principle* reminds us that clinical decisions should be values-based as well. This values-plus-evidence approach is the basis of the shared decision-making underpinning contemporary person-centered clinical care.

Chapter 25, "A Cross-Cultural Values-Based Approach to the Diagnosis and Treatment of Dissociative (Conversion) Disorders," by Bulgarian psychiatrists, Anna Todeva and Assen Beshkov of the Medical University of Plovdiv, illustrates the clinical importance of the Two Feet Principle applying to decisions about diagnosis as well as treatment. The story they describe is of A.A., a woman of Roma origin, who presents with recurrent dissociative symptoms (bodily symptoms due to psychological causes). She eventually responds to evidence-based interventions but only when these are used with due regard to the cultural and other values impacting on her presenting symptoms.

A.A.'s story in chapter 25, can helpfully be read in conjunction with that of Ms. Suzuki in the next chapter, chapter 26, "Treatment of Social Anxiety Disorder or

Neuroenhancement of Socially Accepted Modesty? The Case of Ms. Suzuki" (see below), in that both focus on the role of values specifically in diagnostic assessment (broadly conceived as how a problem is understood) as distinct from treatment (broadly conceived as how a problem is dealt with). This twin dependence of diagnostic assessment, on values as well as on evidence, is important in all areas of health care—recall the story from surgical care of Mrs. Jones' Knee in chapter 1, "Surprised by Values: An Introduction to Values-Based Practice and the Use of Personal Narratives in this Book." That this twin dependence is no less (and may be more) important in psychiatry even than in surgery is well demonstrated by the stories in chapters 25, "A Cross-Cultural Values-Based Approach to the Diagnosis and Treatment of Dissociative (Conversion) Disorders" and 26, "Treatment of Social Anxiety Disorder or Neuroenhancement of Socially Accepted Modesty? The Case of Ms. Suzuki." We return to this point below (see Sect. 4, Values in Psychiatric Diagnosis).

24.1.2 The Squeaky Wheel Principle

The *Squeaky Wheel Principle* states that *we notice values when they cause difficulties (like the squeaky wheel) but (like the wheel that doesn't squeak) they are always there and operative. The principle has counterpart implications for evidence.*

Chapters 26, "Treatment of Social Anxiety Disorder or Neuroenhancement of Socially Accepted Modesty? The Case of Ms. Suzuki" and 27, "Nontraditional Religion, Hyper-religiosity, and Psychopathology: The Story of Ivan from Bulgaria" in this Part exemplify the two sides of the Squeaky Wheel Principle: chapter 26 is concerned with its implications for values, and chapter 27 is concerned with its counterpart implications for evidence. In chapter 26, Eisuke Sakakibara, a neuropsychiatrist at the University Hospital in Tokyo, recounts the story of Ms. Suzuki, a Japanese woman in her middle years, who is referred to a psychiatrist for treatment of social anxiety. This raises troubling ethical questions for the psychiatrist: is this merely neuroenhancement or legitimate treatment of a genuine disorder? Here then, consistent with the Squeaky Wheel Principle, our attention is drawn to the cultural and other values in play because they are conflicting (notably the ethical values in this instance) are 'squeaking.'

The next chapter, chapter 27, "Nontraditional Religion, Hyper-religiosity, and Psychopathology: The Story of Ivan from Bulgaria," by Ivo Mitrev and Mladen Mantarkov from the Medical University of Plovdiv in Bulgaria, provides yet a further illustration of the importance of values in psychiatric diagnosis, this time through the prism of the counterpart implications of the Squeaky Wheel principle, i.e., for evidence. Like chapter 26, chapter 27 exemplifies the Squeaky Wheel principle. But where chapter 26 exemplified the Squeaky Wheel principle as applied to values, chapter 27 exemplifies the principle as applied to evidence. Chapter 26 says 'when the values are visible ('squeaking') don't forget about the evidence.' Chapter 27 says 'when the evidence is visible ('squeaking') don't forget about the values.'

Ivan, the subject of Mitrev and Mantarkov's case narrative, converts to Orthodox Judaism as a young man. This is so unusual in his native culture that he ends up being treated in a psychiatric institution. Once there, however, differences of opinion emerge about whether there is anything psychiatrically wrong with him. Resolving these differences is where values come into play diagnostically. The issues in this instance turn on how the DSM[1]'s 'criteria of clinical significance' are interpreted and applied diagnostically. Key to this, as Mitrev and Mantarkov show through Ivan's story, is a series of cultural and other values.

This is how the argument goes. For an experience or behavior to be 'clinically significant' in DSM's terms, it must be associated with dysfunction in one or more social areas such as 'work, interpersonal relations or self-care.'[2] But what counts as *dys*function in these areas varies from one culture to another according to the values of the culture concerned. Hence, consistent with the Two Feet Principle of values-based practice and notwithstanding the DSM's claim to be a descriptive (hence value free) diagnostic classification (see Footnote 1), this crucial aspect of the differential diagnosis between hyper-religiosity and psychopathology turns critically on balancing a series of contested values. If therefore even the (supposedly) descriptive DSM requires in its application to diagnostic assessment, a process of balancing contested values, it seems likely that something of the same balancing of values will be required across psychiatric diagnosis as a whole.

24.1.3 The Science Driven Principle

The *Science Driven Principle* asserts that *advances in medical science drive the need for VBP (as well as EBP) because they open up choices and with choices go values*

The Science Driven principle takes the links between values and evidence in the delivery of health care to a whole new level. Where the Two Feet and Squeaky Wheel principles emphasize different aspects of the twin requirement for both

---

[1] The DSM is the American Psychiatric Association's Diagnostic and Statistical Manual [1]. Adopted in many countries as the 'bible' of scientific psychiatry, its aim is to place psychiatric diagnosis on a firmly evidence-based footing. For more on the DSM and values, see the Guide to Further information at the end of this chapter.

[2] DSM's 'criteria of clinical significance', as they are called, all take broadly the same form. For schizophrenia, the required criterion is 'Criterion B'. With value words italicized, this reads: 'For a significant portion of the time since the onset of the disturbance, level of functioning in one or more major areas, such as work, interpersonal relations, or self-care, is markedly *below* the level achieved prior to the onset (or when the onset is in childhood or adolescence, there is *failure* to achieve expected level of interpersonal, academic, or occupational functioning' [1, p 99].

values and evidence in health care, the Science Driven principle identifies the origins of this twin requirement in the very progress of medical science.

Thus, it is well recognized that advances in medical science drive the need for evidence-based practice: without the meta-analyses and other resources of evidence-based practice, we are simply unable to keep up with the rate of these advances. Less well recognized though is that the same advances are driving the need also for values-based practice: this, the Science Driven Principle reminds us, is because the impact of these advances in clinical practice is to widen the choices available to patients and with choices go values.

The Science Driven principle, it is important to emphasize, applies across the board in medicine—it applies in surgery no less than in psychiatry. But that the principle is of particular importance in psychiatry is well illustrated by David Crepaz-Keay, Jehannine Austin, and Lauren Weeks in chapter 28, "Journey into Genes: Cultural Values and the (Near) Future of Genetic Counselling in Mental Health" with their science fiction 'Journey into Genes'. The story in this chapter is set in the near future and examines through a fictional genetic psychiatric counseling session, with 'Jim Smith', the way advances in psychiatric genetics already in the scientific pipeline are likely to impact practice. In Jim Smith's story, advances in genetics do indeed offer answers to some of the questions that currently come up in genetic counseling. But on closer inspection, we find that consistent with the Science Driven Principle, such answers as are provided by these advances come at the cost of a whole series of further questions arising from the new choices for patients that come with them.

The authors of this chapter are uniquely well placed between them to understand the impact on practice of advances in psychiatric genetics. The lead author, David Crepaz-Keay, besides being Head of Empowerment at the Mental Health Foundation, is a member of the Ethics Committee of the International Society of Psychiatric Genetics. The committee's remit includes considering the implications for mental health stakeholders of current advances in genetics. Jehannine Austin, the second author, is a professional geneticist and genetic counselor. Like David, she is a member of the Ethics Committee of the International Society of Psychiatric Genetics. David and third author, Lauren Weeks, are collaborating on a pilot program for the Mental Health Foundation exploring the perspectives of mental health service users on genetic advances.[3]

24.2   The Values Tool Kit

The next three chapters illustrate some of the resources for linking science with people available from what we called, in chapter 1, "Surprised by Values: An Introduction to Values-Based Practice and the Use of Personal Narratives in this Book," the 'values tool kit'. These resources are represented here by African philosophy, by transcultural ethics, and by anthropology, respectively. This selection of

---

[3] For more on this study, see the Guide to Further Information at the end of chapter 28, "Journey into Genes: Cultural Values and the (Near) Future of Genetic Counselling in Mental Health."

'values tools' is of course far from exhaustive. But we hope that it serves to indicate the now very wide range of resources available for working with cultural and other values in mental health.

First, then, with Samuel Ujewe's and Werdie van Staden's chapter 29, "Policy-Making Indabas to Prevent "Not Listening": An Added Recommendation from the Life Esidimeni Tragedy," on the administrative indaba, we return to a theme high-lighted in earlier Parts, the resources offered by African thought and practice for health care. Complementing van Staden's chapter 21, ""Thinking Too much": A Clash of Legitimate Values in Clinical Practice Calls for an Indaba Guided by African Values-Based Practice," on the 'clinical indaba,' this chapter illustrates through a real (and widely publicized) story, the tragic consequences that followed from a failure of health service managers adequately to engage in an 'administrative indaba' involving not just the service users who were the recipients of their deci-sions but also their families and the communities from which they came. Ujewe and van Staden show how deep this failure ran. It was particularly acute in an African context in which one's very identity is inextricably woven together with one's social context. But there is surely a wider message here about the importance of genuine consultation for the administration of mental health services in any part of the world and about the 'administrative indaba' as a model for implementation.

The importance of ethics in the values tool kit is well illustrated in chap-ter 30, "Covert Treatment in a Cross-Cultural Setting" by Neil Pickering's nuanced account of the interaction between values-based practice and transcultural ethics in the context of covert (or involuntary) treatment. Combining these two approaches as in Neil's chapter provides a balanced approach that avoids abusive uses of psychia-try developing across very different (and to an extent conflicting) sets of cultural values. Chapter 31, "Discouragement Towards Seeking Health Care of Older People in Rural China: The Influence of Culture and Structural Constraints" continues the challenge of balancing differences of values, this time between generations, with Xiang Zou's anthropological study of elderly health seeking behavior in rural China. Xiang's work provides a powerful illustration of the role of anthropological and other empirical social science methods in promoting cross-cultural understanding of the otherwise hidden cultural values impacting on health care.

24.3   StAR Values and Recovery

It is natural that in health care, the focus should be on negative values. The very point of health care, after all, is to deal with health *problems*. But the crucial impor-tance of focusing also on the positives, on what are called in values-based practice 'StAR values' (Strengths, Aspirations, and Resources), is well illustrated by the final chapter in this Part, Waldo Roeg's autobiographical chapter 32, "Discovering Myself, a Journey of Rediscovery." As Waldo's story graphically illustrates, the problems he has faced as a mental health service user have been all too evident. But recovery, the processes involved in dealing with these problems effectively, required, as Waldo puts it, genuinely recognizing "… the strengths and contribution that everyone can make."

The importance of focusing on strengths as well as problems in mental health assessment became clear in a program on values-based practice supported by the UK's Department of Health in the early years of this century. Called the 'The 3 Keys programme' [2, 3], one of the eponymous three keys to mental health assessment was that it should be strengths-based.[4] It was from this program that the StAR values of values-based practice were later developed. The importance of the StAR values for recovery runs through Waldo's story and the inspiring work of the Recovery College movement of which he is now a part. The 3 Keys programme is also being taken forward through the Bristol Co-production Group to which the authors of the dialogue in chapter 23, "Recovery and Cultural Values: On Our Own Terms (A Dialogue)," Justine and Rick, both belong. Waldo, Justine, and Rick recently collaborated on a short film bringing together their experience of the realities of coproduction (there is a link to this in the Guide to Further Information at the end of chapter 32, "Discovering Myself, a Journey of Rediscovery").

24.4 Values in Diagnostic Assessment

We make no apology for the emphasis on diagnostic values in this Part. Diagnosis is regarded by many of those committed to what they take to be an exclusively scientific view of medicine, as being value free. Decisions about treatment, this view acknowledges, may indeed bring values together with evidence. But diagnostic assessment, the processes involved in coming to an understanding of a problem as distinct from decisions about how that problem should be treated, is, so this view insists, a matter of fact to be decided by value-free science.

To do justice to this value-free view of diagnosis would take us into the long-running debate about whether health concepts (disease, illness, dysfunction, and the like) are, or may be redefined to be, value-free. Values-based practice, as has repeatedly been said, is committed to a scientific view of medicine. The theory guiding values-based practice suggests however a rather different understanding of what exactly is entailed by a *scientific view of medicine*. It suggests that, whatever may or may not be the merits of a value-free view of the nature of science (see below, Sect. 5), when it comes to linking science with people in the context of clinical decision-making (including decisions about diagnosis), values inevitably come into play.

We saw values coming into play clinically in the last Part in relation to the shared decision-making of contemporary person-centered practice. We see them coming together again, here in this Part, in the various principles linking values with evidence (chapters 25, "A Cross-Cultural Values-Based Approach to the Diagnosis and Treatment of Dissociative (Conversion) Disorders," 26, "Treatment of Social Anxiety Disorder or Neuroenhancement of Socially Accepted Modesty? The Case of Ms. Suzuki," 27, "Nontraditional Religion, Hyper-religiosity, and Psychopathology: The Story of Ivan from Bulgaria,"

---

[4] The other two keys, consistent with the program's focus on values-based practice, were that assessment should be person-centered and multidisciplinary. For more on the program, please see the Guide to Further Information at the end of the Chapter.

and 28, "Journey into Genes: Cultural Values and the (Near) Future of Genetic Counselling in Mental Health"), in the resources of the values tool kit (chapters 29, "Policy-Making Indabas to Prevent "Not Listening": An Added Recommendation from the Life Esidimeni Tragedy," 30, "Covert Treatment in a Cross-Cultural Setting," and 31, "Discouragement Towards Seeking Health Care of Older People in Rural China: The Influence of Culture and Structural Constraints"), and, above all, in the importance of looking at strengths (StAR values) as well as problems in any approach to diagnostic assessment that is pertinent to the demands of recovery practice (chapter 32, "Discovering Myself, a Journey of Rediscovery").

24.4.1 Three Ways of Understanding Diagnostic Values in Mental Health

Diagnostic values, although discernable in other areas of health care,[5] are particularly strongly evident in mental health. It is only in mental health, for example, that values are explicitly expressed in its diagnostic manuals (see [5], for a detailed linguistic analysis of the extent and variety of values evident in the American Psychiatric Association's DSM, [1]).

The prominence of diagnostic values in psychiatry has been variously understood. Some have taken this to show that mental health is a scientifically underdeveloped area of medicine (for an early and authoritative statement of this view, see [6]); others that mental illness itself is a myth [7]. The theory underpinning values-based practice suggests instead a third and very different interpretation [8]. This draws on work on the language of values by the Oxford philosopher, RM Hare [9]. Summed up aphoristically this Hare-inspired interpretation is that *'visible values = diverse values'*. In other words, the visibility of diagnostic values in mental health reflects the *relative diversity of the individual values* involved in the areas of human experience and behavior (such as emotion, desire, volition, belief, sexuality, and so forth) with which mental health is concerned.

Thus, in bodily medicine, the values involved are generally shared between clinician and patient. In Mrs Jones' story (chapter 1, "Surprised by Values: An Introduction to Values-Based Practice and the Use of Personal Narratives in this Book"), for instance, the operative values (pain and mobility) were shared between her and the surgeon, Mr Patel. In mental health, on the other hand, as the stories throughout this book so richly illustrate, the corresponding values, involving as they do areas such as emotion, desire, volition, belief, sexuality, and so forth, are highly diverse. Our values in these areas vary not only between clinician and patient but also from one person to the next. Small wonder then that if 'visible values = diverse values' the values involved in psychiatric diagnostic assessment should be more visible than their counterparts in bodily medicine.

---

[5] See for example the story of Mrs Jones' Knee in chapter 1, "Surprised by Values: An Introduction to Values-Based Practice and the Use of Personal Narratives in this Book"; for another example, see [4].

24.4.2 'Visible Values = Diverse Values' and the Three Principles

This Hare-inspired third way of understanding diagnostic values runs through and illuminates the three principles of values-based practice linking science with people. First, it is directly reflected in the Two Feet Principle—the 'two feet' of values and evidence underpin *all* decisions this principle states, including decisions about diagnosis. Then, second, 'visible values = diverse values' is itself an instance of the Squeaky Wheel Principle—the visibility of values in diagnostic assessment in mental health is an instance of the diverse values in question coming to our attention or, in the terms of the principle, 'squeaking'.

Third, 'visible values = diverse values' is reflected (this time in anticipation) in the Science Driven Principle. Diagnostic values that is to say may for now be relatively invisible (because relatively homogeneous) in bodily medicine; but with the new choices opened up by advances in medical science and technology, the Science Driven Principle suggests that diagnostic values may well become as visible in bodily medicine (because they will become as diverse) as they are already in mental health. Infertility treatment is one such area where this has already happened [10]. That mental health is not immune to the effect of such advances is well shown by chapter 28, "Journey into Genes: Cultural Values and the (Near) Future of Genetic Counselling in Mental Health" in this Part—David Crepaz-Keay and colleagues' science-fiction journey into the near future of psychiatric genetics illustrates how advances in medical science and technology by opening up new choices, far from driving values out of mental health, actually drive them even further in.

The 'visible values = diverse values' interpretation, it is worth adding finally, has a particular resonance in mental health, in part negatively, as a foil against abusive practices (as shown notably by Ivan's story in chapter 27, "Nontraditional Religion, Hyper-religiosity, and Psychopathology: The Story of Ivan from Bulgaria," this Part) and, in part positively, as a resource for recovery (as shown notably by Waldo's story in the closing chapter of this Part, chapter 32, "Discovering Myself, a Journey of Rediscovery"). Like other areas of values-based practice, the importance of diagnostic values in both these respects (negative and positive) has in the past been understood largely in terms of individual values [8]. The contributions to this Part extend our understanding of the importance of diagnostic values in mental health to include cultural values as well.

24.5   Conclusions

We have outlined how the contributions to this Part explore some of the ways in which cultural values support an enriched model of the role of values-based practice in linking science with people. Cultural values enrich understanding of the three principles of values-based practice that together spell out key aspects of the relationship between values and evidence in health care, the Two Feet principle (chapter 25, "A Cross-Cultural Values-Based Approach to the Diagnosis and Treatment of Dissociative (Conversion) Disorders"), the Squeaky Wheel

Principle (chapters 26, "Treatment of Social Anxiety Disorder or Neuroenhancement of Socially Accepted Modesty? The Case of Ms. Suzuki" and 27, "Nontraditional Religion, Hyper-religiosity, and Psychopathology: The Story of Ivan from Bulgaria"), and the Science Driven principle (chapter 28, "Journey into Genes: Cultural Values and the (Near) Future of Genetic Counselling in Mental Health"); cultural values also enrich understanding of other tools in medicine's values tool kit, illustrated here with the 'administrative indaba' of African philosophy (chapter 29, "Policy-Making Indabas to Prevent "Not Listening": An Added Recommendation from the Life Esidimeni Tragedy"), transcultural ethics (chapter 30, "Covert Treatment in a Cross-Cultural Setting"), and anthropology (chapter 31, "Discouragement Towards Seeking Health Care of Older People in Rural China: The Influence of Culture and Structural Constraints"); and cultural values come at the heart of the strengths and other values supporting recovery (chapter 32, "Discovering Myself, a Journey of Rediscovery"). We explored the importance of cultural values particularly in diagnostic assessment in mental health.

24.5.1 Cultural Values and Scientific Research

In this Part, we have followed established convention in focusing on the role of values-based practice in linking science with people specifically in the clinical encounter. But the clinical encounter, as Steve Gillard indicates in his contribution to chapter 46, "Beyond the Color Bar: sharing narratives in order to promote a clearer understanding of mental health issues across cultural and racial boundaries", is only the last in a long chain of connections between science and people. The links in this chain include the selection of research priorities and the administration of research funding, several aspects of the planning and execution of research (including the identification of 'variables of interest', the recruitment of research subjects, and the analysis and interpretation of data), peer review and publication, the development of evidence-based guidelines, and the gateway processes of regulation.

Cultural and other values play crucial if largely unacknowledged roles in each and every one of the links in this chain. Only by making these values explicit, as the contributions to this Part make them explicit in clinical decision-making, will we truly be in a position to link science effectively with people in mental health or indeed in any other area of health care.

24.6   Guide to Further Information

For a comprehensive analysis of the pervasiveness and diversity of values in the DSM (the American Psychiatric Association's *Diagnostic and Statistical Manual*), see John Sadler's book on 'Values and Psychiatric Diagnosis' [5].

For further reading on all aspects of diagnostic values, please see the Reading Guide and other sources available on the website for the Collaborating Centre for Values-based Practice in Oxford at: valuesbasedpractice.org/More about VBP.

This part of the website includes a free-to-download full text PDF of the '3 Keys' publication [2].

References

1. American Psychiatric Association. Diagnostic and statistical manual of mental disorders (5th ed, DSM-5). Washington, DC: American Psychiatric Association; 2013.
2. The National Institute for Mental Health in England (NIMHE) and the Care Services Improvement Partnership. 3 Keys to a shared approach in mental health assessment. London: Department of Health; 2008. Also available as a full text download from the website of the Collaborating centre for Values-based Practice in Oxford – see Guide to Further Information, below.
3. Fulford KWM, Duhig L, Hankin J, Hicks J, Keeble J. Values-based assessment in mental health: the 3 keys to a shared approach between service users and service providers, Ch 73. In: Sadler JZ, van Staden W, Fulford KWM, editors. The Oxford handbook of psychiatric ethics. Oxford: Oxford University Press; 2015.
4. Fulford KWM, Peile E, Carroll H. The reluctant hypertensive: think evidence, think values too! Ch 10, Element 7: The two-feet principle. In: Fulford KWM, Peile E, Carroll H, editors. Essential values-based practice: clinical stories linking science with people. Cambridge: Cambridge University Press; 2012. p. 133–42.
5. Sadler JZ. Values and psychiatric diagnosis. Oxford: Oxford University Press; 2005.
6. Kendell RE. The concept of disease and its implications for psychiatry. Br J Psychiatry. 1975;127:305–15.
7. Szasz TS. The myth of mental illness. Am Psychol. 1960;15:113–8.
8. KWM F. Moral theory and medical practice. Cambridge: Cambridge University Press; 1989, reprinted 1995 and 1999.
9. Hare RM. The language of morals. Oxford: Oxford University Press; 1952.
10. Fulford KWM, Peile E, Carroll H. Elective fertility: think high-tech, think evidence *and* values too!' Ch 12, Element 9: The science driven principle. In: Fulford KWM, Peile E, Carroll H, editors. Essential values-based practice: clinical stories linking science with people. Cambridge: Cambridge University Press; 2012. p. 151–62.

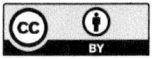

A Cross-Cultural Values-Based Approach to the Diagnosis and Treatment of Dissociative (Conversion) Disorders

Anna Todeva-Radneva and Asen Beshkov

25.1 Introduction

Psychiatric diagnosis is in itself an art, incorporating the architectural accuracy of valid diagnostic criteria and the abstract poetry of patients' values and culture, which change the shapes and shades of every disorder. It is precisely these value-laden characteristics that many take to undermine the status of psychiatry as a science in the contemporary world of evidence-based medicine. However, in reality, they uncover the unrealized complexity of the nature of psychiatric conditions.

Dissociative (Conversion) disorders are some of the disorders presenting with the most polymorphic symptomatology. The difficulties of diagnosis arise not only in the necessity for numerous tests to exclude somatic (bodily) conditions (in the case of conversion predominantly neurological because of the frequent pseudoneurological presentation) but also in the fact that both the patient's (very often culturally rooted) personal understanding of and beliefs about the concept of "disease" can significantly alter the clinical presentation. This in turn may result in misinterpretation, misdiagnosis, and incorrect treatment. This is why it is of major significance for a doctor to take the time to understand the social and cultural background, as well as the contemporary social context and cultural milieu, of the patient and to use this understanding in the diagnostic process and in decisions about treatment.

As the following story of 'A.A' illustrates, when it comes to curing the person, bearing in mind the values and culture of the person in question, and not just the disease, means that medical treatments such as pharmacological therapies are usually not enough.

A. Todeva-Radneva (✉) · A. Beshkov
Department of Psychiatry and Medical Psychology, Medical University of Plovdiv, Plovdiv, Bulgaria
e-mail: anna.todeva@mu-plovdiv.bg; asen.beshkov@mu-plovdiv.bg

25.2   A.A.: A Woman Trapped Not Only by Her Own Mind but also by the Invisible Boundaries Within Contemporary Medical Practice

A.A. (not her real initials) is a 34-year-old Bulgarian woman of Romani descent, suffering from "Mixed dissociative (conversion) disorder". She has only elementary education and is unemployed. She lives with her husband, who she reports to be an abusive alcohol drinker with a tendency to aggressive behaviour when in an intoxicated state, and their two children.

A.A. has been admitted several times to the same psychiatric ward over the years with relapses of her condition. The main reason for the frequent relapses is lack of compliance with the prescribed therapy. Her medical and family histories were unremarkable before the onset of her illness and there is no evidence of physical or psychological trauma in her childhood and adolescence.

The first symptoms occurred after she lost a significant amount of weight in 2011 (35 kg over 9 months). She had no appetite and her mind was preoccupied with persistent thoughts of having stomach cancer. She felt on edge, anxious, futureless and tearful, and even admitted having thoughts of committing suicide.

In 2014 A.A. made a suicide attempt by cutting the veins in her wrists. Following this she was admitted to a hospital where she presented with anxiety, fear of various diseases and death, palpitations, shortness of breath, dizziness and faintness. The latter symptoms intensified even more her anxiety and the level of her fixation upon the significance of her symptoms. Whenever a "crisis" with autonomic nervous system symptoms occurred she would call an emergency unit.

The most recent hospitalization was in December 2018 when her condition worsened again. She presented with anxiety, fear of "going mad", tearfulness and numerous bodily symptoms, some of which she tried to fake. On admission her appearance was neglected, she kept underwear tied in a knot underneath her blouse, which according to her was charmed and protected her against black magic. She was also agitated, tense, spoke in a loud voice and could not stand still for a moment. Excoriation marks from attempts to hurt herself were visible. Her thinking process was accelerated but without delusions, and depersonalization phenomena were also noted. There was no insight on her part.

After all the tests necessary to exclude a number of possible bodily conditions, treatment was initiated with antidepressants (trazodone and escitalopram) and benzodiazepines (diazepam) but there was no improvement in her symptoms. On the tenth day, indeed, after starting treatment, her condition actually deteriorated—she expressed fears of dying, and had numbness and shortness of breath. After a thorough examination she admitted that she had spat out the medication given to her over the last 2 or 3 days. This led to the decision of disciplinary discharge from the hospital due to lack of compliance.

However, even though A.A's relatives were informed, they did not come to the hospital to take responsibility for her and her stay was in consequence prolonged. At that time she said that if she had been discharged she would have come back. During her extended stay another attempt to establish compliance was made, this time successfully. However, the compliant attitude of the patient was only directed at the medicating process in accordance with the hospital rules. We may speculate that the motivation behind it was the doctor's decision to continue her treatment in the hospital despite her previous devious behavior, but there is no conclusive data on the matter. A.A's condition gradually improved and about 5 weeks later she was discharged from the hospital and her relatives finally took her home.

25.3 Commentary

This case is one of the majorities one can find, because nowadays, the focus is shifted toward medication use and not what happens to patients after they leave the hospital with a prescription. A lot more could be uncovered if the usual framework was reshaped. For example, the role of the husband's habits and behavior was never placed into the social context of family status. Was current family environment a part of the reasons for the relapse or was it a different personal psychological experience unknown to the family members? Were the lower education, the language, and cultural gap, all of them creating communication difficulties between patient and doctor, a valid excuse to use the safe, well-known evidence-based approach? And to what degree would the outcome have been different, had there a cross-cultural connection between the doctor and the patient been established?

These questions may remain unanswered in the context of the current case, but their explanation may change the general framework we confide ourselves in as doctors. It is difficult to establish a productive collaboration with a patient whose behavior is influenced not only by their current condition but also by lack of education, language barrier, and different cultural views.

In the contemporary materialistic world, Roma people often face discriminative attitude, since their lifestyle differs significantly. Subsequently, it is a common phenomenon for mental health issues as a contributing factor to such attitude to be underrated and reported at a delayed stage, which has a negative impact on the treatment outcome [1]. Inside this frame of reference, we cannot be certain whether the perception of the impaired mental state of this young woman as a stigma did not influence the time of diagnosis and the course of treatment.

The status of Roma people within the society is not only a reflection of their cultural traditions but also a possible explanation for their different behavior of illness. A study by Vorvolakos et al. showed higher prevalence of some psychiatric disorders in Roma women, compared to their majority counterparts, further supplemented by the discrepancy in the structural/categorical distribution of psychiatric disorders between these groups, namely, the low frequency of more severe diagnoses such as psychosis or bipolar disorder among Roma women [2]. The same study presented a significant contrast in the socioeconomic circumstances of Roma women, which are characterized with higher social pressure in terms of familial issues such as child raising and lack of cultural independence.

Considering these findings in the context of sources of distress sheds new light on the observed behavior of illness of both Roma patients in general and our particular case. However, since the family dynamics was neither investigated, nor targeted in the therapeutic approach, the specific cultural and transcultural interactions were not clarified. Thus, we can only speculate about the role of the family customs and traditions as a source of distress for A.A. and as a predicament for sustaining the patient's compliance.

These are only a few of the numerous more examples why the patient's cultural beliefs and personality traits are at the core of a successful treatment. Unlike all other specialties, psychiatric disorders are hardly ever cured purely by means of psychopharmacology. And even though great progress has been made in understanding the mechanisms through which psychopharmacological medications act in the processes and causes underlining psychiatric conditions, what defines the success of treatment is still a matter of providing care for the person behind the disease in the context of their culture and traditions.

25.4   The Values Arising in this Story

If we review this case within the framework of a conventional evidence-based medical approach, we may conclude that it was handled correctly—a thorough medical and family history was obtained, followed by examination and various tests, a therapeutic approach was specified and subsequently altered, according to the course of the disorder, and a significant improvement of the patient's condition was observed as the outcome. If, however, we step outside this conventional medical frame and change the perspective, we may see an entirely different image, one less colorful and at best half-finished.

When one reads this story between the lines, they will see many questions left unanswered. For example, is it possible for A.A. to perceive her illness as an escape from her addicted husband? If so, is it her choice to stay with him and what are the fundamental values behind such a decision? What triggered the excessive alcohol consumption of her husband—was it her condition or something else? And whatever the reason is, have his values deteriorated beyond repair or can he still be a source of support, not fear, for his wife? The answers to these could have provided yet another tool to understand and treat A.A's illness, but they were not obtained.

When it comes to the treatment plan, even more questions arise, because it remained strictly evidence-based, purely pharmacological and value-free. Do we attribute this decision to the doctor's values or to the framework that medicine understood as not more than a science has created? Perhaps it is a combination of both, since following the guidelines is safe and well grounded; however, the choice whether to stay within these boundaries belonged to the doctor alone. Yet, the choice to let A.A. stay and continue the treatment even after she was subject to disciplinary discharge is extremely value-laden, because it was not made due to following a set of rules, but for the single purpose to help.

Another "side effect" of the evidence-based treatment of a woman with such a value-laden cultural inheritance is that it can never establish the necessary trust and respect between the doctor and the patient, and hence, it couldn't be and remained unsuccessful in that her compliance continued only within the four walls of the hospital with her treatment remaining purely pharmacological and dependent on the constant supervision of medical personnel. It is not medications that the Romani believe in, but their rituals for purification. Therefore, compliance with the treatment may have been ensured, if it was supplemented with a method directed to changing those particular psychological barriers, set by the patient's beliefs (for example, hypnosis or a religious ritual for purification). It is worth adding that the psychiatric department where A.A. was hospitalized has previous experience in applying methods such as hypnosis, but it was not included in her documented treatment plan.

Some of the reasons for her failed treatment are worth emphasizing. This was essentially because A.A.'s symptoms were not perceived as culturally influenced. Thus, the therapeutic approach undertaken couldn't be and remained unsuccessful because it was directed only toward those symptoms and their probable biological underpinnings, and not to their cultural cause. Consequently, The medical specialists deprived themselves of a valuable accessory therapeutic mechanism by neglecting the significance of investigating the family dynamics within their Roma cultural context and how including the family members in the diagnostic and treatment processes might have influenced the course of the illness. If in this case, the relatives perceived the doctor's efforts to observe and value their traditions as part of the therapy, while at the same time, they were well acquainted with the signs and symptoms of the disorder and how it was likely to progress, they might have supported the patient's treatment not only by ensuring that she was regularly medicated but also by taking part in the arrangement of any culturally appropriate rituals that would have satisfied the patient's psychological attitude and understanding. When the family members realize the association between conflicts, emotions, and symptoms (the importance of specific cultural, regional, ethnic, etc., language expressions such as "nerves, nerve attack, crisis"), they may at least try to change their attitude to the patient and be more accepting, considerate, tolerant, forgiving, less critical, and demanding.

The reactively chosen medical approach may be understood as an expression of the "value blindness" concept of values-based practice. The doctor listens to the patient, trying to find a combination of symptoms, defining a particular diagnosis, but at the same time fails to recognize the values driving these symptoms. This "values blindness" may reflect an existing educational gap and/or a language barrier.

It is very important to recognize the necessity of maintaining a balance between science and values not only in psychiatry but also in medical practice as a whole, because the cause, development, and treatment of every medical condition are deeply influenced by cultural inheritance and personal values.

25.5 The Influences of Culture on this Story

We know that somatization and conversion are frequently resultant superficial manifestations of suppressed/repressed emotional conflicts, specifically related in most cases to interpersonal (family, relatives, and friends) conflicts and tension, especially when suffering individuals are suggestible and alexithymic or when these are culturally accepted idioms of distress. For the Romani, the origins of illness are "pollution", lack of good fortune, etc. It is their firm belief that the larger a person is, the healthier, luckier, and happier that person will be [3]. In this context, the onset of the patient's disorder is related to the loss of weight that in her culture, it is perceived as loss of good fortune. Most of her symptoms were most likely related to this loss and were a presentation of a culturally specific distress.

If we look at the history of the Romani people, we might find ourselves astonished at how much of their current differences can be rooted in their life in the past. This is a nomadic population who was often persecuted and discriminated against (discrimination is still a relevant hindrance for their integration to western culture nations), and for that reason, their most sacred relationships are those within the so-called extended family. This can also relate to their lower educational status. It was essential for their survival in the past to stay united and supportive of each other during their long journeys from place to place, mastering abilities that could provide them with the daily bread, which can hardly fit in the contemporary view of proper education. This has also led to the immense diversity of the professed religions of the Romani people, which, however, does not undermine the influence these religious and familial identities have on their well-being and their perception of such [4]. Also, religious beliefs and values are known to have a major effect on mental health and behavior in every individual [5].

The Roma traditions and beliefs have a deep influence over their behavior that in turn they are trying to change because nowadays they lead a settled life. It may be impossible for an outsider to fully comprehend the complexity of the meaning of their traditions because these incorporate both the endowment of their ancestors and the endeavor to preserve their sacred and rich history within the new world they are trying to fit in.

25.6   Conclusions

The main purpose of medicine and psychiatry is to not only treat the symptoms of a disease but also to improve the patient's quality of life, which necessitates the application of an integrative approach combining state-of-the-art scientific findings with the ancient cultural inheritance of every human being. In order to accomplish a paradigm shift toward personalized and values-based medical approaches, we need to realize the complex cross-cultural interactions in the doctor-patient relationship. Moreover, we should try to gain a unique perspective on every single patient as opposed to the current tendency to reduce all individuals to the common denominator of their disease and expand our range of knowledge beyond conventional therapeutic guidelines.

Acknowledgements The story of A.A. was kindly submitted by Valentina Milkovska, M.D.—State Psychiatric Hospital, Pazardzhik, Bulgaria.

25.7   Guide to Further Sources

For a more extensive account of the elements of values-based practice and the cross-cultural characteristics of the Romani people, see Ref. 2.

References

1. Lee EJ, Keyes K, Bitfoi A, Mihova Z, Pez O, Yoon E, Masfety VK. Mental health disparities between Roma and non-Roma children in Romania and Bulgaria. BMC Psychiatry. 2014;14:297.
2. Vorvolakos T, Samakouri M, Tripsianis G, Tsatalmpasidou E, Arvaniti A, Terzoudi A, Livaditis M. Sociodemographic and clinical characteristics of Roma and non-Roma psychiatric outpatients in Greece. Ethn Health. 2012;17(1–2):161–9.
3. Vivian C, Dundes L. The crossroads of culture and health among the Roma (Gypsies). J Nurs Scholarsh. 2004;36(1):86–91.
4. Dimitrova R, Chasiotis A, Bender M, van de Vijver FJ. Collective identity and well-being of Bulgarian Roma adolescents and their mothers. J Youth Adolesc. 2014;43(3):375–86.
5. Bhugra D. Commentary: Religion, religious attitudes and suicide. Int J Epidemiol. 2010;39(6):1496–8.

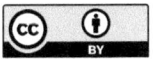

Treatment of Social Anxiety Disorder or Neuroenhancement of Socially Accepted Modesty? The Case of Ms. Suzuki

26

Eisuke Sakakibara

26.1 Introduction

People see psychiatrists for various reasons, and their willingness to treat their disorders also varies. Negative or ambivalent attitudes toward psychiatric treatment are not uncommon among patients with psychotic disorders, which present moral dilemmas for mental health professionals. However, such situations are not restricted to psychotic disorders. There are cases where a person makes a psychiatric visit to have a psychiatrist arbitrate which party should yield when there is a gap between what she can do and what those who surround her expect her to do. The psychiatrist's role in such cases may be unproblematic if the diagnosis of mental disorder is obvious, but when the case lies on the border between normality and pathology, it is not clear how psychiatrists as mental health professionals should behave.

In this chapter, I will illustrate the issues arising in such cases with the story of Ms. Suzuki, a fictitious case narrative but one based on multiple cases I have experienced. As will be seen, it is natural that those concerned seek to resolve their difficulties by reference to factual norms of psychiatric diagnosis from which to draw an ethical guidance. But I will argue that this disguises value judgments for matters of fact, and I will illuminate how the patient's and the clinician's values impact on clinical decision making.

E. Sakakibara (✉)
Department of Neuropsychiatry, The University of Tokyo Hospital, Tokyo, Japan

© The Author(s) 2021
D. Stoyanov et al. (eds.), *International Perspectives in Values-Based Mental Health Practice*, https://doi.org/10.1007/978-3-030-47852-0_26

26.2 Case Narrative

Ms. Suzuki was 43 years old when she first visited a psychiatrist. She was a small Japanese woman who lived in the urban district with her husband. When she first visited the clinic in Tokyo, she wore neat clothes and sat down in the chair softly looking at the psychiatrist with downcast eyes.

She had been experiencing nervousness in front of others since she was in the fifth grade. In elementary school, teachers sometimes selected pupils to read from the textbook. She disliked reading aloud in the class; her heart used to flutter with anxiety lest she be picked to read. This concern clouded her school life, but she stayed in school. As she got older, she became very considerate—sometimes too considerate—for others. For example, she always walked in the street so attentively as not to bother the other pedestrians. When she went to the supermarket, it was onerous for her to ask a salesclerk about the merchandise because she took a long time waiting for the best time to call a salesclerk so as not to impose on their time unnecessarily. Others who noticed her sensitivity sometimes appreciated her attentiveness. She was prone to gloominess, but she was generally emotionally stable and had never suffered from a prolonged depressive state.

She entered a middle-ranked university and majored in literature. After graduation, she started work as a clerk in the office of a company dealing in furniture. Making a phone call and picking up the phone made her nervous. Yet her careful way of doing her job and sensitivity in interpersonal relationship were positively evaluated by her boss and colleagues in most cases. She was rather inconspicuous in her workplace because she rarely expressed her own opinion. She had once made an appointment with a psychotherapist of a behavioral cognitive orientation and received psychotherapy for 6 months, which helped her to overcome her hardship in her mid-twenties. Her social anxiety, however, was not greatly ameliorated.

When she was 28 years of age, she received a proposal of marriage from a man she had known since she was a university student and they married. She and her husband tried to have a child until she was in her thirties, in the end without success. Her relationship with her husband was satisfactory. Because her husband also had a job, she lived in financial comfort. In Japan, women who marry tend to leave work after the first child is born. She kept working in the same company because she had not borne a child.

Her situation changed when, now aged 43, she received a promotion. The personnel department decided to promote her because, as is often the case in Japan, an employee of her age and with 20 years of service with the company was expected to undertake an administrative post. After her promotion, she managed three subordinates and had to make presentations to executives. When she made these presentations, she fretted over the trembling of her hands and stuttering of her voice, wondering if she looked strange to her colleagues. She frequently regretted that she behaved inappropriately after she had talked to others. One of her subordinates reported her problem to her supervisor. The supervisor recommended that she see a psychiatrist, whereupon she reluctantly made an appointment for a psychiatric visit.

Although her job performance seemed unsatisfactory, her capacity for clerical business was intact. She was doing well with her husband. She had no physical health issues. She never smoked or took alcohol. As for her family history, her mother went to a psychiatric clinic regularly and took minor tranquilizers.

She clearly had some of the symptoms of social anxiety disorder (SAD), but it was uncertain whether she met the diagnostic criteria. Her adaptation to social life had been good until she was 43 and her functional impairment was restricted to certain types of tasks that were associated with her promotion, rendering the satisfaction of the "clinically significant distress or impairment" clause questionable. Her attitude towards psychiatric treatment was ambivalent; while she did not want to visit the clinic regularly and receive treatment, she did want to improve her situation.

26.3   The Values Arising in this Story

The psychiatrist was faced with the dilemma of what to do. On the one hand, Ms. Suzuki had sought help for a potentially remediable condition. However, this was at her boss's instigation, and Ms. Suzuki did not satisfy widely accepted norms for the relevant diagnostic category (SAD). So, what should the psychiatrist do? To refuse to help might put her work situation and hence other aspects of her personal well-being at risk, but treatment in this situation might amount to an abusive use of psychiatry, since it seems to serve social rather than medical ends.

The number of prescriptions of antidepressants and psychostimulants has been increasing in recent years [1]. The expansion of pharmacotherapy is occurring where the borderline between normality and pathology is ambiguous, such as neurodevelopmental disorders, mood disorders, and anxiety disorders. To elucidate the problems associated with the expansion of pharmacotherapy for these disorders, it is helpful to refer to the ethical debates on what has come to be called "neuroenhancement"—applying biomedical technologies to improve cognitive or emotional capacities beyond therapeutic purposes—because neuroenhancement is continuous with the treatment of these disorders.

Discussions of the use of psychotropic agents for nontreatment purposes make explicit hitherto unnoticed values in psychiatric practice. The ethical concerns associated with neuroenhancement are as follows [2, 3].

- *Safety/efficacy*: The safety and efficacy of psychotropic agents for the healthy should be all the better and more securely established than for patients with mental disorders because healthy people do not have urgent reasons to take them.
- *Coercion*: Coercion is a situation where individuals unwillingly take neuroenhancing medication in response to direct or indirect pressure from the people around them, even if they use this type of drugs formally of their own free will. Those who belong to an organization are especially vulnerable to coercion from their colleagues. Coercion to use enhancing drugs is not uncommon among professional athletes.

- *Complicity*: What kind of change is recognized as enhancing human capacity depends on the culture and the period in which one is embedded and is relative to the values of the people surrounding them. Therefore, neuroenhancement has the possibility of entrenching the dominant values of the time that are arbitrary and sometimes unjust. For example, a cosmetic surgeon's performing skin whitening for black people in a region with discrimination against blacks reinforces the racist idea that white skin is more valuable than black skin [4].
- *Authenticity*: Authenticity is "being true to oneself." The use of psychotropic drugs is often considered as threatening one's true self. In the world of professional sports, a performance achieved with the aid of a drug is considered counterfeit. In addition, a person's decisions made under the influence a drug are often questioned as being truly hers. Quite a few people fear taking psychotropic drugs because their personality might change.

Ms. Suzuki was ambivalent toward pharmacotherapy because she held mutually competing values. She was proud that she had carried out her responsibility in her workplace and her home, which made her hesitant to rely on medications. Although she had been impeded by her social anxiety, her interpersonal subtlety and social anxiety were two sides of the same coin. The former sometimes made a positive contribution to her relationship with others and was part of her identity. Therefore, she was not sure whether getting rid of it would spoil her "true" self or instead help her to become her true self, as described by "Tess" in Kramer's *Listening to Prozac* [5]. Her attitude toward her promotion was also equivocal. She thought that she did not need the promotion because it entailed tasks she was not good at (i.e., more assertiveness and leadership). At the same time, she wanted to meet the expectations of the company she had belonged to for so many years.

From the viewpoint of the psychiatrist, it was perplexing whether to treat her case as a psychiatric disorder because he also had values pulling him for opposing directions. Most psychiatrists have will to help anyone in psychological difficulty. At the same time, they often observe the policy that a physician should devote herself to the treatment of "true" illnesses and refrain from engaging in the "enhancement" of those who are troubled but healthy. The latter intention is especially strong when they attend patients under the coverage of national health insurance, for it in principle presupposes that an individual has been diagnosed with a particular disorder before receiving treatment. Daniels distinguished these two values or ethoses among physicians and called the "expansive" and "hard-line" views of medicine [6].

In addition, in the case of Ms. Suzuki, the psychiatrist was anxious about violating her autonomy by diagnosing her as suffering from SAD and treating her because she had been prompted to see a psychiatrist. Treating a person who is not fully willing to receive treatment but has been urged to see a psychiatrist by those around her or who cannot refuse to accept medication because of the situation in which she is embedded is a milder form of coercion.

If the status of her disorder had been unquestionable, the psychiatrist would have straightforwardly recommended treatment for her without much deliberation based on the general idea that "a disorder should be treated." In borderline cases like Ms.

Suzuki's, however, one can infer nothing from such a general idea. In such cases, clinicians actually consider whether the patient should be treated in the first place. They then add a factual judgment of whether or not she has a mental disorder in accordance with the primary value judgment, as if the former is inferable from the latter. Synofzik indicates that the diagnosis in such cases is a "cryptonormative rhetoric move" that disguises a value judgment for a judgment of fact [7]. As discussed further in Chap. 27, even the DSM's "criteria of clinical significance," although assumed by many to be descriptive (being part of a descriptive classification), require making a number of value judgments when applying them in a given clinical situation. Trying to reduce the problem to a matter of proper diagnosis thus disguises a value judgment as a judgment of fact and neglects the complicated entanglement of values of those involved. In other words, in cases such as Ms. Suzuki's, we should not evade wrestling with the conflict of values when deciding whether to treat the individual in front of us.

26.4   The Influences of Culture on this Story

The consideration of values in this case is complicated by the culture of the company to which Ms. Suzuki belonged and the culture of Japan of which she is a member. In regard to her company, this had adopted a wage system based on seniority, which is common in Japan. Therefore, as their employees get older, they are assigned heavier duties and are expected to do more supervisory and administrative jobs. That Ms. Suzuki had begun to suffer hard times in her forties was at least partly due to the expectations of her company.

In regard to her country, on the other hand, Japanese culture has been called "a culture of shame," and shyness, reserve, and nonassertiveness are accepted as the norm. Nonassertiveness has been thought of as a virtue of women in the past, and these cultural values have survived until today. As such, they are considered by many to be part of a continuing Japanese culture of oppression of women. For instance, the proportion of women in management positions in Japan is about 12%, the lowest among developed countries [8]. This might be related to the epidemiological finding that the prevalence rate of SAD is *lower* in Japan than in the United States [9, 10]. Because it is unlikely that Americans are more socially anxious than the Japanese, a possible explanation of this difference is that social anxiety with a severity that is pathologized in the US is normalized in Japan, where women's exclusion from management positions in the workplace is a norm rather than an exception. This is the context where Kramer's suggestion that SSRIs are "feminist drugs" is understandable, for they liberate and empower women [5].

From the viewpoint of psychiatry's complicity with culture, we can observe a tug of-war between the values of the mesosocial culture—her company—and the values of the macrosocial culture, namely, those of Japan. On the one hand, diagnosing Ms. Suzuki with social anxiety disorder and treating her accordingly seems to endorse the culture of her company, which practices a seniority system that disregards individual differences in aptitudes for posts. On the other hand, denying her disorder status and refraining from treating her would indirectly affirm Japanese culture's oppressiveness to women, hindering the advancement of woman's social status.

Finally, cultural differences have an influence not only on value judgments but also on the interpretation of the most factual part of psychiatry, namely, the scientific evidence of pharmacotherapy for SAD. The evidence of the efficacy of SSRIs for the treatment of SAD is abundant, whereas that for neuroenhancement is scarce. However, Japanese psychiatrists should consider the fact that SAD diagnoses are less frequent in Japan than in western countries, where most of the randomized controlled trials have been performed. This allows us to interpret the "neuroenhancement" of socially accepted modesty in Japan as pharmacologically equivalent to the "treatment" of SAD in western cultures, for which we have abundant evidence for the efficacy of SSRIs.

26.5 Conclusions

In this chapter, we have explored the influence of values in psychiatric practice through the fictitious case narrative of Ms. Suzuki, a Japanese woman with substantial anxiety in interpersonal situations, but whose diagnosis of SAD is questionable. The Two-Feet Principle of Values-Based Practice indicates that both values and facts are essential for clinical decision-making. In terms of the dichotomy of facts and values, it is usually thought that a diagnosis may be categorized as a matter of fact. However, the case presented in this chapter illustrates that the principle is applicable not only to treatment choice but also to the diagnosis of a mental disorder itself. A diagnosis of mental disorder has a value component that is sometimes influenced by the surrounding culture. This implies that the Two-Feet Principle cannot be fully materialized by grafting the discussion of values related to treatment options onto the psychiatrist's diagnosis, the latter of which is considered a purely factual judgment. To make better clinical decisions on diagnosis and treatment, we should explicitly state the conflicting values of those involved and the cultural influences on them.

Acknowledgements This study was supported by the Uehiro Foundation on Ethics and Education (http://www.rinri.or.jp). The foundation had no role in the design of the study. I also thank Bill Fulford for insightful comments and advice for completing the chapter.

References

1. Olfson M, Marcus SC. National patterns in antidepressant medication treatment. Arch Gen Psychiatry. 2009;66(8):848–56.
2. Farah MJ, Illes J, Cook-Deegan R, Gardner H, Kandel E, King P, et al. Neurocognitive enhancement: what can we do and what should we do? Nat Rev Neurosci. 2004;5(5):421–5.
3. Parens E. Is better always good?: the enhancement project. In: Parens E, editor. Enhancing human traits. Washington, DC: Georgetown University Press; 1998. p. 1–28.

4. Little MO. Cosmetic surgery, suspect norms, and ethics. In: Parens E, editor. Enhancing human traits. Washington, DC: Georgetown University Press; 1998. p. 162–76.
5. Kramer PD. Listening to Prozac: a psychiatrist explores antidepressant drugs and the remaking of the self. New York: Viking; 1993.
6. Sabin JE, Daniels N. Determining "medical necessity" in mental health practice. Hast Cent Rep. 1994;24(6):5–13.
7. Synofzik M. Ethically justified, clinically applicable criteria for physician decision-making in psychopharmacological enhancement. Neuroethics. 2009;2(2):89–102.
8. International Labour Organization. Women in business and management: the business case for change; 2019.
9. Kessler RC, Chiu WT, Demler O, Merikangas KR, Walters EE. Prevalence, severity, and comorbidity of 12-month DSM-IV disorders in the National Comorbidity Survey Replication. Arch Gen Psychiatry. 2005;62(6):617–27.
10. Ishikawa H, Kawakami N, Kessler RC, World Mental Health Japan Survey Collaborators. Lifetime and 12-month prevalence, severity and unmet need for treatment of common mental disorders in Japan: results from the final dataset of World Mental Health Japan Survey. Epidemiol Psychiatr Sci. 2016;25(3):217–29.

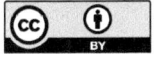

Non-traditional Religion, Hyper-Religiosity and Psychopathology: The Story of Ivan from Bulgaria

I. Mitrev and M. Y. Mantarkov

27.1   Introduction

The relationship between religion and psychiatry remains a difficult and contentious area [1]. There is a widespread view that religion boosts mental stability. However, in certain cases, extreme religiosity may undermine mental health [2]. Then again, psychotic disorders can present with religious delusions. In order to define a religious idea as delusional, it should exceed what is within the expected beliefs for an individual's background, including culture and education.

Hyper-religiosity may be considered a psychiatric disturbance at least according to the American Psychiatric Association's *Diagnostic and Statistical Manual* (the DSM), when it interferes with normal functioning. DSM offers what it describes as a descriptive (hence value-free) way of assessing mental health issues. Yet as the story of Ivan presented in this chapter illustrates, the judgments of dysfunction on which DSM's differentiation between normal hyper-religiosity and religious delusions critically depends are essentially *value* judgments. As such, as Ivan's story further illustrates, the differential diagnosis is considerably influenced by culture. The influence of cultural values is further complicated by the fact that in certain cases, religion or denomination is related to nationalism and there is thus a substitution of faith for identity.

We present, then, the story of Ivan, a young Bulgarian man, who converted to Orthodox Judaism, a religious denomination highly unusual in his country of birth.

I. Mitrev (✉) · M. Y. Mantarkov
Department of Psychiatry and Medical Psychology, Medical University of Plovdiv, Plovdiv, Bulgaria

Clinic of Psychiatry and Medical Psychology, University Multiprofile Hospital for Active Treatment "Sveti Georgi", Plovdiv, Bulgaria
e-mail: ivomitrev@gmail.com; mantarkov@gmail.com

27.2   Case History

Ivan (not his real name) was an 18-year-old Bulgarian man, who completed only his elementary education and was currently unemployed.

Family history: Ivan had a paternal first cousin with schizophrenia; and his father was described as impulsive and explosive.

Bad habits: none reported.

Social conditions: Ivan's social conditions were adequate. He was currently living with his parents. They were not particularly religious Eastern Orthodox Christians; Ivan himself did not receive a religious education. He was an only child.

He was born at 37 weeks of gestation of a first normal pregnancy. His birth weight was 3000 g. He was kept in a neonatal intensive care unit for 5 days. Neonatal jaundice was suspected. He started walking before the age of one and spoke his first words before 18 months. He was sent to nursery school at the age of two, where he adapted well. At three, he went to kindergarten, where he refused to participate in formal celebrations (some of them religious in nature, such as Christmas and Easter; but most of them secular). In his 2 years of preschool education he generally kept to himself.

He started school at seven together with his peers. He graduated from primary school (grades 1–4) with top marks. From grade 5 onwards his academic performance dropped drastically. He found school meaningless and often failed to do his homework assignments. He played a lot of computer games and wanted to become a professional player. From grade 2 through grade 7 he refused to eat meat. After his 7th grade he was admitted to a Vocational-technical school to study computer programming. He finished his 8th grade with passing grades. He did not complete his 9th grade.

During his school years, although never showing signs of mental health issues, he exhibited a number of behavioural oddiites. As early as his first years of school he was described as squeamish and fastidious about food. He showered with baking soda, as he believed that soap was harmful. In his 5th grade he refused to wear underwear because it was too restrictive. He started wearing tracksuit bottoms instead.

In his 7th grade he became annoyed with his father's cough and yawns. He also became annoyed when people touched their eyes. He refused to be touched. After a conflict with his father he broke the television set and the remote control. On account of his refusal to attend school, the family saw an outpatient psychiatrist. Antipsychotic treatment with Haloperidol 1.5 mg/day PO was prescribed but Ivan refused to take the medication. Consequently another outpatient psychiatrist prescribed antipsychotic treatment (initially with Aripiprazole, followed by Risperidone). No significant effect was observed. He became vegan. After a conflict with his father, he and his mother moved out to live with his grandmother. Consequently he started living alone, because after a series of domestic conflicts, both his parents moved out. He hardly ever left the home. In the autumn of 2016 he was hospitalized in a psychiatric clinic and treated with Aripiprazole 10 mg/day PO. He was discharged with the diagnosis Schizotypal personality disorder, "calm, often with loose associations and a tendency to form magical and symbolic thinking". The recommended outpatient treatment was Omega-3 fatty acids and CBT (Cognitive Behavioral Therapy).

After discharge, he took no further psychotropic medications. Fear of death inspired an interest in religion. His interest in Christianity lasted a day; his interest in Islam—2 months. He even considered converting to Islam. Later that year, he became interested in Judaism; gradually his interest became stronger and he adhered with increasing rigor to religious rules. He became a follower of the Orthodox Jewish movement, seen by some as a sect.

He now only eats kosher foods. A year ago he threw away a keychain of his father's with a cross. He confided that he wanted to go to Israel to study Judaism in Yeshiva living on donations. Because of his identification with Orthodox Judaism, Ivan has not had his hair cut or shaved his beard ever since his conversion. He has avoided touching or even looking at women. He has spent most of his time reading religious texts and watching religious videos on the internet. In the past 6 months he has not socialized with anyone other than his parents outside his religion. He has been in touch with rabbis on the internet.

Ever since, Ivan has had hyper-religious and possibly delusional ideas about food. He holds that food had to be prepared in the daylight "against daemons." He spends hours preparing food so it is not "contaminated" and eats separately. This has to be done, because a mezuzah (a piece of parchment with holy writings that repels evil) had not been fixed to the door.

He has shown other hyper-religious behaviors. For example, he broke an icon in the office of an outpatient psychiatrist, which he did not regret, claiming it depicted "idols". The outpatient psychiatrist diagnosed him with paranoid schizophrenia and recommended to Ivan's parents compulsory treatment in a psychiatric clinic. However, when they met with the inpatient psychiatrist, they came to the shared decision that voluntary hospitalization in the clinic would be more appropriate. Ivan consequently signed an informed consent form. He explained: "I am here, because I don't want to study and work." He agreed to take one tablet of an antipsychotic medication daily.

Psychological assessments of personality, thought, emotions and volition were conducted in the clinic: "Results from the personality questionnaire (Minnesota Multiphasic Personality Inventory—MMPI-2): due to high scores on one of the validity scales, which is interpreted as a sign of strong defenses, the profile is considered invalid. Thought: no notable disturbances in the rate and form of thought; the content of thought is dominated by religious beliefs and attitudes belonging to an orthodox movement in Judaism, which are not in keeping with the local religious and sociocultural background.

It is in terms of his religion that Ivan explains his thinking and behavior, including the adherence to certain rules and laws about bodily and social functioning that are significantly different from those of modern Bulgarian society. He believes he is governed by high moral standards and denies any hostility or negative impulses to others whatsoever. He denies delusional, depressive, aggressive and suicidal ideas. Abstract thinking: he finds no difficulties with the formation of antonyms, the interpretation of proverbs and with arithmetic operations. Emotions: results from Zung

Self-Rating Depression Scale— no evidence of depression; results from Hamilton Anxiety Rating Scale—no evidence of anxiety.

A conversation with Ivan's father revealed information about conflicts and difficulties in Ivan's upbringing as well as elements of controversy and inconsistency in his thinking and behavior in his childhood, with a tendency to manipulate and be manipulated.

Conclusion: Ivan gives the impression of a young man looking for answers to existential questions as well as for intimacy, security and belongingness as part of identifying the parameters of his own identity. He declares insight. He confides that he intends and plans to join a religious community and shows flexibility with different ways of coping under different circumstances. Family therapy was recommended."

Laboratory findings: mild alimentary anemia.

Computed tomography scanning of the head and posterior cranial fossa without contrast: normal.

In the clinic Ivan was treated with Olanzapine 10 mg/day PO. No significant change in his mental condition was observed. During his hospital stay Ivan avoided eye contact with the other patients and refused to eat any of the hospital food. He asked: "What are you treating me for? Are you treating my religion?" He stated: "This is the only religion without mistakes." However, as to the 'mistakes' of other religions, he could only point out minor inconsistencies, such as the incorrect chronology of an event or a misnomer of a town in their holy books.

In a clinical staff meeting the diagnoses Schizoid personality disorder, Schizotypal personality disorder, Delusional disorder and Paranoid schizophrenia, were discussed and Schizotypal personality disorder was accepted.

This story has no happy ending at least as yet. By the time of discharge the clinicians had not been able to form a working diagnostic and therapeutic alliance with Ivan. On discharge he refused family therapy and said: "Now, I am going to be even more religious, and I am going to Israel."

27.3 The Values Arising in This Story

The principal and arguably only value held by Ivan was his religion; he was obsessed with it. To defend this value, he went to extremes, for example, by breaking the icon in the office of the outpatient psychiatrist in an act of iconoclasm. He refused to work and did not want to study anything but the religion to which he had converted.

As to the values of Ivan's parents, they wanted their only child to stay in Bulgaria, to study and to work. They thought their son needed to take psychotropic medications. On account of this and on the advice of the outpatient psychiatrist, they considered compulsory treatment, which would have seriously compromised the principle of autonomy.

The psychiatrist viewed breaking the icon as a sign of severe psychopathology. In this, he was thinking of the DSM's criteria of clinical significance as offering an evidence-based   way   of   differentiating   psychopathology   from   normal hyper-religiosity. But his diagnostic assessment was influenced by value judgments. The relevant DSM criterion is in this instance 'impairment of social functioning': surely, the psychiatrist assumed, breaking my icon is a sign of social dysfunction! But in this, he was drawing without recognizing it on (mainly implicit) value judgments. To take a related example, someone who leaves his home and work and goes off to meditate in the desert may be thought to be functioning well in a society that values religious retreat, but to be functioning badly in a society that is more work-oriented. One implication of this, relevant to the outcome of Ivan's story is that maybe he will function better in another environment – why not a religious community in Israel?

Interestingly, the values of the clinical psychologist in this respect were different from those of the psychiatrist. As he (the psychologist) put it: "Ivan is not the typical young man of today, but I don't think he has a mental disorder." This is important because it underscores the significance of multidisciplinary assessment in coming to a balanced judgment between conflicting diagnostic values in a given case (see Introduction to this Part).

Overall, therefor, there are a number of conflicting values in play here that crucially influence how Ivan's story is understood and what is done about it. The outpatient psychiatrist—influenced in his application of DSM's criteria of clinical significance by his own implicit values—diagnosed Ivan with paranoid schizophrenia, which necessitates antipsychotic therapy, even at the (potential) cost of compulsory treatment. Guided by his own religious values, Ivan did not think he had a mental disorder, and so he refused to take medications (later as a compromise he agreed to take one pill a day for a limited period of time). The inpatient psychiatrist sought to balance these conflicting values by offering Ivan and his parents a compromise solution—voluntary inpatient treatment in a psychiatric clinic.

With regard to treatment, the inpatient psychiatrist was hesitant whether to prescribe antipsychotic therapy, as he did not expect it to be particularly effective in a patient with a personality disorder; he nonetheless prescribed an antipsychotic for the duration of Ivan's hospitalization. The clinical psychologist, who did not think that Ivan had a mental disorder, recommended family therapy, but Ivan refused to attend. His parents were outraged by the psychologist's opinion: they commented, "He said, there is nothing wrong with him". True, they were surprised by the lack of efficacy of antipsychotic therapy. But their reaction to this was that they expected the psychiatrist and psychologist to "persuade" Ivan "to not be a religious fanatic."

27.4 The Influences of Culture on This Story

Bulgarian society is not particularly religious [3]. Over-engagement in religious activities is not approved by society. Most Bulgarians describe themselves as Eastern Orthodox Christians, abide by traditional ritual practices, but do not live an orthodox way of life [4]. Ivan's hyper-religiosity was thus naturally seen as falling outside accepted norms of behavior.

In Bulgaria, it is accepted that presenting oneself as Orthodox (Christian) is a sign of national identity. The Bulgarian Orthodox Church was a factor in the survival of the Bulgarian people under the Ottoman rule (1396 to 1878) as well as in the Bulgarian national liberation movement (mid 1850s–1878[1]). The Orthodox Church has thus invariably been associated with nationalism and the state [5]. In 1879, the Tarnovo Constitution formally established the Bulgarian Orthodox Church as the national religion of the nation. Judaism, on the other hand, is usually considered the ethnic religion of the Jewish people. It could be argued that this substitution of faith for national identity was responsible for the mainly negative attitudes to Ivan.

A further cultural factor driving these negative attitudes is likely to have been the generally unfavorable attitude of the Bulgarian Orthodox Church to other religions and religious denominations. Recently, the Pope visited Bulgaria. The Holy Synod and the patriarch welcomed him coldly. A metropolitan bishop stated: "The visit of the Roman Pope is a political act. Its aim is to unite all churches around Rome so that when the Antichrist comes, the Pope can meet him." Bulgarian society as a whole does not approve of conversion to religions that are not traditional for the country. Again, then, Ivan was very much out of step with his society.

Being out of step in this way came to a head when Ivan broke the icon in the outpatient psychiatrist's office. The psychiatrist in question found it appropriate to put an orthodox icon in his office as "a spiritual symbol" even though it was visited by patients of different religions and denominations, as well as by atheists. A religious belief can be classified as delusional when it is idiosyncratic, rather than accepted within a particular culture or subculture. This undoubtedly contributed to the outpatient psychiatrist's view that Ivan had religious delusions.

There were also wider Bulgarian values in play. First, as to their children, Bulgarians have always strived to give them the best possible education. Ivan's unwillingness to study in a secular school was thus considered by his parents, in line with the majority of society and some psychiatrists, to be a sign of psychopathology. Second, as to work, it can generally be argued that Bulgarian society is work-oriented and disapproves of people who do not work. Again, Ivan found himself at odds with this widely held cultural value, thus adding to the evaluation of his behavior as abnormal.

27.5   Conclusions

It is evident that Bulgarian cultural values influence the way people (including mental health professionals); see the story of Ivan. The diagnostic judgments of mental health professionals are considerably influenced by culture. Diagnostic differences attest to the significance of multidisciplinary assessment in coming to a balanced judgment between conflicting diagnostic values.

---

[1]After the Crimean War the Bulgarian struggle for liberation evolved into a national liberation movement. In the late 1860s it entered a new, higher stage.

The story of Ivan also illustrates that the judgments of dysfunction on which DSM's differentiation between normal hyper-religiosity and religious delusions critically depends are essentially *value* judgments.

References

1. Fulford KWM. Religion and psychiatry: extending the limits of tolerance. In: Bhugra D, editor. Psychiatry and religion: context, consensus and controversies. London: Routledge and Kegan Paul; 1996.
2. Van Praag HM. God's champions and adversaries: about the borders between normal and abnormal religiosity. In: Verhagen PJ, Van Praag HM, López-Ibor JJ, Cox J, Moussaoui D, editors. Religion and psychiatry: beyond boundaries. Hoboken, NJ: Wiley; 2010.
3. Nazarska G, Shapkalova S. Study of religious values in present Bulgaria. In: Krikoryan R, Slavcheva K, Penou S, editors. Humanism, science, religion—values, paradigms and challenges in interreligious relations. Sofia; 2015.
4. Витанов Р. Религиозността на съвременния българин. In: Омарчевски А, Макариев П, editors. Християнство и философия. София: Парадигма; 2014. (Vitanov R. The Religiousness of Modern Bulgarians. In: Omarchevski A, Makariev P, editors. Christianity and Philosophy. II. Sofia: Paradigm; 2014).
5. Kushelieva Z. Развитие на отношенията между църквата и държавата в България. Kritische Zeitschrift für überkonfessionelles Kirchenrecht. 2016;3:39–44. (Kushelieva Z. Development of the Relations between the Church and the State in Bulgaria. Kritische Zeitschrift für überkonfessionelles Kirchenrecht. 2016(3):39–44).

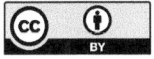

Journey into Genes: Cultural Values and the (Near) Future of Genetic Counselling in Mental Health

David Crepaz-Keay, Jehannine Austin, and Lauren Weeks

28.1 Introduction

Our understanding of the role of genetics in individual vulnerability to mental ill-health and response to treatment is increasing every day. Correlatively, the cost of genetic testing[1] is decreasing and will soon reach the point where an individual's genetic profile will become a normal part of doctor patient consultations. Not only that but it is now possible to buy for around £100 a range of kits that purport to offer DNA[2]-based personalised health solutions, thus theoretically empowering people to take more control of their health-related decisions.

Although not yet routinely part of everyday health consultations, these developments in the science of genetic medicine are sufficiently advanced as to have become the subject of anticipatory health planning in many parts of the world. In the UK, they are the subject of a recent (2019) Government Green Paper,[3] 'Advancing our health: prevention in the 2020s' [1]. This sets out a clear agenda for genetics and

---

[1] The term genetic testing covers a range of techniques designed to identify individuals' unique genetic make-up and how this might relate to their risk of particular conditions and their likely responses to treatments.

[2] DNA is an abbreviation for deoxyribonucleic acid. This is the molecule that contains the genetic code of organisms.

[3] A Green Paper is a consultation paper circulated for comment before moving to specific proposals in a White Paper and from there to implementation (in some cases including parliamentary processes of producing enabling legislation).

D. Crepaz-Keay (✉) · L. Weeks
Mental Health Foundation, London, UK

J. Austin
UBC Departments of Psychiatry and Medical Genetics, Vancouver, BC, Canada

© The Author(s) 2021
D. Stoyanov et al. (eds.), *International Perspectives in Values-Based Mental Health Practice*, https://doi.org/10.1007/978-3-030-47852-0_28

Table 28.1 Extract from the Government Green Paper (2019) 'Advancing our health: prevention in the 2020s'

In the 2020s, people will not be passive recipients of care. They will be co-creators of their own health. The challenge is to equip them with the skills, knowledge and confidence they need to help themselves
We are: • Embedding genomics in routine healthcare and making the UK the home of the genomic revolution   • Reviewing the NHS health check and setting out a bold future vision for NHS screening   • Launching phase 1 of a predictive prevention work programme from Public Health England (PHE)

Table 28.2 Patient and public engagement in psychiatric genetics: a summary of the Mental Health Foundation Research

Patient and public engagement in psychiatric genetics—Mental Health Foundation research
Aim: Explore thoughts, feelings and opinions of psychiatric genetic testing and any personal insights into this subject area. Psychiatric genetic testing has the potential to develop more personalised treatment, yet there are many ethical considerations
Ethical considerations: Access to information (e.g. police, employers, family), how much information individual receives, length information is stored for and potential mental health impact of testing (e.g. if person receives result of higher mental health vulnerability will information enable them developing said mental health difficulty, also potential impact on family and family choices)
Participants: Individuals ranging in age, ethnicity and gender with lived experience
Method: Qualitative, interactive discussion groups discussing three subject areas: Psychiatric genetic testing; mental health impact of non-psychiatric genetic testing; and pharmacogenomics
Results: Indicates how personal the decision-making process is for genetic testing and was mixed in views of for and again such testing. Many factors were considered, however there was unanimous decision that the choice for whether you get genetic testing should remain a free choice and not something imposed upon you. Research like this is important as it puts the voice of lived experience at the forefront, which is crucial for developing future mental health treatment options

genomic medicine to become integral to public health within the coming few years. An extract from the Green Paper illustrating the level of commitment already being made to this agenda is given in Table 28.1.

The following case narrative illustrates the impact of these anticipated developments on mental health through an imaginary consultation set in the near future when the aspirations of the 2019 Green Paper have become incorporated into everyday practice, it is also informed by the Mental Health Foundation's on-going research summarised in Table 28.2.[4]

The consultation is of course fictional, but the scientific developments assumed by those concerned are all within the reach of current technologies—so the case

---

[4] Further details of this research are given in the Guide to Further Information at the end of this chapter.

narrative is fiction but not *science* fiction. The science is indeed real and (almost) upon us. Note however that the actual risk and probability scores used are illustrative only and should not be read as actual scores for the conditions or treatments mentioned.

28.2   Case Narrative: *'Come In and Sit Down'*: A Doctor/ Patient Consultation

The patient, Jim Smith, is in his early twenties. He has been experiencing particular forms of visions and voices consistent with a diagnosis of schizophrenia. There is a family history of mental ill-health: this has not been discussed in detail among family members but a grandmother is talked about in a way that suggests she spent a number of spells in psychiatric hospitals. Jim Smith had been referred to a psychiatrist who gave a provisional diagnosis of schizophrenia. This is the follow up consultation that will by then be required under the new personalised medicine policy introduced (so the story line assumes) following the 2019 Green Paper and its subsequent development and implementation in UK health policy and law.

The doctor, Helen Jones, is well versed in psychiatric genetics (as a medical student she did a genetics research project and had been encouraged to follow a career in this field). After inviting the patient to 'come in and sit down', she starts by reminding Jim Smith of his diagnosis of schizophrenia based on reported and observed symptoms. She then outlines the established intervention recommended by NICE Guidelines[5] for schizophrenia and reminds him of the informed consent process. She explains that the recommended first treatment achieves the desired therapeutic effect for approximately one third of people with this diagnosis; has a marginal therapeutic effect with some adverse reactions for another third; and has no therapeutic benefit and significant adverse effects for the remaining third. Only through trial and error can the best therapeutic outcome with the minimal adverse impact be established; the process could take many months; and there is no way to tell in advance which of the various treatment options will do good or harm until the good or harm has been done.

Under the personalised medicine policy (now newly introduced), she then offers Jim Smith the option of his genome being sequenced. If he accepts this, Dr Jones explains, it will entitle him to an enhanced personal treatment plan (EPTP) based on his genotype. Although the EPTP is free it is contingent on enrolling into the UK National Biobank Programme (see Guide to Further Information), a project that

---

[5] NICE is an independent body, the National Institutes for Health and Care Excellence, set up by the UK government to commission regular reviews of treatment options for different conditions and, on the basis of these, to publish evidence-based treatment guidelines.

aims to improve the prevention, diagnosis and treatment of a wide range of serious and life-threatening conditions with a view to improving personalised medicine.[6]

Dr Jones goes on to explain the role of the Biobank to Jim Smith, spelling out that the more complete the Biobank becomes, the more of the population it is able to include, the more effective it will be in meeting its aims. She explains that on current best evidence an EPTP for schizophrenia improves the likelihood of therapeutic benefit to 80% and reduces the risk of significant adverse effects to about 5% (as noted above, these figures are at the time of writing fictitious and used for narrative purposes only).

There are two further considerations to bear in mind, she continues, before reaching a decision about genomic screening: first, how much more health information (i.e. over and above likely response to treatment) does he (Jim Smith) want to be reported and shared, and with whom; and, second, bearing in mind the fast moving nature of the field, how far would he be happy with possible developments in the use of Biobank data currently being considered, for example by academic researchers, the police, credit agencies, insurance companies, DVLA, employers, and benefits agencies.

28.3 Discussion

In this discussion, we review the above consultation from the perspective of the values issues arising (individual and cultural) and how these interact with the scientific and medical advances assumed to have taken place. The discussion is in part informed by our experience with a small series of discussion groups (see Acknowledgements) exploring patients' perspectives emerging practice in psychiatric genetics. Although the details are still being analysed, one clear message from these discussions is the individuality of personal values. For example, some people in the discussion group were very clear that they would not want to know anything about their genetic make-up or any risks, whereas others would want to know everything.

28.3.1 Developments in Psychiatric Genetics

Other than for the specifics of the risks mentioned, the above consultation draws on established findings of the growing field of psychiatric genetics. To the best of

---

[6] Terminology is sometimes confusing here. The term 'personalised medicine' is generally used to mean medicine that is geared to the particular biological make up of the individual – their genetic profile is particularly important in this respect, we have coined the term "Enhanced Personal Treatment Plan" to reflect this significant increase in how individual treatments may become. 'Person-centred medicine' is different in that it focuses on the particular needs, wishes and expectations of the patient. The 'person-values-centred care' of values-based practice focuses particularly on the values of the patient as an aspect of person-centred care (see chapter "Surprised by Values: an Introduction to Values-based Practice and the Use of Personal Narratives in this Book").

current knowledge, our genetic make-up really does contribute to our risk of being affected by a range of health conditions, including, within mental health, many of those widely described by contemporary psychiatric diagnostic categories. These include, as in the above narrative, Jim Smith's diagnosis of 'schizophrenia' based on the presence of a number of specific forms of experiences (specific forms of 'visions and voices').

Psychiatric diagnostic categories of this kind are not universally accepted not least within the contemporary neuroscience research community (see also Sect. 4, below). Yet notwithstanding the likely scientific limitations of these diagnostic concepts, there is growing evidence of a genetic contribution to individual differences in how people respond to established treatments for conditions so defined. This is why 'pharmacogenomics' as it is called (basing drug treatments on an individual's genetic profile) is becoming an ever more important aspect of personalised medicine.

28.3.2   Scientific Solutions to Values Issues?

On first inspection, the above advances in psychiatric genetics might seem if not to resolve at least to ameliorate the values issues raised by treatment choice in Jim Smith's story. In the first part of his consultation, he is presented with three possible outcomes for the NICE recommended first line treatment for schizophrenia. In deciding whether or not to consent to this recommended treatment, he is in effect asked to take a gamble on the balance of risks and benefits that he will experience (depending on which of the three risk groups described by Dr. Jones he turns out to fall into). Then, in the second part of the consultation, he is offered access to genetic testing that will greatly reduce his gamble. It will give him (in the fictitious numbers given in the story) a large degree of certainty about his likely response to treatment.

Not only that but, to extend the story a little (though again not beyond the immediate future of genetic testing), Jim Smith's test results may well resolve further questions he may have had about specific risks. For example, one recognised risk of the treatments in question is weight gain. This is an outcome of treatment that (carrying as it does a range of aesthetic and health implications) is valued differently by different people. In coming to a shared decision, therefore, as the basis of contemporary best practice and legal rules on consent [2, 3], the risk of weight gain would have to be explored by Dr. Jones with Jim Smith. Such discussion would be better informed with more precise genetics-profile-based information about his likelihood of weight gain to hand.

So, job done? Well, no, because on further inspection, we see that the values issues have been increased rather than reduced by the addition of the option of genetic testing. Certainly, within the terms of reference of the story, genetic testing makes available to Jim Smith better information about the likely balance of harms and benefits of treatment in his case. This is nothing if not extremely helpful both to Jim Smith and to Dr. Jones in coming to a shared decision about how to proceed.

But this information comes at a price. It comes at the price of having to make a whole series of further choices about whether or not to proceed with genetic testing and if so to what extent and for what purposes. For each of these contingent choices, there will be a range of risks and benefits to consider. Thus, in the first place, as Dr. Jones points out, the test is free, but only if Jim Smith agrees to 'sign up' to the Biobank Programme. There are benefits (mainly to others) if he agrees to this but also risks (around the confidentiality of his genetic information now and in respect of future possible uses of the Biobank data by other agencies). In respect of these issues, he, Jim Smith, will have as it were a unique 'values profile' sitting alongside his unique genetic make-up. He will, that is to say, have a unique personal take on what matters or is important to him about these issues. He will have a unique values profile, similarly, about all the further issues concerning what additional genetic information he, Jim Smith, will want reported to him (and/or others) about his own test results over and above his likely response to the proposed treatment for his schizophrenia.

28.3.3   The 'Science Driven' Principle of Values-Based Practice

Jim Smith's story thus illustrates the 'Science Driven' principle of values-based practice, namely, that the impact of advances in medical science and technology is not to diminish but rather to enhance the need for values-based practice as a partner to evidence-based practice in the shared decision-making that underpins contemporary person-centred clinical care (see chapter "Surprised by Values: An Introduction to Values-Based Practice and the Use of Personal Narratives in This Book"). His story shows too why this should be so. For as in Jim Smith's story, the impact of advances in medical science and technology is to widen the range of choices that we (patients and clinicians) have available to us—and with choices go values.

28.3.4   How to Do It

Helen Jones, the doctor in the above narrative, is well aware of the advances in genetic medicine relevant to Jim Smith's condition, and given her research as a medical student, she is better versed in them than many of her colleagues [4]: this is perhaps why Jim Smith's doctor made the referral. Certainly, she makes a good showing of explaining the technical issues to her patient. This as we have seen is not enough for purposes of shared decision-making as the basis of consent to treatment. Nor is it enough, so the evidence suggests [5], for purposes of psychiatric genetic counselling[7] if it is to empower rather than disempower patients.

---

[7]Genetic counselling is the process of "helping people to understand and adapt, to the medical, psychological and familial implications of genetic contributions to disease" [6]. In the psychiatric context, it involves helping people make personal meaning from what is known about how genetic and environmental factors contribute together to the development of mental health difficulties and using this to frame an enhanced understanding of how to protect mental health. The counsellor will help develop strategies for coping with the risk in family, the related uncertainty of testing and help people living with a mental health difficulty.

What more, then, is needed and how is it to be delivered? We do not have space to consider the challenges of delivery in detail here. But it is important at least to be aware of the resources available. There is a generic resource of training and other materials available to support values-based practice in different areas of health care including mental health (see Guide to Further Information below). There is also, specifically in relation to psychiatric genetic counselling, a growing resource, first, of evidence-based information about what is important to patients about the counselling they receive and the counsellor from whom they receive it, and, second, of practical aids to support delivery. Again, we do not have space to describe these resources in detail but will offer two examples with the above consultation particularly in mind (Table 28.3).

First, then, as to the evidence about what works, Table 28.3 is adapted from *The Empowering Encounter* developed using Grounded Theory to study psychiatric genetic counselling [7]. The factors shown are a small subset of those that make up the full *Empowering Encounter*. But they illustrate the range of factors that are

Table 28.3 What matters to patients in psychiatric genetic counselling

Factor	Example patient quote	Dr Helen Jones
Receiving support and information		
• Being heard	*[The genetic counsellor] let me talk, which is something that I think a lot of people don't do… to be able to talk about what I do [to manage my MI], to be heard and be validated was helpful*	NO
• Feeling validated	*I liked that [GC] affirmed a lot of the things that I've been trying to do to manage my mental illness… so its good to know that, like it validates my efforts*	NO
• Knowledge	*Until genetic counselling, no one ever coherently explained to me why I have a mental illness. And I think that's a conversation that needs to be had because most people just think they're having a bad time of it or they just think that they just need to try harder and that's [because] they don't understand that it's an illness*	YES
• Tool for understanding	*I think that the simplified jar analogy* (see text and Fig. 28.1) *was good, it was easy to understand and was presented in a really good way. I thought it was a useful tool*	NO
Characteristics of the genetic counsellor		
• Empathetic	*I just felt that [the genetic counsellor] really understood what I was going through and was really open to connecting*	NO
• Non-judgemental	*I didn't feel like [the genetic counsellor] was judging me, I felt like she genuinely wanted to help me*	YES
• Knowledgeable	*With [the genetic counsellor] there was a lot more knowledge on her part and [it was] evident that she's heard stories and worked with people who have mental health issues that are the same as I have*	YES

important if a consultation in psychiatric genetics counselling is to be empowering for the patient concerned (and thereby effective in motivating health-supporting behaviours). Note that among these factors, giving information and technical competence is indeed highly valued by patients ('knowledgeable' comes up strongly in the *Encounter*—see Table 28.3). But to be effective in empowering patients, giving information competently has to be twinned with a range of what the authors call 'emotional factors', such as (in Table 28.3) the patient feeling that they are 'being heard' and end up 'feeling validated' and that the genetic counsellor is 'empathetic' and 'non-judgemental'.

Understood through the model of values-based practice, the factors that make up the *Empowering Encounter* represent patients' values in the consultation. There will be, as we have seen, further individually unique values that figure crucially in shared decision-making between the clinician and patient. But the factors identified in the *Empowering Encounter* study, representing as they do what matters or is important to patients in the context of psychiatric genetic counselling, are essential as enabling values—they are essential if the counselling is to be effective in engaging with the particular values of the individual patient concerned and hence empower that individual in processes of shared decision-making.

The right hand column of Table 28.3 represents our 'score' for Dr. Jones as represented in the consultation with Jim Smith at the start of the chapter. Her success with the information side of the consultation contrasts with her relative failure in its emotional aspects. And yet as we have seen, both are essential to an effective consultation.

All this of course, as Dr. Jones would no doubt be the first to point out, carries costs—training costs—and, in clinical practice, time costs. These costs we believe should not be overstated. First, there are, at the very least, quick wins to be had. The consultation at the start of this chapter, for example, would have gone very differently if Dr. Jones had introduced herself. Instead of 'Come in and sit down,' she might have said 'Come in and please have a seat, Mr Smith. My name is Dr Jones' (See Guide to Further Information). The time cost of this minimal courtesy would have been negligible and such costs, as there were, would have been amply repaid in terms of enhanced patient engagement and shared decision-making.

Then again, to come to the second of our examples of the resources already available to aid implementation, there are well-validated tools available to support the consultation. The 'metal illness jar' analogy, illustrated in the Fig. 28.1 is a case in point. Derived from practical experience of genetic counselling and developed with input from people with mental health conditions and their family members, the use of this analogy emerged from the *Empowering Encounter* study as a valued resource for meeting the 'understanding' component of an effective counselling experience (see [7]; also Table 28.3).

In offering these brief comments on the resources available to support effective implementation in genetic counselling, we do not wish to be taken to be underestimating the entailed costs. Our point is rather that at least in the case of *psychiatric*

Fig. 28.1 The Mental
Illness Jar Analogy
(see text)

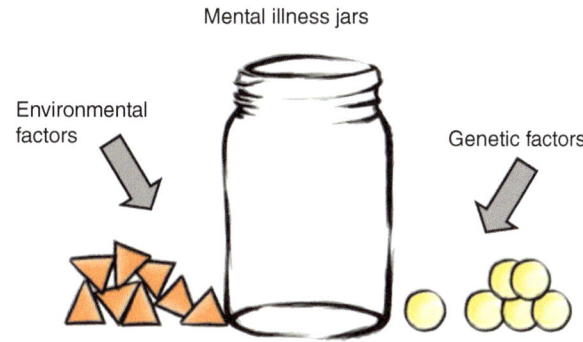

Mental illness jars

Environmental
factors

Genetic factors

genetic counselling, there are resources available that make the costs in principle affordable. Which is good news. For as the story of Jim Smith and his doctor Helen Jones illustrates, the further our journey into genes takes us over the next few years, the more will it become important to attend equally to the values-base as to the evidence-base of this promising but increasingly challenging area of mental health care.

28.4   Conclusions

Our aim in setting the consultation between Dr. Helen Jones and Jim Smith at the start of this chapter in the near future was to anticipate our bottom line, namely, that, as an instance of the wider 'Science Driven' principle of values-based practice, advances in psychiatric genetics, far from resolving the values issues involved in shared decision-making, actually make them ever more acute.

We have focussed here on the implications of the Science Driven principle for practice. But it has in, as it were reverse engineered form, implications for scientific and medical research or at any rate for the translation of such research into improvements in clinical care. Translation of research was the subject of a (2014) blog by Thomas Insel [8], at the time Director of the world's largest neuroscience research funder, the USA's National Institute for Mental Health. Responding to widespread frustration at the failure of the neurosciences to translate into tangible improvements in patient care, Insel launched the RDoC (Research Domain Criteria, [9]) as an alternative to the long-dominant American Psychiatric Associations' DSM (Diagnostic and Statistical Manual). Insel was surely right that the DSM is not the last word in psychiatric diagnostic classification. But the message of the Science Driven principle illustrated by this chapter is that if genetics is any guide, the reasons for the translational failures (with which Insel and others are rightly) concerned have less to do with the deficiencies (real or imagined) of neuroscientific research and more to do with a failure to attend to the factors involved in—to borrow a further phrase from values-based practice (see chapter "Surprised by Values: An Introduction to Values-Based Practice and the Use of Personal Narratives in This Book")—linking science with people.

Acknowledgements The 'mental illness jar analogy in the Fig. 28.1 is based on an illustration by Cindy Campbell-Lashley found in [10]. We are grateful to the Laces Trust for support for the Mental Health Foundation programme exploring patients' perspectives on emerging practice in psychiatric genetics. We would also like to thank our colleagues from the Dragon Cafe for their contribution to this research.

28.5 Guide to Further Information

For more on values-based practice including training resources, please see the website for the Collaborating Centre for Values-based Practice at St Catherine's College, Oxford: valuesbasedpractice.org

Details of the UK Biobank can be found at https://www.ukbiobank.ac.uk/

The 'Hello my name is' campaign website is at: https://www.hellomynameis.org.uk

For further details of the Mental Health Foundation programme exploring patients' perspectives on emerging practice in psychiatric genetics, please see www.mentalhealth.org.uk/our-work/research.

References

1. Department of Health and Social Care. Advancing our health: prevention in the 2020s—consultation document. 2019. https://www.gov.uk/government/consultations/advancing-our-health-prevention-in-the-2020s/advancing-our-health-prevention-in-the2020s-consultation-document.
2. Herring J, Fulford KWM, Dunn D, Handa A. Elbow room for best practice? Montgomery, patients' values, and balanced decision-making in person-centred care. Med Law Rev. 2017;25(4):582–603. https://doi.org/10.1093/medlaw/fwx029. https://academic.oup.com/medlaw/advance-articles. Accessed 19 Jul 2017.
3. Hughes JC, Crepaz-Keay D, Emmett C, Fulford KWM. The Montgomery ruling, individual values and shared decision-making in psychiatry. Br J Psychiatry Adv. 2018;24:93–100. https://doi.org/10.1192/bja.2017.12.
4. Hoop JG, Roberts LW, Hammond KAG, Cox NJ. Psychiatrists' attitudes, knowledge, and experience regarding genetics: a preliminary study. Genet Med. 2008;10(6):439–49. https://www.nature.com/articles/gim200866.pdf.
5. Hollands GJ, French DP, Griffin SJ, Prevost AT, Sutton S, King S, Marteau TM. The impact of communicating genetic risks of disease on risk-reducing health behaviour: systematic review with meta-analysis. Br Med J. 2016;15(352):i1102. https://doi.org/10.1136/bmj.i1102.
6. Resta R, Biesecker BB, Bennett RL, Blum S, Estabrooks Hahn S, Strecker MN, Williams JL. A new definition of genetic counseling: National Society of genetic counselors' task force report. J Genet Couns. 2006;15:77–83. https://doi.org/10.1007/s10897-005-9014-3.
7. Semaka A, Austin J. An "empowering encounter": the process and outcome of psychiatric genetic counseling. J Genet Couns. 2019;28(4):856–8. https://doi.org/10.1002/jgc4.1128.
8. Insel TR. Transforming diagnosis. 2019. www.nimh.nih.gov.

9. Cuthbert BN. The RDoC framework: facilitating transition from ICD/DSM to dimensional approaches that integrate neuroscience and psychopathology. World Psychiatry. 2014;13(1):28–35.
10. Peay HL, Austin JC. How to talk with families about genetics and psychiatric illness. 1st ed. W. W. Norton: New York, NY; 2011.

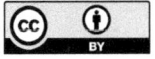

Policy-Making Indabas to Prevent "Not Listening": An Added Recommendation from the Life Esidimeni Tragedy

Samuel Ujewe and Werdie Van Staden

29.1 Introduction

Mental healthcare users, their families, health practitioners and government officials may fear the day that a health policy change turns out to be lethal. This happened in the Life Esidimeni tragedy during 9 months of 2016 and 2017 when more than 140 mental healthcare users died as a consequence of a policy change in a South African province. This chapter summarises and reflects on this tragedy as reported by the Health Ombudsman after a thorough official investigation [1].

One main finding captured as the heading of chapter 10 of the Ombud's report was a "failure to listen". However, none of the recommendations in the report advises that in the future "you should listen". For this reason and averting similar tragedies in the future, we additionally recommend a practical decision-making process by which to listen properly, specifically a policy-making indaba in an African version of values-based practice.

29.2 The Life-Esidimeni Tragedy

In what is arguably the most advanced healthcare system in sub-Saharan Africa, South Africa witnessed a foreseeable consequence of a loosely developed and poorly executed mental healthcare policy in the province of Gauteng. The policy ordered that about 1400 people be moved from Life Esidimeni mental healthcare

S. Ujewe
Canadian Institute for Genomics and Society, Toronto, ON, Canada

W. Van Staden (✉)
Centre for Ethics and Philosophy of Health Sciences, University of Pretoria, South Africa

© The Author(s) 2021
D. Stoyanov et al. (eds.), *International Perspectives in Values-Based Mental Health Practice*, https://doi.org/10.1007/978-3-030-47852-0_29

facilities to multiple care homes of non-governmental organisations (NGOs), resulting in 140 individuals dying over a course of 9 months between 2016 and 2017.
Amidst horrific circumstances, the actual causes of death included thirst and hunger. An autopsy showed two lumps of hard plastic in the stomach of a patient who
had died alone locked up in an outbuilding. Reports indicated furthermore that
many patients were tied up and bundled up into buses and open pick-up vans in
transporting them to their new locations.

The extent of the tragedy became only publically known after a complaint had
been submitted to the Health Ombud. His report presented a deeply concerning situation revealing that all 27 NGOs to which the patients had been transferred operated under invalid licences and that all the deaths occurred under unlawful
circumstances. Unsuitable conditions and incompetence at the NGOs were directly
linked to the high number of deaths among transferred patients.

The Ombud's report showed that for every one death at the Life-Esidimeni care
facilities, there were 19 deaths at the NGOs. This was underscoring that the NGOs
were ill equipped to provide even in the basic needs of the patients they had received.
To add to the problem, at the time of publishing the final Ombud's report, some of
the patients who had been transferred could not be located by the Gauteng
Directorate of Mental Health or their families and the provincial government could
confirm the identities of only 48 of the patients who died. This meant that most of the
families who had lost their loved ones had to wait months to access their bodies,
and others did not even know whether their family members were still alive or dead.

The relocation of patients from the Life Esidimeni healthcare facilities to the
NGOs was ushered by the Gauteng's government's decision to end its long standing
contract with Life Esidimeni Healthcare network. The Gauteng Department of
Health described the move as part of a process to deinstitutionalise patients and
save money. However, the implementation proceeded prematurely with the receiving
institutions accepting patients before they had signed service contracts. This meant
that they went unpaid and were unable to provide adequately for the patients. They
also received patients hastily without clinical records, treatments or health care
plans. As the Ombud report also found, the transfers had been inadequately planned,
chaotic, and rushed.

Before the transfers, the provincial directorate had been forewarned in a couple
of urgent court challenges that the transfers would be unwise, flawed and put
patients' lives at risk. The decision to move the patients out of Life Esidimeni facilities was made against expert advice from professional, user-movement and civil
society stakeholders. The South African Society of Psychiatrists (SASOP) had noted
the risks earlier in 2015 and warned that the transfer would be premature and
highly risky. Likewise, other groups and families of the patients had been very concerned to such an extent that court litigation had been filed against the government.
The court did not proceed with the legal case based on the government's assurance
that patients would not be moved without consent from their families, and that the
facilities and the healthcare would be similar to provisions at the Life-Esidimeni
facilities. These promises were not kept as most affected families were not notified

of, let alone involved in, the transfers. Some only learnt of the transfers and deaths months later.

The Ombud's investigation found that the decision to transfer the patients was a transgression of various laws and a violation of the constitutional human rights of the patients, including a lack of respect for the human dignity of the patients. The latter finding is ironic considering that "esidimeni" is an isiZulu word for "in dignity".

29.3   The Limited Reach of Ombud's Recommendations

Ombud's report concludes with various recommendations. Regarding the past events, these include disciplinary actions, corrective measures, further criminal investigations, legal proceedings, and financial compensation for surviving patients and families. Looking forward to averting the recurrence of similar events, the recommendations are mostly in human rights, regulatory and legal terms. For example, the recommendations are for a systematic and systemic review of human rights compliance and possible violations elsewhere in South Africa, the review of licensing processes, refinements of the relevant laws, and developing checks on legal and regulatory compliance.

Although these recommendations are no less important, their reach is inevitably limited—after all, lives have been lost and the clock cannot be turned back. We want to highlight another limitation, specifically regarding future policy-making. This is, the human rights and regulatory terms of the recommendations do not address one of the key findings of the Ombud, reported as the main finding of its chapter 10. This is "the failure to listen or to take advice", which was of "grave concern".

Instead, the decision to transfer the patients was said to be "final and non-negotiable" and "the project had to be done". The government executive officer "would not listen" and "left no room for engagement". Many employees felt "powerless" and having to implement and deliver the outcome of a project in which they "did not believe", with an outcome they thought "impossible to achieve" and "not do-able within the short time frame". Personnel said they did not "shape the project's evolution", "were not participants in the decision-making processes", and that it was "tough" and "very stressful" to implement. The report alludes to "a general climate and culture of fear and disempowerment" in which families and health workers felt "not being listened to" and "being left out".

The report criticises that the planning process for making the transfers was largely limited to the government officials, without "involving communities and civil society organisations in any credible manner." The failure to listen persisted even when challenged by legal action, going against the warnings and advice of "widespread professional, expert and civil society stakeholders"—warnings that "have sadly come true".

29.4   The Indaba for Listening Properly in Policy-Making

To avert a similar tragedy, we advocate that all stakeholders implied in the formulation and execution of health policy should listen properly to each other. This requirement should extend beyond the reach of rights, laws and regulations, or recommendations in these terms as made in Ombud's report. By analogy, whether and how spouses love each other should generally exceed the reach of matrimonial rights, laws and regulations notwithstanding that these may be relevant potentially.

This means all stakeholders implied in the formulation and execution of health policy should listen properly to each other, not merely in terms of legal and regulatory prescriptions and rights. Although these values may be potentially important, listening to each other would only be done properly when also "listening to" other values of the stakeholders.

An indaba in an African version of values-based practice (A-VBP) is a practical process for stakeholders to listen properly to each other [2]. The isi-Zulu word "indaba" captures a process common in sub-Saharan Africa, described inclusively as a meeting to discuss a matter where individuals and communities have a voice in generating a common story to tell about a matter of concern. Chapter 21 of this volume, titled "Thinking Too Much: A Clash of Legitimate Values in Clinical Practice Calls for an Indaba Guided by African Values-based Practice" illustrates a clinical indaba. An indaba is similarly suited to generate a common story in policy-making.

A policy-making indaba in A-VBP would comprise a meeting during which all the stakeholders implied in the formulation and execution of a health policy listen properly to each other. Indaba participants would listen to what matters to fellow participants, getting to know and understand their values. As described for a clinical indaba in chapter 21 of this volume, listening properly to a fellow participant on what he, she, a community or a society value does not mean that fellow participants have to adopt that value, nor that someone has to compromise or relinquish theirs [3, 4]. Rather, the policy-making indaba would seek to generate a shared story that accounts creatively for differences between values. A key question for leading [3] the policy-making indaba with leadership skills in the Life-Esidimeni situation could for example have been: *how may (the story of) the resulting policy account for the differences between values of the stakeholders without dismissing or changing anyone's values?*

Policy-making indabas in mental health would require that actions of care providers and governing officials create spaces for sustained engagement with the patients, to the extent possible, and their families and/or communities. In the Life Esidimeni case, for instance, the government's decision to terminate the contract or change the nature of care given to the patients should not have been actioned without a family and community indaba. Following this, another indaba to determine where and how to transfer patients should have been undertaken. These indabas could have established common grounds between the government, healthcare providers and the patients' families and communities regarding the conditions of the patients and the nature of care they receive, while also seeking creative ways to account for differences of values among them.

Listening properly to each other in a policy-making indaba may be implored by the human right by which all people are bestowed with dignity, whereby human stakeholders should listen properly to each other. Another perhaps more persuasive reason in an African context is found in an African way of living one's personhood [5]. Personhood in an African context has largely been described in terms of Ubuntu. The idea of Ubuntu situates every individual person within a community or society as inevitably existing in relationship with others around them. Ubuntu also recognises the dependency of a community on its individuals [6]. Thus, a person is a person through other persons, where the individual person is inevitably involved in varied social and moral duties and commitments that focus on the wellbeing of others around them [7]. This means that "the existence of an individual—his/her livelihood, activities, achievements, and burdens—is predicated on those of other individuals, who together share a common social space" [8]. The converse also pertains: the existence of a community is predicated on the existence of its individuals. The relational coexistence derives from the African communal structure that emphasises imperatives for social relationship and vital interdependencies [6, 9]. The ethic, thus, emphasises reciprocal and dual responsibility [9], where individuals are drawn by shared-values towards obligations to each other and to the communities where they belong as well as a responsibility of a community towards anyone of its members.

The nature of African communal and relational personhood means that family or communal participation is crucial in mental health policy-making. Given the social embeddedness of personhood in African settings, the person suffering from a mental disorder would be considered as being compromised in or even losing his/her personhood, owing to the isolation and impaired social functioning commonly associated with mental disorder. When the affected person becomes less a part of his/her network of relationships, the situation is of crucial social consequence, not only for the person affected, but also for their families, communities and entire network of relationships.

The decision to end the care services of Life Esidimeni was initiated through a process that did not recognise the communal embeddedness of their personhood. The emphasis on the financial dimension further buttresses the lack of acknowledgement of the patients' place within their communities, especially by shutting out third-party participation in the process. Instead, a prior indaba process in the Life Esidimeni case could have ensured that decisions recognised these social interdependencies of personhood. Through an indaba, finding harmony among the differing perspectives in the decision-making process might have averted the tragedy that ensued.

29.5 Conclusions

A policy-making indaba within A-VBP provides a practical process in which all stakeholders implied in the formulation and execution of health policy may listen properly to each other. Listening properly to each other entails that the differing values are accounted for in the resulting policy, which is in effect contracting co-authorship and co-responsibility for a health policy. Accordingly, policy-makers are not merely governmental officials and politicians but are extended to all stakeholders implied in the formulation and execution of a health policy. Especially familiar in an African context, this extension may be impelled by an African communal and relational way of living personhood, whereby reciprocal responsibility is taken up for each other among individuals as well as between a community and its individual members [5, 6, 9].

References

1. Makgopa MW. The report into the circumstances surrounding the deaths of mentally ill patients: Gauteng province. Republic of South Africa: Health Ombud; 2017.
2. Van Staden CW, Fulford KWM. The indaba in African values-based practice: respecting diversity of values without ethical relativism or individual liberalism. In: Sadler JZ, van Staden CW, Fulford KWM, editors. Oxford handbook of psychiatric ethics. Oxford: Oxford University Press; 2015.
3. Van Staden CW. Spiritual and other diversities at the heart of invigorating leadership: a South African spark. Int J Leadersh Public Serv. 2010;6:73–7.
4. Van Staden CW. Stuck in the past or heading for flourishing people in diversity. S Afr J Psychiatry. 2010;16:4–6.
5. Van Staden CW. African approaches to an enriched ethics of person-centred health practice. Int J Pers Cent Med. 2011;1:11–7.
6. Crepaz-Keay D, Fulford KWM, Van Staden CW. Putting both a person and people first: interdependence, values-based practice and African Batho Pele as resources for co-production in mental health. In: Sadler JZ, van Staden CW, Fulford KWM, editors. Oxford handbook of psychiatric ethics. Oxford: Oxford University Press; 2015.
7. Munyaka M, Motlhabi M. Ubuntu and its socio-moral significance. In: Murove MF, editor. African ethics: an anthology of comparative and applied ethic. Scottsville: University of KwaZulu-Natal Press; 2009.
8. Ujewe SJ. Just health care in Nigeria – the foundations for an African ethical framework. Preston: University of Central Lancashire; 2016. p. 124–5.
9. Gyekye K. Tradition and modernity: philosophical reflections on the African experience. Oxford: Oxford University Press; 1997.

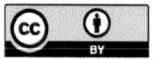

Covert Treatment in a Cross-Cultural Setting

30

Neil Pickering

30.1 Introduction

In the course of the narrative case in this chapter, the ethical question of the use of covert treatment (CT) arises. The parents of a young man (Arjun) have brought him for a consultation with a psychiatrist. The family are from India, but live and work in the UK. The parents have concerns that Arjun has had recurrence of a mental illness, but Arjun refuses to accept this. Rather, he believes that his path and that planned for him by his parents have diverged.

The parents believe that CT may be a solution to the problem that has arisen and relate how Arjun's previous mental health issues were treated in this way, while they were visiting India some years before. The psychiatrist—herself from India—refuses to consider CT for Arjun, citing the local (UK) law. Yet she is torn at least in the sense that her previous experience in India has also shown that CT can be successful, and she fears for Arjun's future without medication. She is also aware of cultural influences on the ethical assessment of CT.

The story is invented but based on published cases [1–3]. The psychiatrist is from India where she trained and first practiced.

30.2 Narrative History

Arjun comes in with his mother and father. It's my first consultation with them and I invite them all to sit at my desk. Arjun seems to prefer to stand, somewhat in the background from my perspective. His parents are neatly dressed, business people (it turns out). They are all of Indian descent—as am I. The three of them moved to the UK from New Delhi 15 years previously. I observe Arjun while his mother and

N. Pickering (✉)
Bioethics Centre, University of Otago, Dunedin, New Zealand

D. Stoyanov et al. (eds.), *International Perspectives in Values-Based Mental Health Practice*, https://doi.org/10.1007/978-3-030-47852-0_30

father talk. He is dressed in casual jeans—slightly dirty looking and torn—a newish t-shirt, and old trainers. He is distinctly unkempt, unshaven, and his teeth look like they could do with a clean. I briefly reflect on my own appearance—much more like the parents' than the son's.

"So, how can I help?" I ask. His father tells me that he and his wife are very worried about Arjun.

"Until about 6 months ago, he seemed to be doing very well—he was studying for an MBA at college. Or so we thought. He is a very bright boy. Then suddenly, we found he had stopped studying 3 months before! We didn't notice anything at the time. We're very busy, we run an import-export business, and we're at work all hours."

"He won't talk to us, Doctor" says Arjun's mother.

"He is our only child" says his father, "and we plan for him to join us in the business. We have spent many thousands of dollars on his education. He has done well—top grades at school and as an undergraduate. But now ..." his voice trails off.

I ask if I can speak to Arjun on his own. "I don't know if you'll get anything much out of him" says his mother as she and her husband leave.

It does take some time to get Arjun's attention, and even then he doesn't seem keen to talk about his health.

"Look, I'm fine" he says eventually. "I just lost interest in my studies, that's all. It happens, right? It was all about business and finance and stuff. But that's all very material, isn't it? Now I'm studying the soul."

"Your parents are worried" I venture.

"That's their soul—you see!" he says. "They're tied up in the details of the world—the material things. They think there's something wrong with me—because I have communications with other souls. But it's not my fault they're deaf to the soul-world."

Now he's talking, he's quite voluble. A picture emerges of a person who has auditory hallucinations—these souls he says he talks to. And he seems to have some delusions related to them, though they're all fairly harmless in themselves. Except, just occasionally as Arjun continues, there's something paranoid—"souls can read souls" he says, a little darkly. "Nothing can be hidden in the soul-verse."

After around 15 min, I invite his parents back in and Arjun goes out for a smoke.

"Well," I say cautiously, "I'd need to see him for longer to be sure, but in my judgement he's hearing voices and he's got some minor delusions. There's just a touch of paranoia."

"Can you give him something, doctor?" asks Arjun's father. "Something to get him back on track."

"Not without his consent" I reply.

"We've tried that" says his father. "He doesn't even see there's anything wrong with him."

"When we were visiting India about 6 or 7 years ago" says Arjun's mother "they gave him something—he didn't know"

"Was he unwell then, too?" I ask.

"Yes," says the father, "it was before he went to university, and we took him on a trip back to New Delhi; he suddenly started talking to himself all the time, and he got a bit aggressive with his mother. But he wouldn't accept help—just like now. Well, my wife's uncle is a doctor in that part of India, and he suggested giving him some medicine in his tea. He was back to normal in no time."

I hesitate—covert medication was something that I'd used in India myself, before I came to the UK. But its use was a matter of lively debate. What about individual choice? Well—there was scepticism about the sort of Western bioethical ideas that we'd all heard of—autonomy, individual patient rights, and so on. Fine in a rich country like the UK. Anyway, wasn't Indian society characterised by a sense of family and community? A debate on the same lines was going on in the Indian psychiatry journals at that very time [4]. Sometimes, family comes first— that this was our Indian heritage, our culture. Individualism and bioethics principles based on it were foreign. In the actual case where I used covert treatment, it'd seemed to work—in not dissimilar circumstances to those of Arjun. The patient was a young woman who had been training to be a teacher; suddenly, she'd said she'd been told to take a different path—but some anti-psychotics in her food had sorted all that out.

"I can't support giving him medicine without his agreement," I said after a moment. "You can't do that here—it's against the law. We'll have to try and persuade him he needs help."

"Good luck with that" Arjun's father says bitterly.

Arjun re-joins us, but after some conversation, where I give my professional view, he is clearly not budging. "Look, I'm moving on" he says.

"You'll be moving out" says his father, "if you don't sort yourself out."

"Whatever" replies Arjun.

Where might this be going? Parents getting more and more worried, rows about Arjun not paying his way, doing something with his life; him pushing back. He'll perhaps end up leaving home—couch surfing, at least until his friends get sick of him? Meanwhile, his untreated state of mind is likely to deteriorate. And then …. The uncle in India—when they were on holiday there—he acted quickly, sorting out Arjun's first psychotic episode. Set him on track for a place in the community. But Arjun's trajectory here in the UK is likely to be rather different—into social isolation, a life in fragments. It's not certain, of course: but it's a good bet. What would really be wrong with giving him the help he needs but won't ask for—now, before he ends up in the system, before he estranges his family and friends? Isn't that what I'm here for? True, at this stage, he's able to decide for himself—yet even now, when the delusions are still harmless enough, isn't he already not himself? And what of the family—of which he is a part, which has brought him up? Isn't that an important and real part of the picture?

"So, what do we do now?" asks Arjun's mother, with desperation in her voice.

The only response I have is to advise them to keep talking to him, persuading him, helping him see what's happening. "Make another appointment, for two weeks' time" I say. As I usher them out, my next patient is waiting.

30.3   Values Arising in This Story

In the following analysis, at first, a general assessment of the values at play will be given, before the focus falls on CT and the legitimacy of the value differences at play.

Value-Based Medicine (VBM) focuses on the values in play in narratives where there are differences of view about what to do. We can take values in the wide sense of what matters or is important to those concerned in the story. Two features are strongly expressed in the narrative:

1. Value of education and study, the ethic of work
2. Value of individual freedom—self-expression

(These two values also link to others—see below.)

The first of these—the value placed in education, study and work—is explicitly stated by Arjun's parents. One can imagine that the psychiatrist implicitly endorses these values too. But Arjun implicitly endorses the value of individual freedom—of choosing a path for himself, one different to that his parents have embraced and have desired for him. These two values, of education, study and work, and individual expression, while they do not necessarily conflict with one another, have in the narrative become a focus of difference and disagreement.

A number of other values can also be found in the narrative—some of these are clearly related in various ways to the first two. These include:

3. Value of family—of continuing a line, perhaps of giving back, building the future
4. Value of independence—of being able to support oneself, and ultimately give back
5. Value of social acceptance and social connectedness—having friends, a place in the society, and the fear of isolation
6. Value of appearance—how you present yourself (with associated values of neatness, cleanliness and so on)
7. Value of culture—of what matters to a group, which ties it back to its roots, which it can appeal to
8. Value of health—as an enabler of other things or as a value in itself
9. Value of mental stability and coherence, capacity to decide, perhaps relatedly, authenticity and identity
10. Value of autonomy—conceived abstractly as an expression of an individual's capacity to make authentic decisions and his or her right to be free
11. The values of beneficence and non-maleficence which (like autonomy) are abstracted conceptions, in this case capturing concerns about people's well-being
12. The overt values of a profession, such as the profession of psychiatry (which may vary in different cultural contexts) but might include: patient centred care, least restrictive methods of treatment, restoring health and preventing ill health

Some of these values are part of the background—they are values against which paths and states of human lives can be gauged, including ones against which a person's health can be judged. Others seem perhaps to be more in the foreground, setting the problems by which the immediate situation is characterized. Some values seem to unite and some seem to divide—and this includes concrete values around day-to-day appearance and behavior, as well as the more abstract ideas such as the value of work, or of finding one's own way, discussed earlier.

30.4 Covert Treatment (CT)

Briefly, CT can be defined as treating someone in such a way as to deliberately prevent them from knowing that they are being treated. There is a substantial but quite fragmented literature on this practice (see further reading).

30.5 Cultural Values and CT

Cultural values can be identified as those shared by and transmitted through groups of people. In the sense of a set or sets of shared (group) beliefs and values, which play an explicit or implicit guiding role in their behavior, everyone has a culture or cultures.

Relatedly, in the literature on CT—especially in its use with those with mental health problems—a cultural divide has been identified. There are cultures where the focus is more on the family or community, and where CT may be seen as justified for mental health problems, and cultures where the focus is more on the autonomy of the individual, and where CT for mental health may not be seen as acceptable [5, 6].

Arjun's family's request for CT may well be associated with the values perspective of their Indian culture. This perspective—sometimes generalized even further to 'the East'—is often presented as being focused on family and community, to which the individual is said (descriptively) to be subordinate.

> In an Indian family life, one's individuality is subordinated to collective solidarity, and one's ego is submerged into the collective ego of the family and one's community. Consequently, when a problem—financial, medical, psychiatric, or whatever—affects an individual, it affects the entire family. ... [7]

This should be taken in a slightly more radical way than simply that the family is affected by the illness of one of its members. Arjun's family expect Arjun to share their plans for him; and these plans reflect the continuity of the family's shared identity inter alia in the business they run. Arjun's illness has effects on the family through its impact on these shared plans, and not only through the parents' concern for him as an individual suffering from a disease.

This has significant normative implications for the individual:

> It is expected for an individual to stay part of the family and of the community, the individual will submit to communal norms and will not deviate to an extent where it becomes necessary for the deviant to be ostracized. ... [7]

Given this background, CT may seem sometimes to be justified. This justification may not be (as it might appear to 'western' eyes) merely a rationalization of an imposition of conformity, or paternalism. Rather, it may be a means by which the ostracism of an individual can be avoided, where avoiding this is justified by the perceived significance of group membership to individuals.

On the other hand, individual autonomy can be conceived (in traditional and abstract bioethical terms) as an achievement and right (as in the right to respect for autonomy). In this form, autonomy has become foundational in contemporary 'Western' bioethics. From this 'Western' perspective, it is natural to assume that respect for Arjun's autonomy is the key guiding value in the story.

The adherence to individualistic notions of autonomy may lead to CT being seen as fundamentally an insult to the self-determination of individuals. Indeed, it has been argued that it is inherently self-defeating to deploy CT to attempt to treat someone with a psychiatric problem, since the aim of treatment is to return autonomy to an individual person. This aim is fundamentally undermined by a method that relies on taking autonomy away [8].

30.6   Cultural Values and Value-Based Medicine (VBM)

VBM invites us to attend to the values that may underlie disagreement and tensions amongst people and between health professionals and their patients and patients' families.

These differences of values are explicitly recognised in the multiperspective principle of VBM:

> In VBM, conflicts of values are resolved primarily, not by reference to a rule that prescribes a "right" outcome but by processes designed to support a balance of legitimately different perspectives ... [9].

The use of the term 'legitimate' here suggests that there are criteria for distinguishing legitimately different from nonlegitimately different values perspectives. But this is misleading—in fact the scope of legitimate value differences is the same as the scope of value differences.

> That our values are not only different but legitimately different also follows analytically from the separation of fact and value (or, more exactly, of description and evaluation) insisted on by "nondescriptivism" in philosophical value theory [9].

The argument is that different value perspectives are legitimately different because there is not necessarily a right value perspective. In contrast, in cases of differences over facts (description) one can assume that there is a right description, and there are means for moving to consensus. For example, doctors and families might disagree about whether a particular drug can help the patient or not—but a consensus is in principle achievable (e.g. by trying the patient on the drug). But an ethical disagreement about whether CT is an acceptable approach to treatment may represent an irresolvable dissensus.

However, the narrative is set in within the wider UK cultural context. The setting does seem to give a particular weight to the values supporting the individual's rights as against those of the group. Indeed, it might be said that this value is so widely shared in the UK that it would fall under the category of a value that is rightly supported by regulation [9].

30.7   Transcultural Ethical Perspective

The transcultural approach to ethics [10] seeks to challenge a simplistic assumption of cultural homogeneity.

There has been a tendency amongst anthropologists, for example, to exaggerate and emphasize cultural difference, constructing cultures as 'radical others'. One assumption underlying the notion that cultures represent 'radical others' is that cultures are homogeneous, having, for example, a single mind set (or mentality). In contrast, transcultural approaches draw attention to the internal variety of cultures and the resulting complexity of commonalities and differences between cultures.

For example, the widely cited contrast between communalistic/family oriented cultures and individualistically oriented cultures might be thought to underlie and determine different attitudes to CT in those cultures. But, within a culture, the relationship of the individual to the wider group may be discussed and perhaps contested, and the claims of both may be explored and questioned.

In the UK, this internal variability presents itself through the significance placed on decision-making competence. This is the site of a fundamental disagreement, about whether and to what extent a poor decision (as judged by community standards) is systematically linked to faulty decision making processes, that is to decision making incompetence. What hangs on this judgement is the point at which the individual loses authority over his or her own decisions.

While there is no space to go into the detail about the disagreements on this point, the heterogeneity at issue is most obviously expressed in the contending views taken on what is called asymmetry. Asymmetry is the view that while a person may have the capacity to choose to accept a treatment that the same person may simultaneously lack the capacity to refuse the very same treatment. Asymmetry in effect provides a means by which autonomy may be limited to those whose choice conforms to that expected by or approved by society.

But asymmetry is not accepted by all. Within the UK, there is a significant division of opinion, suggesting variability rather than homogeneity of values or at least of the weight to be placed upon values.

30.8 Conclusions

VBM supports the idea that differing value perspectives are inherently worthy of consideration—that they are legitimate.

Transcultural ethics tends to offer support for the legitimacy of different value perspectives. It recognises, for example, that within a culture there may be significant variability. As a result, a practice, such as CT, can become the focus of considerable debate within a cultural group, as well as cross-culturally.

In the UK, however, a dominant value—that of individual autonomy—receives strong legal support. In view of this, the case for CT for Arjun doesn't seem to have cultural legitimacy. It is ruled out, whatever the values may be that support it.

Yet, even in the UK, the value of autonomy may be tempered through the mechanism of capacity assessment. In the UK, competence is a central judgement. It is related to the potential harmfulness of a person's choice through the idea of asymmetry. CT for mental health patients may not seem to be a legitimate option in the UK. However, the urge, expressed by Arjun's parents and psychiatrist, to prevent any further decline in his health and avoid a feared future of social isolation is also expressed in the malleability of capacity judgements.

Acknowledgements My grateful thanks to the editors of this volume, Taryn Knox, attendees at the 2018 INPP Conference (Hong Kong) and Bioethics Centre seminar (2019), and the members of the Bioethics Centre Postgraduate Forum, all of whom commented on various earlier versions of this paper.

30.9 Guide to Further Sources

In addition to the Indian Journal of Psychiatry issue [4] and [1–3, 5, 6, 8], a case discussion of CT was published in the Asian Bioethics Review (Pickering NJ. (ed.) 2013. Case Scenario 2: Covert Treatment of Violent Patients. *Asian Bioethics Review* 5(3):198-223). For articles on Transcultural approaches to ethics see [10] and the other articles in that special edition of the Kennedy Institute Journal of Ethics.

References

1. Khurshid KA. A tale of two cities. Am J Psychiatry. 2006;163(8):1335–6.
2. Wong JGWS, Poon Y, Hui EC. Clinical ethics "I can put the medicine in his soup, Doctor!". J Med Ethics. 2005;31:262–5. https://doi.org/10.1136/jme.2003.007336.
3. Kala AK. Covert medication; the last option: a case for taking it out of the closet and using it selectively. Indian J Psychiatry. 2012;54(3):257–65. https://doi.org/10.4103/0019-5545.102427. PMCID: PMC3512364.
4. Sathyanarayana Rao TS, Kallilvayalil RA', Andrade C, Kala AK, Antony JT, Murthy RS, Sarin A, Ramachandran P, Rangaswamy T, Srinivasan N, Srinivasan T. Editorial and Special Theme. Indian J Psychiatry. 2012;54(3):203–5, 257–79.

5. Srinivasan T, Thara R. At issue: management of medication noncompliance in schizophrenia by families in India. Schizophr Bull. 2002;28:531–5.
6. Stroup S, Swartz M, Appelbaum P. Concealed medicines for people with schizophrenia: a U.S perspective. Schizophr Bull. 2002;28:537–42.
7. Laungani P. Mental illness in India and Britain: theory and practice. Med Law. 1997;16:509–40.
8. Aherne L, van Tosh L. Taking issue: the irreversible damage caused by surreptitious prescribing. Psychiatr Serv. 2005;56:383.
9. Fulford, KWM (2009) Facts/Values: Ten Principles of Values-Based Medicine . In Radden J (ed.) The Philosophy of Psychiatry: A Companion Published to Oxford Scholarship Online: January 2009 https://doi.org/10.1093/acprof:oso/9780195149531.001.0001. https://doi.org/10.1093/acprof:oso/9780195149531.003.0017.
10. Nie J-B, Fitzgerald RP. Connecting the east and the west, the local and the universal: the methodological elements of a transcultural approach to bioethics. Kennedy Inst Ethics J. 2016;26(3):219–47.

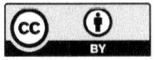

Discouragement Towards Seeking Health Care of Older People in Rural China: The Influence of Culture and Structural Constraints

Xiang Zou

31.1 Introduction

Within contemporary bioethical writing, ethical deliberations about patients' health-seeking behaviours have long been centred on issues of patients' rights, agency and autonomy. This right-based ethical paradigm, however, is incomplete, as it conveys by and large the values of those privileged patients in developed social settings—i.e. those who tend to be autonomous, who have relatively better access to quality medical care resources and who are able to navigate institutional structures proactively. In contrast, values regarding the health-seeking behaviours of patients in underdeveloped sociocultural contexts have long been omitted.

This chapter speaks to the values of and perspectives towards seeking health care among older patients in Chinese rural settings. Those concerned are in general financially disadvantaged, highly dependent and hence less autonomous and lack proper access to health care. This chapter portrays the discouraged, despairing attitudes about the elderly seeking health care in rural China, as internalised by older patients themselves and expressed by their families and the public. Underlying this discouragement is a widespread cultural value, namely the social expectation that people should endure suffering and hence that the importance of seeking elderly health care should be downplayed. Additionally, this discouraged attitude mirrors the lack of proper access to commodified health care of rural patients as an aspect of the rural-urban structural divide.

Drawing upon empirical data collected from 6 months of field work in a Chinese rural hospital, Qincun Hospital, in 2016, this chapter illustrates the discouraged attitude towards older patients seeking health care through the story of Aunt Chen, an older mother who was hospitalized in Qincun Hospital during the time of the current study, to obtain hospital care and the reactions of her family. Oral informed

X. Zou (✉)
Department of Medical Humanities, Southeast University, Nanjing, China
e-mail: xiang.zou@hotmail.com

consent was given by the family involved in the case study published below. To protect the confidentiality of the research participants, all identifying information was removed. For example, the names used in this chapter—including those of interviewees and locations—are pseudonyms. The Human Ethics Committee of the University of Otago in New Zealand approved the research (Reference No. 15/106).

31.2 Aunt Chen's Story

Aunt Chen, an 83-year-old widow, suffered from multiple chronic symptoms. Over the past decade she had been heavily reliant on inpatient treatment for pain relief. Like most rural residents over 60 years of age in China, Aunt Chen did not have any formal source of income to secure medical care. Given this situation, the responsibility for her long-term care and treatment-related decision-making fell on her family—that is, her three children. Additionally, due to the lack of access to quality health care resources (most of which were located in urban settings), the Qincun Hospital was sought as the most affordable solution to her health care needs.

Over the past decade of health seeking, Aunt Chen's symptoms had continued to progress with much of her care and treatment proving futile. Her family thus felt discouraged and became reluctant to continue support for her medical care. Discouragement was further exacerbated by the fact that her three children had migrated to city areas for employment. Aunt Chen however remained proactive about seeking hospital care and treatment despite these discouragements. The family process of negotiating medical care and family support led to severe conflicts between the two generations. For example, during the current study, there was an occasion that Aunt Chen suffered from a recurrence of coronary heart problems and requested her children to send her to Qincun Hospital. Her family, however, rejected her request since, at that time, the whole family was involved in the preparations for a young family member's wedding ceremony, asserting that nobody had the time or energy to accompany her on a hospital visit. Seeing there was no way out, Aunt Chen threatened to commit suicide during the wedding if her family still rejected her request for a hospital visit: "Don't be busy with the wedding, prepare for my funeral!"

Aunt Chen's threat worked and she was sent over to the hospital where medical drips were promptly offered. The threat, on the other hand, heightened her children's annoyance. For example, Aunt Chen's third son once made a comment about her persistent health seeking and preoccupation with longevity—he saw this as "unreasonable" and said it was "because she was too scared of death". "If you don't [bring her to the hospital], she threatens she will die or will tell other people we children are not filial…Which older person does not have some pain? Does it really need hospital treatment? She had seen her 83rd already. Why can't she just let it go?" The moral concern of being accused as "un-filial" pressure the family to continue their support with Aunt Chen's hospital care and medications.

This view was shared by other people in their circle who agreed that, as an older person, Aunt Chen had asked "too much", and that it was wrong of her to pursue health care and longevity. For instance, Aunt Wang, another 80-year-old mother who was also hospitalised, narrated her own experiences and encouraged Aunt Chen to be "reasonable" in the face of family neglect: "Every time I was sick, my children just pretended that they had no idea about it. But that's all right. Being an older person, you need to be content [zhizu] with what you've got!" The view that Aunt Chen was in the wrong was also expressed by a doctor from Qincun Hospital, who said: "You know she [Aunt Chen] will never to be able to get well. It is unwise to be always clinging to life and devote much to medical care…At her age, it is not worth treating that seriously…"

Aunt Chen was just in her 50s when her husband died. To raise her four children, she endured enormous hardships and suffering working as a farm labourer. These hardships and suffering, she believed, were the cause of her ill condition, "I worked too hard, that's why I became so sick when I got old"- an interpretation morally justified her chronic conditions that deserved proper care and support from her children in repayment. Her family's negligence and public accusations made her feel wounded. She resisted them by revealing a strong will to live: "everyone said I should come back home and wait for death. But I'm not prepared for it yet!"

On the other hand, Aunt Chen also internalised the public discouragements, expressing a deep concern of being accused as "greedy" and her family's reluctance to take on the heavy burden of support for her long-term health care: "I know they were so fed up with me. If I continue living in the hospital, they will get very angry and stop offering me anything…"

The result was that Aunt Chen managed to cut short the length of her inpatient stay. After only a few days of treatment, she requested to be discharged and to return home for rehabilitation. It was unknown how she would be treated at home.

31.3 The Values Arising in This Case

Aunt Chen's story highlights the prevailing discouraging attitude towards seeking elderly health care in a Chinese rural locality. This discouraging attitude was expressed by Aunt Chen's family and came to be particularly prominent when the family prioritised the younger member's wedding ceremony over seeking for Aunt Chen hospital care and treatment. Discouragement is also revealed in the attitudes of local people who accused Aunt Chen of being immoral for asking "too much" in the way of medical care. Underpinning these discouragements is the value that older people's health was "unworthy of care and treatment" and therefore their proactive health-seeking behaviours are morally "inappropriate" and culturally unacceptable. Instead, what is "appropriate" for an older people is to be self-restrained with seeking health care, being good at enduring chronic pain and suffering, and to consciously reduce the burden of health care on their families. This local perception is in direct opposition to the conventional (in Western medical ethics) positive understanding of "ideal" patients who proactively engage in health-seeking and pursuing personal well-being.

A set of contradictory values arises from her attempts to sustain medical care and family support; however, her struggle with unfavourable values and conventions discourages her from doing so. As a patient, Aunt Chen revealed a strong will in pursuing her desire for personal health and longevity. As an older family member, on the other hand, she also bore the moral expectation of being self-restrained and reasonable, prioritising the interests of the whole family and reducing the burden of medical care on them. Torn between these contradictory values, her case provides a lens on what really mattered for Aunt Chen, as a patient or a socially accepted older person, when accommodating these different values and priorities and seeking a middle-way out. It also encourages us to ask what kind of social, cultural and structural backdrop shapes the circumstances that discourages and devalues health care seeking for older people. It is to this that I turn next.

31.4 The Social, Cultural and Structural Backdrop of Aunt Chen's Story

The public discouragement illustrated by Aunt Chen's story mirrors cultural values common in many rural regions, that view enduring pain and suffering as being morally "upright" personal virtues. As reported in contemporary literature, personal characteristics such as maintaining thrifty and self-constrained lifestyles, and being good at enduring hardships and conscious of reducing their adult children's financial burdens, are usually perceived as morally upright and positive for older people in rural China [1–3]. These cultural values encourage older people to be self-restrained with seeking health and much needed care for themselves since they view these as the behaviours "appropriate" for older people and wish to become socially recognised virtuous members of their society.

Related to these cultural values, a discourse of "worthlessness" and ageist discriminations, constructed under the influence of a market economy, also contribute to the devalued significance of care for the aged in China. In the traditional Chinese society, most older people enjoyed a high gerontological status and were honoured for their mastery of wisdom and representation of high moral standards of the society [4]. Throughout the economic reforms of the past three decades, marketization and privatisation have created a new image of self-actualising and self-reliant individuals, under which people were encouraged to bear their own responsibilities for health care and late-age support. Just as the market economy prioritised independence and competitiveness, so it also problematized the image of Aunt Chen, and other older people who like her were frail, feeble and sick, relying on external care and support to survive. Older people had seen a decreased gerontological status from experiencing socioeconomic transformations in China, and their health needs were perceived as a "worthless" socioeconomic burden. Both the state and individual families become reluctant to support aged care. Unwillingness to care is heightened by the massive outwards migration of rural populations to urban areas to seek employment, from which rural families experienced comprised capacities and resources to assist health-seeking for their older members.

Another social force that contributes to the discouragement of health seeking behaviour among the elderly is the lack of access to health care resources that has been a product of the persistent rural-urban divide. The Chinese household registration policy (*hukou* system) [5, 6] designated all Chinese residents to one of two types of households, either rural or urban, based on the types of for the aged employment they were entitled. Based on this divide, rural residents were granted with inferior access to social welfare, such as insurance coverage and social pension systems (in contrast to urban dwellers). The lack of institutional support means rural older residents had to rely on their families to secure health care and late-age support constrained as they were by structural obstacles. Additionally, the *hukou* system also constructs a sense of inferiority amongst rural residents that by labelling them as "second-class", "backward peasants" [1, 7]. This social discourse is highly discriminated and further discourages health-seeking of rural older people.

Discouragement to seeking support in old age was further intensified by a lack of trust in the commodified health care industry in China. Since China started market economy reforms in the 1980s, the government gradually withdrew its funding from social welfare systems. The public hospitals became underfunded, and health provides increasingly reliant on revenues generated by fees for high-tech interventions and (often excessive) prescriptions [8]. Meanwhile, as much for the aged of expenditures were devoted to the development of larger hospitals in urban areas, rural hospitals suffered from severe staff and compromised quality of medical care facilities [9]. These institutional changes resulted in heightened financial barriers of accessing hospital care that further disadvantaged rural older people who were of lower socioeconomic status. Discouragement to support elderly health care was further heightened by the public pessimism about the curability and recovery of older people's chronic symptoms, making the public refusal and the perception of elderly health-seeking as a waste of resources culturally legitimated.

31.5 Conclusions

Drawing upon the case of health-seeking of Aunt Chen's family collected from a 6-month field work in a rural primary hospital, this chapter portrays a discouraged, dispiriting attitude towards health-seeking of rural older people in China. Underpinning this discouragement is the prevalence of discriminatory attitudes that by downplaying the significance of elderly health care as "worthless" socioeconomic burden. The construction of this "worthless" perception is not only culture-related but also structure-induced. The cultural belief is that morally prioritising older people's good endurance of pain and suffering and self-restrained personal characteristics significantly contributes to the public discouragements towards elderly health-seeking. In addition, the structural reality of rural-urban divide and socioeconomic deprivations compounds the public discouragements and devaluation. In this respect, this discouraged attitude not only reflects the influence of cultural values but also suggests rural residents' dissatisfaction with the state-based social welfare system in contemporary rural China.

Acknowledgements The author is in debt to all of the participants in the study.

31.6   Guide to Further Sources

1. The Chinese term *zhizu* literately can be translated as "the feeling of being content" in English. In the Chinese social context, *zhizu* indicates a disposition that encourages people to be self-restrained with and actively low their expectations on pursuing personal interests and desires for achieving the ends of happiness and welfare. Keeping *zhizu* has been perceived as a type of personal virtue and thus morally upright and culturally encouraged.
2. For more details about the geographic information of the field site, Chengcun Town (程 村 镇), where the Qingcun Hospital was located, see: https://baike. baidu.com/item/ (in Chinese), access on 15th November, 2019.

References

1. Long Y, Li LW. "How would we deserve better?" Rural–urban dichotomy in health seeking for the chronically ill elderly in China. Qual Health Res. 2016;26(12):1689–704.
2. Lora-Wainwright A. 'If you can walk and eat, you don't go to hospital': the quest for healthcare in rural Sichuan. In: Duckett J, editor. China's changing welfare mix local perspectives. 1st ed. New York: Taylor and Francis; 2011.
3. Lora-Wainwright A. Fighting for breath: living morally and dying of cancer in a Chinese village. Honolulu: University of Hawaii Press; 2013.
4. Benjamin D, Brandt L, Rozelle S. Aging, wellbeing, and social security in rural northern China. Popul Dev Rev. 2000;26:89–116.
5. Chan KW, Zhang L. The Hukou system and rural-urban migration in China: processes and changes. China Q. 1999;160:818–48.
6. Zhang Z, Treiman DJ. Social origins, hukou conversion, and the wellbeing of urban residents in contemporary China. Soc Sci Res. 2013;42(1):71–89.
7. Zhang L, Ong A. Privatizing China: socialism from afar. Ithaca: Cornell University Press; 2008.
8. Yip WC, Hsiao WC, Chen W, Hu S, Ma J, Maynard A. Early appraisal of China's huge and complex health-care reforms. Lancet. 2012;379(9818):833–42.
9. Zou X, Nie J-B. Access to care by older rural people in a post-reform Chinese hospital: an ethical evaluation of anthropological findings. Asian Bioeth Rev. 2019;11(1):57–68.

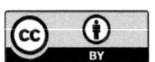

Discovering Myself, a Journey of Rediscovery

Waldo Roeg

32.1 Introduction

I currently work as a Peer Recovery Trainer at Central North West London NHS Foundation Trust (CNWL) Recovery College. I am also a consultant for Implementing Recovery through Organizational Change (ImROC). But my life was not always so. Indeed, I have used services now for over 35 years, both for my drug and substance misuse and for my mental health. In this chapter, I tell the story of my recovery: of the many wonderful people who supported me in my journey; and of how my experience is now helping me in my current role working with others towards their own recovery.

32.2 Homeless and Without Hope

It all started when I was a teenager. I came from an affluent family, had a good career in films for 25 years ... and learned how to hide my problems. Well that couldn't last. It ended 17 years ago now when I had a major breakdown and lost everything. I became bankrupt, so lost my home. I lost my career as I had been 'found out'. I lost my partner, family, dignity and status in society. But most of all I lost myself.

I ended up living on the street with only the clothes I stood up in. I moved from one dealer to another, doing odd jobs for them for measly bits of drugs and the crumbs from their tables, turning to petty crime to fund my meager existence. I

W. Roeg (✉)
Central and North-West London Recovery and Wellbeing College, Central and North West NHS Foundation Trust, London, UK

© The Author(s) 2021
D. Stoyanov et al. (eds.), *International Perspectives in Values-Based Mental Health Practice*, https://doi.org/10.1007/978-3-030-47852-0_32

ended up in constant conflict with law enforcement and in and out of police cells. My only goal was to survive. My existence was so precarious that I feared that trying to improve my situation—risk what little I had—might rebound badly on me. I learned that any efforts that I made did little to improve my situation. I felt I had become worthless and became very cautious about making any efforts to move on.

32.3 Point Zero

All the stigma associated with my mental health and substance misuse was heightened 100% by being in such poverty and so reliant on state aid as my only income … and a very small income it was because I was of 'no fixed abode'. I was made to feel utterly useless by services who saw me only as another worthless mad junkie on the streets. They tried to mitigate my symptoms with medication and it made me believe that was all there was going to be for me. My interaction with services at the time was minimal—just enough to ensure a supply of medication.

I did just enough to survive and became acclimatized to it. My own sense of shame and stigma was such that I adopted the way of the street just to be able to identify with something. I worked out that it was easier to stop short of doing anything to better myself as I thought it would not yield sufficient gain to outweigh the extra effort. This gave people the impression I was lazy. I lost any thought of being accepted in wider society. My expectations of myself were zero and the expectations of everyone around me were zero.

I was so lost I felt as though all the possibilities of life were far beyond my reach. I told myself that, at 42, I had 'semi retired'. I had been going in and out of hospital and after my last admission I finally surrendered: gave myself up entirely to services agreeing to anything they demanded of me. They agreed to put me into a hostel.

32.4 Housing First

This was the first stable roof I had for 2 years. It also meant I could claim state benefits and have a small but steady income. They started the process of rehousing me. I was very lucky because I met another resident while I was at the hostel. She was the first person in years who didn't view me as just a 'mad junkie on the streets'. She was utterly non-judgmental and actually seemed to be impressed by me. We had a baby whilst we were in the hostel. After 2 years in the hostel we went into temporary housing for another 2 years: it was a place of our own and it made a huge difference.

This stability allowed me to get on top of my drug taking but not my mental health. I was still struggling daily and isolating myself indoors. The constant struggle to survive sapped all hope. There were times when the constant worry about benefits, finding the rent, the possibility of losing our flat and whether or not there would be enough for us to eat, was almost as bad for my mental health as being on the street. It was having a baby to look after that gave me something to live for.

32.5   Opportunity

We were finally rehoused permanently in 2005. I continued to use services but it felt I was on a treadmill going nowhere. Expectations around what I could do were very low. I had left school with no qualifications and had only worked in the 'arts' so felt I had been left on the shelf of possibilities. Eventually I was asked if I wanted to do a work placement. The low expectations I had of myself meant that I only agreed to do this if they guaranteed it would not lead to me having to take work. The thought of what working might do to my state benefits—the risk that I might be worse off financially by working—terrified me. They agreed to my conditions and I went to a work placement in Community Day Services supporting a gardening group in the afternoons.

32.6   Control

I was given a set of keys to the building as soon as I arrived. This was the first time in a very long time that I felt trusted—especially with a building full of computers. It was the first time I felt I was being valued and treated with dignity and respect. What is more, other staff listened to me when I spoke up. I was really made to feel a part of the team. This very different relationship cost very little but had huge implications for me.

32.7   Hope

It was not long before I moved on to volunteering for 3 days a week at the Day Centre and really working as a Peer Support Worker. I was using my own experiences to model a sense of hope that recovery could be a possibility for people using the Centre. Being able to do this really fired my enthusiasm and passion and I soon found myself with a determined goal. I had been on the receiving end of help for so long that I had forgotten just how powerful being in a position to help others could be, even if this was just making someone a cup of tea.

The volunteer work gave me access to training and I started accessing the mental health training for staff within the local authority where I now work (CNWL, Camden and North West London). I also had my first experience with 'Wellness Recovery Action Plans' (WRAP, [1]). I found there were so many strategies I had been using to survive without realizing it. Having a plan and being conscious of my aspirations allowed me to start to thrive rather than just survive. I began to learn how to manage my own difficulties and get the best out of my situation.

32.8   Recovery

Getting involved with WRAP led to my first real experience in coproduction. A group of staff members and people who used the service collaborated to create our own 'Health and Wellbeing Plans'. These are now used across CNWL have led to all sorts of opportunities for me.

Finally, in peer support I had found something I wanted to do and felt I was good at. I was able to access the first Peer Support Training programme at CNWL. This was the first time I had ever undertaken any sort of academic training and I completed it! I was asked to be a part of CNWL's bid to become part of the initial Implementing Recovery through Organisational Change programme (ImROC, [2]). As part of ImROC, CNWL started to develop Peer Support Worker positions in services; set up a Recovery College and looked at recovery education; and developed a more recovery-focused approach to risk. Involvement with these endeavors at a Trust level led to me becoming a consultant with the ImROC team providing support to other organisations across the UK in their quest to develop more recovery-focused services.

Finally I took the plunge and went back to work as a Peer Recovery Trainer when CNWL opened our Recovery and Wellbeing College in 2012. This is not a sheltered position. I was recruited like any other member of staff, however I was supported in finding the right amount of hours so that I was assured of being better off financially in work.

This opened a new horizon for me with a host of new opportunities. It has given me a new sense of hope and, although I don't earn a great deal, it is enough to help enable me to thrive. I am now a contributing citizen putting the skills I have to good use. I am building on what is strong in me, rather than what is wrong with me. I still take medication, and find some things a real struggle, but now I am someone who both uses services and helps to deliver services. In both of these roles I have witnessed many changes both in services and in myself.

32.9   What I Have Learned

I was once asked to write a list of the things that have helped in my own recovery journey. The list is quite long! But I would not wish to shorten it. Each in different ways has contributed. Together they make an unbeatable combination:

1. Acceptance.
2. Feeling a part of the community both at home and at work: the feeling that you belong.

3. A feeling of independence.
4. A self-management plan.
5. Being confident to advocate for myself.
6. Being valued for what I can contribute: moving from feeling grateful to people to discovering I have qualities that are valued.
7. Stable housing.
8. Being an active citizen and feeling my social status is not less than the people who support me.
9. Overcoming my own stigma and shame.
10. Gaining a sense of momentum.
11. Having a small group of people that looked at me differently that helped me to look at myself differently.
12. Changing attitudes.
13. Use of a different language—the language of recovery.

Most of these things cost nothing extra. For the most part, they are about a different sort of interaction and different relationships. The Recovery College where I work, and others like it, embody so many of the things that have helped me in my journey of recovery. 'Patients' become 'students' and relationships are transformed through coproduction. They challenge stigma and genuinely recognize the strengths and contribution that everyone can make.

32.10 Conclusions

In this chapter, I have told the story of my own experience of recovery from mental health problems complicated by drug misuse. I have also offered a brief reflection on how I am now building on what I learned from that experience in my current work supporting others in their recovery.

Recovery is a contested term [3]. We use it in the recovery movement to mean *recovering a good quality of life as defined by what is important to the person concerned* (i.e. that person's *individual values*). So defined, the factors that contribute to an individual's recovery journey are necessarily very diverse. There are correspondingly many theories of recovery [4]. I indicated in the last section above the long list of factors that contributed to my own recovery. But if I had to choose just three factors that in my experience and the experience of others, seem essential, they would be the three by which the very culture of the recovery college movement is defined, hope, control and opportunity.

Acknowledgements In my current roles, both as a peer trainer in recovery and as a consultant for ImROC (see introduction), I have had the opportunity to work alongside some of the best people I have ever worked with. Sharing their passion has been a huge part of what has inspired me in my own recovery over the last few years.

My story as told in this chapter was published originally in the journal *Mental Health and Social Inclusion* [5]. I am very grateful to Mental Health and Social Inclusion and to its editor, Rachel Perkins, for permission to reproduce it here.

32.11 Guide to Further Sources

For further information on the recovery movement please see:

Meddings, S., McGregor, J., Roeg, W. and Shepherd, G. (2015), "Recovery colleges: quality and outcomes", Mental Health and Social Inclusion, Vol. 19 No. 4, pp. 212–221. https://doi.org/10.1108/MHSI-08-2015-0035

Slade, M., Oades, L., and Jarden A., (eds) (2017) Wellbeing, Recovery and Mental Health (2017) (eds). Cambridge: Publisher Cambridge University Press. ISBN1107543053, 9781107543058

And a recently released film on recovery by the author at: https://www.youtube.com/watch?v=9iO4D0j_0A8

References

1. Copeland ME. Wellness Recovery Action Plan (WRAP). 1997. www.mentalhealthrecovery.com.
2. http://www.imroc.org/about-us/.
3. Slade M, Amering M, Farkas M, Hamilton B, O'Hagan M, Panther G, Perkins R, Shepherd G, Tse S, Whitley R. Uses and abuses of recovery: implementing recovery-oriented practices in mental health systems. World Psychiatry. 2014;13:12–20.
4. Slade M. Personal recovery and mental illness: a guide for mental health professionals (values-based medicine). Cambridge: Cambridge University Press; 2009.
5. Roeg W. Discovering myself, a journey of rediscovery. Ment Health Soc Incl. 2016;20(4): 217–20. https://doi.org/10.1108/MHSI-04-2016-0013.

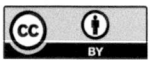

Part V
Training

Training for Task: An Introduction to Part V, Training

33

Bill Fulford

With this penultimate part of the book, we come to the sharp end of values-based practice, namely the clinical skills that form the bedrock of the process on which it relies in supporting balanced decision-making on values in the context of clinical care. As described in chapter 1, "Surprised by Values: An Introduction to Values-based Practice and the Use of Personal Narratives in This Book", values-based practice builds on four main areas of learnable clinical skills, awareness, knowledge, reasoning, and communication skills. In this chapter, we fill out our descriptions of these skills areas and indicate how they are extended and enriched by the cultural values illustrated by the contributions to this Part (Table 33.1).

The training methods on which values-based practice has relied to date are derived largely from its original theoretical base in ordinary language philosophy. Part II, Theory, illustrated how the theory underpinning values-based practice could be much enriched by opening it up to other philosophical traditions, including those of non-Western cultures. The next two Parts explored aspects of this culturally enriched form of values-based practice, by way, respectively, of its model of service delivery (Part III, Practice) and of its role in linking science with people (Part IV, Science). The contributions to this Part explore aspects of this same cultural enrichment for the task of training for values-based practice. As we will see engaging with cultural values, while bringing with it new challenges for skills training, at the same time offers a much enriched resource base for the required training.

Authors
The editors with input from the contributors to Part V

B. Fulford (✉)
St Catherine's College, University of Oxford, Oxford, UK
e-mail: kwmf@kwmfulford.com

D. Stoyanov et al. (eds.), *International Perspectives in Values-Based Mental Health Practice*, https://doi.org/10.1007/978-3-030-47852-0_33

Table 33.1 Annotated Table of Contents for Part V, Training

33.1 Awareness of Values

We start this Part with the first and foundational skills area for values-based practice, viz., raised awareness of values, and of the (often surprising) diversity of values.

The two brief exercises we included in chapter 1, "Surprised by Values: An Introduction to Values-Based Practice and the Use of Personal Narratives in This Book"—the 'three words exercise' and the 'forced choice exercise'—are illustrative of what has become the standard approach to awareness training in values-based practice. Developed originally by Kim Woodbridge-Dodd (the first author of chapter 44, "Reflections on the Impact of Mental Health Ward Staff Training in Race Equality and Values-Based Practice"), this was the approach adopted in the first training manual for values-based practice ('Whose Values?', [1]). Inspired by ordinary language philosophy [2, 3], the approach has subsequently been adopted across a range of clinical areas (see Guide to Further Information below). Powerful however as the approach has proved to be, that there remains much scope for improvement is evident, if in no other ways, from our own failure of self-awareness of values within values-based practice noted in chapter 1 (see section, 'Why now?').

The first two chapters in this Part illustrate the scope for further strengthening of values awareness within a culturally enriched form of values-based practice. Rosalind Austin (chapter 34, "Values-Based Practice When Engaging with Voice-Hearers") illustrates the importance in this respect of personal narratives through the stories of two voice hearers, Paul and Mary. The two narratives, taken together, draw out an important feature of voice hearing that although neglected by services, is transparently self-evident within the cultural context of voice hearing.

The neglected point in essence is this: that voice hearing although indeed sometimes a negatively evaluated experience (as it was for Mary) may sometimes come with distinct positive aspects as well (as it did for Paul). These positive aspects may as we have indicated be surprising to those (notably within services) for whom voice hearing is assumed to be a 'symptom' and hence necessarily a negative experience. But that this assumption of negativity may be clinically harmful is evident from Paul and Mary's stories. For as Rosalind goes on to show in her chapter, understanding the balance of positive and negative values attached to voice hearing for a given individual is vital to a recovery-oriented approach to clinical care.

The effectiveness of Rosalind and David Crepaz-Keay's work in the Educational Voice Hearers Network is one reason why in this book we based our approach so firmly on personal narratives. By allowing us to engage across and between cultures, personal narratives provide a powerful resource for establishing a culturally enriched form of values-based practice. Connecting with traditions in which the heuristic power of personal narratives has not been forgotten may facilitate this. In Part I, professional storyteller, Olusola Adebiye, with co-authors Tutiette Thomas and Temitope Ademosu, illustrated the healing power of storytelling in African culture with their chapter 11, on Madness, Mythopoetry and Medicine.

Chapter 35, "Dharma Therapy: A Buddhist Counselling Approach to Acknowledging and Enhancing Perspectives, Attitudes and Values" illustrates another such resource in this case represented by a Buddhist approach to mental health called Dharma Therapy. Mindfulness is of course nowadays familiar in Western mental health settings. But as Buddhist authors, Venerable Sik Hin Hung and Jennifer Yim, point out, mindfulness as it is currently practiced in Western mental health has, to its loss, become disconnected from its roots in Buddhist philosophy and practice. Their story of Peter Chan shows how Dharma therapy provides a more joined up approach. They emphasise that like any other therapy this is not for everyone. But where Dharma therapy works, an essential contribution to its effectiveness is the way that it helps to raise awareness of, and thus put those concerned in touch with, their true values, with what really matters in their lives.

33.2 Knowledge of Values

With the next three chapters, we move from awareness to knowledge of values. Before turning to individual contributions, there are two general points to bear in mind about knowledge of cultural values. The first is that—to put it bluntly—it is possible to get it. It is sometimes assumed that 'evidence of values' is somehow beyond the scope of empirical methods of enquiry. To the contrary, however, there are available a whole range of both qualitative and quantitative (and combined) methods available from the social and anthropological sciences for exploring the values of—for exploring what is important or matters to—this or that given group. We noted one such method in the introduction to Part III, Practice: the combined methodology adopted by Anthony Colombo and colleagues for exploring the implicit values of different professional groups within multidisciplinary mental health teams (chapter 15, "Vectors of Best Practice: An Introduction to Part III, Practice"). The contributions to this Part add further examples (see below).

With cultures, then, as with individuals, we should avoid just assuming that we know what is important to them. We have to, and we can, find out. But the second general point that is important to bear in mind about knowledge of cultural values is that such knowledge, however robustly derived, should never trump the values of a given individual. Recall the mantra about knowledge of values from chapter 1 that in values-based practice everyone is an 'n of 1'. Everyone, that is to say, however firmly embedded in his or her culture of origin, has a unique 'values finger-print'. Knowledge of cultural values does have a proper role to play. It provides hints of or nudges towards what is *likely* to be important or matters to someone from a particular background or in a particular situation (a patient, for example, presenting with a given condition). But it is still important in any particular situation to find out what is in fact important or matters to the individual concerned. (We return to how this is done below, see 'communication skills').

Turning now to the contributions to this Part, three chapters illustrate in different ways how the resources of the social sciences can be harnessed to provide well-grounded knowledge of cultural values. First, ethnography (chapter 36, "Dangerous Liaisons: Science, Tradition, and Qur'anic Healing in the Dakhla Oasis of Egypt") as used by Mohammed Rashid and Werdie van Staden in the former's study in the Dakhla oasis. Mohammed's deep immersion in the area over an extended period provides remarkable insights into the tensions of values between Western and non-Western approaches to healing as these came together in the striking figure of a respected local Qur'anic healer, Sheikh Rayyes. The next chapter (chapter 37, "Know Thyself: Jane Discovers the Value of Her Depression"), based on its author's (Tamara K Browne's) study of people with depression, shows the power of the social sciences as reflected in an interview study. Echoing Rosalind Austin's work with voice hearers (chapter 34, "Values-Based Practice When Engaging with Voice-Hearers") Tamara shows through the story of one of her participants how depression, although for most people a deeply negative experience, may nonetheless come with positive aspects. There are pointers to this in historical work on depression (or its cognates, [4]). But in contemporary contexts, as Tamara's work illustrates, it is from the social sciences that we are able to derive fine-grained and reliable information as the basis of person-centred clinical care.

With the third chapter on knowledge, Michael Bennet's (chapter 38, "Case Studies in the Culture of Professional Football Players and Mental Welfare and Wellbeing") work with professional footballers, we come to a novel and positive resolution of the tension between individual and cultural values. Michael's study uses discourse analysis to explore the findings from his interviews with a number of players from different clubs in the UK professional football league. In this chapter, he describes one of a number of emerging themes, called by one of his interviewees 'The Snowball Effect'.

So described, the study, although presenting novel and important findings, may appear unremarkable as an application of social science methods. But the study is innovative at a number of levels. It is the first in-depth qualitative study of what matters or is important to professional footballers. There have been many rather superficial quantitative studies. But Michael's is the first to dig below the surface to provide well-grounded understanding of the issues. It is also the first such study to be carried out with clinical interventions explicitly in mind—as a qualified therapist and Head of Welfare for the game's governing body in the UK, the PFA (Professional Footballers Association), Michael was motivated in part by the fact that to date professional football has been a neglected area of mental health. And, Michael being himself an ex-professional footballer, it is the first such study to combine rigorous social science methods with personal experience of the field of study.

It is in this third respect, in the combination his study offers of rigorous methods with personal experience, that Michael provides a resolution of the tension between individual and cultural values. His approach is highly rigorous methodologically. But as an ex-professional footballer himself, his approach is not that merely of a detached researcher. There are of course methodological pitfalls in adopting an engaged rather than detached perspective in work of this kind. But there are methodological pitfalls too in being detached. This is why combining his personal experience with the use of a rigorous social science method makes Michael's study so important. It means that he brings a unique combination of expertise by training and expertise by experience to his work. The result is a rigorous qualitative social science study of the culture of professional football that is informed and filled out by Michael's personal experience as a former professional footballer. Uniquely illuminating, it provides insights into the values of people working within a culture to which most of us have either no access from personal experience or, worse, the potentially misleading access provided by media coverage. In Michael's hands, moreover, the study provides these crucial insights explicitly in the service of guiding therapeutic interventions.

33.3 Reasoning About Values

Reasoning about values has a long tradition in moral philosophy on which contemporary bioethics has drawn freely. Values-based practice, too, has drawn on the same traditions of moral reasoning but with an important difference. Where bioethics has (in the main) used the traditions of moral reasoning as a way of getting 'right answers', values-based practice has drawn on these traditions with the more modest aim of broadening understanding of the values in play in the situation in question.

The difference we should say straight away is not as stark as we have drawn it here. In early editions, for example, of the seminal *Four Principles of Biomedical Ethics*, its authors (the philosopher Tom Beauchamp and the theologian James Childress) emphasised that their eponymous four principles were intended to provide a framework, no more and no less, for mapping out the dimensions of an ethical issue in medicine [5]. This is exactly how 'principles reasoning' is used in values-based practice, to map out the values in play. For example, a values-based approach to the use of mental health legislation in the UK used principles reasoning in this 'mapping out' way [6]. As in bioethics again, so also in values-based practice, the top-down approach of principles reasoning has to be balanced with the bottom-up approach of case-based reasoning (or casuistry). The latter connects with our point in chapter 1, about the power of narrative to illuminate values. Philosophers, Albert Jonsen and Stephen Toulmin, reintroducing casuistry to medical ethics [7], noted how the appeal to concrete case examples tapped into our implicit understanding of a situation.

Values-based practice, in drawing on traditional forms of moral reasoning in this 'mapping out' way, connects with other approaches in the 'values tool kit'. It follows, for example, the precedent set by Oxford's first Professor of Medical Ethics, Tony Hope, working with Bill Fulford, in the Oxford Practice Skills Project [8]. This project established the general approach of partnership between ethics/values and science in clinical decision-making that now underpins values-based practice. As a teaching resource for medical students, it brought together for the first time, ethics, law, and communication skills with evidence-based medicine as the basis of clinical decision-making. Values-based practice also has parallels with contemporary movements in bioethics towards developing practical resources for problem-solving (as distinct from prescriptive ethics). These movements are called variously 'clinical ethics' or 'practical ethics' (see, for example, [9]).

In this Part, we have included two chapters that between them illustrate the resources of traditional forms of moral reasoning applied to cultural values. Taryn Knox' detailed case study (chapter 39, "Sexual Orientation Change Efforts and VBP") makes the point for case-based reasoning in her powerful explication of the conflicting cultural and other values involved in decisions about conversion therapy for homosexuality. The story in this chapter shows just how sensitive such decisions are to the specific contingencies presented by the particular situation. The balance of considerations in her target case as Taryn points out, might have come out very differently if, say, contrary to current realities, there were a form of conversion therapy available of proven safety and effectiveness.

Case-based reasoning may be used to good effect in isolation. Combining it with other methods can however boost its powers of explication. One such method, as Michael Wong, from the University of Hong Kong, illustrates in chapter 40, "Values, Meanings, Hermeneutics and Mental Health", is hermeneutic analysis. His narrative case study is of 'Mary', a woman in her middle years, who is referred to the local Neuropsychiatry Clinic for assessment of persistent abnormal movements believed to be secondary to the medication she had been prescribed for a pre-existing condition (depression with psychotic features). Her management followed standard medical protocols. But these proved effective only when combined with hermeneutic analysis used to deepen understanding of the cultural and other values driving her medical presentation.

33.4   Communication Skills

Values-based practice as has been said is 'nothing without communication skills' ([10], chapter 7). Communication skills are important to values-based practice in two specific respects: for eliciting values (recall the listening skills shown by the surgeon in the story of Mrs. Jones' knee in chapter 1, "Surprised by Values: An Introduction to Values-Based Practice and the Use of Personal Narratives in This Book") and for conflict resolution.

As with other areas of values-based practice, its relationship with communication skills is that of a two-way partnership. Communication skills contribute in these two specific (and other general) ways to values-based practice. Values-based practice in turn contributes content to communication skills. The values-based concept of StAR values (Strengths, Aspirations, and Resources), as used in teaching, for example, is combined with the ICE (Ideas, Concerns, and Expectations) of standard communication skills training, to give the mnemonic ICEStAR. This reminds students to explore positives (StAR values) as well as negatives (ICE) with their patients.

The final two chapters in this Part show the potential contributions of culturally enriched forms of values-based practice for both aspects of values-based communication skills: for eliciting values (chapter 41, "Disha: Building Bridges-Removing Barriers: Where Excluded and Privileged Young Adults Meet") and for conflict resolution (chapter 42, "Online Counseling 'the World Without a Label'"). Reporting from Pune in India, Sadhana Natu (chapter 41) describes their innovative Disha programme. Through case studies and personal testimonies, she illustrates how bringing students together from diverse backgrounds within peer support groups provides a powerful way for participants to become more aware of their own and others' values. The Disha programme is thus a model for the 'open society of stakeholders' that, as we describe in our concluding chapter (chapter 47, "Co-Writing Values: What We Did and Why We Did It") and After Word, it is the ultimate aim of this book to establish.

Chapter 42, "Online Counseling 'the World Without a Label'", by Irma Dobrinjic and colleagues, from the University of Tuzla in Bosnia and Herzegovina, illustrates the potential of new technology in support of the communication skills for conflict resolution in values-based practice. Conflict resolution is well developed for face-to-face encounters. But coming face-to-face is precisely what the conflicts in Irma Dobrinjic and colleagues' group of clients (adolescents and their families) are all about. Through the story of Adnan and his family, they show how effective their online counselling service may be in helping to manage the conflicts of values arising between young people with behavioural problems and their parents over engagement with services. The young people in question, as their case narrative illustrates, are brought to services by their parents but reject help for fear of being stuck with a label. Computer literate however as these young people invariably are, they engage readily and often to good effect when counselling is offered in an online form. Such counselling is available at a time of the young person's choosing and being anonymous it comes literally, as their title has it, 'without a label'.

As with Sadhana Natu's Disha programme, there are lessons from Irma Dobrinjic and colleagues' online counselling service for the "open society of stakeholders" that, as we describe in our concluding chapter (Chapter 47) and After Word, it is the ultimate aim of this book to establish. They indeed comment on the potential for developing similar online counselling services in other situations around the world. As an exercise in conflict resolution, the effectiveness of their approach is all the more impressive for the fact that it has been developed in the challenging post-war circumstances currently obtaining in Bosnia and Herzegovina.

33.5   Conclusions

This Part of the book is concerned with the training implications for a culturally enriched form of values-based practice. In each of the areas covered—awareness, knowledge, reasoning, and communication skills—the implications cut both ways. Engaging with cultural values raises new challenges for training in the skills for values-based practice. But such engagement also offers new assets for and models of training.

The communication skills for values-based practice, the topic of the last two chapters in the Part, provide particularly powerful illustrations of this two-way cut. Sadhana Natu's Disha programme in Pune (chapter 41, "Disha: Building Bridges-Removing Barriers: Where Excluded and Privileged Young Adults Meet") and Irma Dobrinjic and colleagues' online counselling service in Tuzla, Bosnia and Herzegovina (chapter 42, "Online Counseling 'the World Without a Label'"), have both been developed in challenging local circumstances, respectively, extreme economic and social differences among students, and post-war conflict. Yet both have developed effective ways of delivering culturally appropriate values-based mental health services. Their examples thus show that challenging as training for the task of delivering a culturally enriched form of values-based practice may be, it is a task that can nonetheless be done.

33.6   Guide to Further Information

For more on skills training in values-based practice, please see the website for the Collaborating Centre for Values-based Practice in Oxford at: valuesbasedpractice. org/More about VBP.

This includes a number of exemplar training materials that are available as free full-text downloads.

References

1. Woodbridge K, Fulford KWM. Whose values? In: A workbook for values-based practice in mental health care. London: The Sainsbury Centre for Mental Health; 2004.
2. Fulford KWM. Moral theory and medical practice. Cambridge: Cambridge University Press; 1989. (Reprinted 1995 and 1999).

3. Fulford KWM. Living with uncertainty: a first-person-plural response to eleven commentaries on values-based practice, chapter 13. In: Loughlin M, editor. Debates in values-based practice: arguments for and against. Cambridge: Cambridge University Press; 2014.
4. Fulford, KWM, Crepaz-Keay D, Stanghellini, G. Depressions Plural: pathology and the challenge of values. Chapter 14, pps 141–158 in charles foster and jonathan herring (eds) depression: law and ethics. Oxford: Oxford University Press
5. Beauchamp TL, Childress JF. Principles of biomedical ethics. 3rd ed. Oxford: Oxford University Press; 1989.
6. Fulford KWM, Dewey S, King M. Values-based involuntary seclusion and treatment: value pluralism and the UK's Mental Health Act 2007. Chap. 60. In: Sadler JZ, van Staden W, Fulford KWM, editors. The oxford handbook of psychiatric ethics. Oxford: Oxford University Press; 2015.
7. Jonsen AR, Toulmin S. The abuse of casuistry: a history of moral reasoning. California: University of California Press; 1988.
8. Hope T, Fulford KWM, Yates A. The Oxford practice skills course: ethics, law and communication skills in health care education. Oxford: The Oxford University Press; 1996.
9. Persson I, Savulescu J. Unfit for the future: the need for moral enhancement (Uehiro series in practical ethics). Oxford: Oxford University Press; 2012.
10. Fulford KWM, Peile E, Carroll H. Essential values-based practice: clinical stories linking science with people. Cambridge: Cambridge University Press; 2012; Japanese edition, Medical Sciences International 2016; French edition, John Libbey Eurotext, 2017.

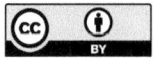

Values-Based Practice When Engaging with Voice-Hearers

34

Rosalind Austin

34.1 Introduction

This chapter draws on the stories of two people, Paul and Mary, to explore the values arising in voice-hearing and how they may be addressed through the resources of values-based practice.

I met Paul and Mary and heard their stories as part of my doctorate work with Durham University's 'Hearing the Voice' project, a large interdisciplinary research team that seeks to explore the widest possible interpretation of what it is to hear voices. For my doctoral project, I interviewed 30 voice-hearers, who I largely recruited from two community mental health centres in North-East England and South-East England. Paul and Mary were two of these. This chapter describes in their own words their very different experiences of voice-hearing and what these experiences meant to them. Employing the inclusive definition of values adopted in values-based practice (as what matters or is important to those concerned, see introductory chap. 1), the chapter explores what mattered or was important respectively to Paul and Mary about their voice-hearing, and the influences on them of their respective cultural contexts.

In mental health contexts, voice-hearing is often treated merely as a negatively evaluated symptom to be treated as a disease. Conversely, among mental health advocacy organisations, voice-hearing is sometimes celebrated as a positive and rewarding experience. The headline finding from my study was that the realities of voice-hearing are far more complicated than either of these extremes. It involves complex and sometimes conflicting values, of the person concerned, and of others around them. Paul and Mary's stories illustrate this reality.

R. Austin (✉)
Collaborating Centre for Values-Based Practice, St Catherine's College, University of Oxford, Oxford, UK

© The Author(s) 2021
D. Stoyanov et al. (eds.), *International Perspectives in Values-Based Mental Health Practice*, https://doi.org/10.1007/978-3-030-47852-0_34

34.2 Paul's Story

Paul, an ex-soldier in his early 30s who is now unemployed, hears the voice of a defined character he calls 'the Captain'. In the interview, Paul said:

A lot of other voice-hearers have 'a voice'. It is somebody different from themselves. With me, it is just myself. I visualise him as me but with a scruffier beard and different attire and things like that [...] He looks different to me. He's quite aggressive, quite an old-school man's man. That's how he comes across [...] It's just there 24/7, always talking away to myself, getting replies and all this. That's just the way it is now. Some voice-hearers can put their voices away. Some tell them, 'I don't want to speak to you at this moment, could you come back later on?' With mine, it's just part of me, I'm like a Siamese twin, but on the inside.

Paul views his voice at times as being like a person. It is a characterful voice, 'an old-school man's man', who has his own distinct appearance, dress sense, and emotive aspect, with the voice being aggressive. It thus offers an example of a voice that has a distinct character with internally individualised agency, one of four levels of agent-representation in auditory hallucinations, or voices, described by the psychologists Wilkinson and Bell's [1] exploration of voices as social agents [2].

Paul draws attention to how his voice is internalised: it is 'just part of me'. He emphasises this connection by saying that the voice is 'a Siamese twin [...] on the inside'. The logic of the 'twin' here suggests that Paul has an intimate relationship with the voice, viewing it as internal and conjoined to him. Notably, he earlier claimed that it is 'my own voice but in different tones', which also suggests that he understands himself to be having a relationship with a voice that is at some level part of himself.

Later in the interview, Paul develops the image of the voice by saying that it *'was the captain of the ship really'*. Such a characterisation has links to Paul's military background, and it is a military image that he uses to invoke the imbalance of power in his relationship with 'the Captain'. The latter's voice triggers fear and anxiety; Paul said, *'He [the Captain] was on the bow, making all the decisions and I was just there in the background watching him.'* Here, Paul is describing an intimidating relationship where the voice has the power to watch him in a spectatorial way. Paul does not seem able to establish any firm boundary with the voice, where he might manage to get control, and he listens to it all day long. As Marius Romme (a psychiatrist) and Mervyn Morris (a psychiatric nurse) suggest, many voice-hearers who become psychiatric patients 'were afraid of their voices, overwhelmed by them, and felt powerless' [3, p. 2].

Paul took antipsychotic medication, but continued to hear the voice of the Captain. He sets aside times to listen to the voice, as it provides companionship for him. In my interview with him, he told me that he spent time doing different activities—such as fishing—when he would time-share with the voice. Paul understands fishing in a creative way, as within the context of doing this activity, he is able to engage in a dialogic relationship with the voice, so that he is less afraid of it. Noticing that the voice enjoys fishing too, Paul is distracted by it to the point where he would 'miss a bite' of a fish on the line. Despite his irritation, Paul is relieved that he has found *'something that we both enjoy'*. Until now, there has been little common ground with his voice, so fishing is helpful in that it offers Paul a way of relating to his voice differently as he 'sit[s] on a bank'. The Captain's protective role, which is to 'stop me getting bullied in the future', switches to one of being a companion, and is described by Paul as being a *'family member you love to hate'*. This reduces Paul's anxiety, so that he can have *'a good laugh'*. This suggests again that the voice is a person-like entity who in fact benefits from being entertained.

The voice came to have importance to Paul. It is clear in the context of the interview that the voice mattered a good deal to him. What mattered to Paul was to be able to share a joke with the voice, and for it to function as a companion.

34.3 Values in Paul's story

A number of important values are evident or implied in this story, both Paul's values and the values of other people.

34.3.1 Paul's Values

As to Paul's values—as to what mattered or was important to him—it is clear from the story above that The Captain was at least in part a positive aspect of his life. Moreover, when I met Paul during the interview, it seemed that the voice caused him no problems with other people, at least with the general public. For example, Paul sometimes reacted to the voice by talking to it out loud when he was shopping in his town—but this had no untoward consequences in terms of other people's reactions.

That people's voices are often (as with Paul) benign or even sometimes positive is widely ignored even though the evidence has been available for many years [4]. It is clear from Paul's story that while he wished to listen to and respond to his voice on a regular basis, this was perceived negatively by many of those around him.

34.3.2 Other People's Values

Paul nonetheless did have problems in other areas reflecting other people's negative evaluations of voice-hearing. In another part of the interview, for example, he recounted how he was denied custody of his child; and his ex-wife used his mental health as a reason for barring him access. Similar views about frequent voice-hearing being unacceptable are widely adopted in mainstream Western society. This is why Paul's ex-wife was supported by his medical team and the family court in considering that Paul needed to have medical treatment to suppress or eliminate his voices; and they argued that when Paul is actively hearing voices, his ability to care for his young daughter is compromised. Paul was sad that he was not trusted with the care of his daughter.

But if Paul's talking back to his voice really 'caused no problems', was it ethical (or legal) to restrict Paul's responsibilities, including his parenting rights? Did Paul's ex-wife and the family court find Paul's verbalised to-and-fro conversation with his voice alarming? Were the lawyers and medical staff who wrote reports being pressurised 'to do something about' Paul's voice-hearing experience? Were there significant safeguarding issues regarding Paul having custody of his child? Any or all of such negative values are likely to have been in play.

Yet staff must have been well intentioned in the actions they took. In professions like psychiatry, this generally means treating voice-hearing as a hallmark symptom of schizophrenia or some other form of psychosis [5]. It is thus assumed to be a bad thing whatever the person concerned thinks.

These considerations remind us of the practical impact of The Two Feet Principle of values-based practice, that values as well as evidence are important in all aspects of health care decision-making: this includes, often crucially, as in Paul's story, diagnostic assessment [2, 6]. What this means in practice is that even if a medical model were an appropriate way of understanding Paul's story, understanding what mattered or was important to him about his 'symptoms' would still have been vital to any decision about how to 'treat' them.

34.4 Mary's Story

Mary is in her late 50s and is a retired staff nurse. She worked as a nurse for 30 years. For 12 of these years, she heard voices at times when she was working on a medical ward in a busy hospital. Mary is very reflective about the way that she consciously shut down her emotions when she was working in a highly stressful working environment where 'people die'. She said:

Once I was engrossed in work, I could keep going. But it was difficult. I mean, you shut down your emotions because you've got people working on a medical ward, and people die. They die. But you've got to get on with your job. So you can't be emotionless, but you've got to shut it out somewhere. And I was shutting down completely. I did what I had to, you know, tell relatives or whatever. But I had nowhere to go with that as a nurse. And all these emotions built up and up and up. So by the time I had the operation in 1999, they were there…they were at their height.

Mary is here describing a strategy widely adopted by staff working on medical wards to keep their emotions in check so that they can do their jobs. Deaths on the ward are expected, and as Mary puts it, 'you've got to get on with your job'. However, in Mary's case, she was 'shutting down' her emotions completely. Given that she frequently worked nights and was the nurse in charge of the ward, she found it helpful to feel in control of the space as far as was possible, by having *'the door shut'*, as she didn't *'want people walking in and all the rest of it'*. She would also *'stick to a routine'*, when dispensing medication to patients. Mary recalls that if *'I had it all organised I knew I could cope with it, and that way I could keep my emotions at bay, suppressed, because that's it, I've got everything organised'*. Later in the interview, she said that *'the best way I've seen it [the shutting down] ever explained, was someone explained it to me as Data in Star Trek. The robot who wants his emotions.'*

This particular robotic image that Mary selects indicates a perceived fundamental lack of emotions. Mary reflects that *'when I was working, I didn't realise how much I was suppressing'*. In the above extract, Mary said that her 'emotions built up and up and up', and yet she had no one with whom to share her feelings. She said that *'one of my bugbears of let's say adult nursing is that they don't get any debrief'*.

However, it was not until her late 30s when she experienced an *'acute stressor'* in the form of undergoing life-threatening, major surgery, that Mary started to hear voices. There can be a 'sleeper effect' of trauma [7], where the person does not process the trauma emotionally at the time it actually takes place. In Mary's case, the stress of undergoing *'two major operations, which nearly killed me'* was compounded by her being in a vulnerable, dependent state as she *'couldn't move off the bed, and I was being fed'*. She was also on morphine, which altered her mental state. Many people experience delirium in intensive care units ([8, 9]). In Mary's story, the situation was further complicated by what she later revealed about her *'childhood trauma'* of being sexually abused by *'a very respected member of the community'* when she was a young girl.

Mary's story is in this respect consistent with the psychiatrist Judith Herman's [10] observation that survivors of abuse may successfully cope with adult life until defensive structures break down due to a very stressful event (like the operation). Mary was later encouraged by a psychiatrist to make the connection between her childhood experience of abuse and the voices that she hears. Following a change of diagnosis from schizophrenia to personality disorder, Mary went on to have 3 years of intense psychological support by attending group therapy run by a psychologist, organised by a Complex Needs Service.

34.5   Values in Mary's story

As with Paul's story, it is helpful to consider Mary's values and how these interacted with those of others around her.

34.5.1 Mary's Values

Although a very different narrative from Paul's, Mary's story raises many of the same considerations from the point of view of values-based practice: the importance of the values of others, of attending carefully to what matters or is important to the person concerned, and of balanced decision-making A central difference however is that where Paul valued his voice positively, Mary valued her voices negatively.

Mary identified how one of the male voices that she heard represented the anger that she was unable to feel or articulate. She suggested that her suppressed emotion came out in this voice, and she calls it 'Mr Angry'. Mary acted out how *'Mr Angry's with me today'*, by storming around looking angry. Thus, where Paul's voice was internalised, Mary describes her voice as having an external reality, in that she conceptualises it as being like a person who accompanies her. Mary said that other members of the complex needs group she joined (who knew that Mary was a voice-hearer, and permitted her to 'bring her voices into the group') were relieved that she was able to make this connection between her emotion and her voice, as it explained her behaviour.

34.5.2 Other People's Values

Mary's story highlights a further crucial set of values for values-based practice, namely of the multidisciplinary team, specifically, in Mary's story, the complex needs team. In values-based practice, different team members (i.e. a psychiatrist and a psychologist) bring to clinical care not only a range of knowledge and skills but also a range of values [11]. This range of values is important as a resource for meeting the corresponding range of values presented by patients. This in turn contributes to balanced decision-making on person-values-centred care.

The 'team' in values-based practice though is not limited to health and social care professionals, but may include many others with a role to play in a given situation. Thus, housing, education, and other professionals may often have key contributions to make (for examples, see ref. [12]). Crucial, though, in addition, may be the contributions of peers with shared experience. In Mary's story, the members of the complex need group with whom she worked included 'peers'. In this, Mary's voice-hearing was accepted thus normalising her voices, in stark contrast to the hospital setting, where Mary suppressed her voices and emotions so that she could work effectively as a nurse. When Mary first began to hear voices, as a patient in the intensive care ward after her operation, she felt that it was not safe to share this (as she perceived it) stigmatised experience.

Rather strikingly, however, as she reported, none of the peer members of her Complex Needs Group actually shared her experience of hearing voices. There was thus no 'shared' peer knowledge of coping strategies for voice-hearing of the kind to which Mary would have had access had she attended a hearing voices group. (For more on Hearing Voices Groups please see the Guide to Further Sources, below.)

34.6   Conclusions

In this chapter, I have explored through the stories of two voice-hearers, Paul and Mary, the wide range of values raised by voice-hearing and the correspondingly wide range of applications of values-based practice. I began with a close reading of Paul's story to bring out the key values involved in terms of how voice-hearing is understood and worked with. This illustrated the practical impact of the Two Feet

Principle of values-based practice that values are important in all aspects of health care decision-making. The second close reading of Mary's story then raised awareness of the diversity of voice-hearing, and why it is important to engage effectively with individual values. In this individual case, the skills and values of the multidisciplinary 'team' were required, and then, the values of a complex needs group, which led to Mary feeling that her experience of voice-hearing has been normalised. In this setting, she has learnt to live well with her voices and her emotions, which in her opinion are inextricably bound together.

Acknowledgements I am grateful to Durham University's 'Hearing the Voice' project for the grant that I received from them to fund this doctoral research.

34.7   Guide to Further Sources

Please find below links to websites that give further information on voice-hearing, and what support is available. These resources are helpful for those who hear voices, as well as for mental health professionals and researchers.

Educational Voice-hearing Network, Collaborating Centre of Values-based Practice, St Catherine's College, Oxford University—https://valuesbasedpractice.org/what-do-we-do/networks/educational-voice-hearing-network/

Soundscape with voice-hearers—https://valuesbasedpractice.org/what-do-we-do/networks/educational-voice-hearing-network/soundscape-with-voice-hearers/

Durham University's 'Understanding Voices' website—https://www.dur.ac.uk/imh/understandingvoices/

Durham University's 'Hearing the Voice' website—https://hearingthevoice.org/

London Hearing Voices Network website—http://www.mindincamden.org.uk/services/lhvn

34.7.1 Hearing Voices Groups

Voice-hearers seek support from peer support groups for voice-hearers, known as 'hearing voices groups'. The Hearing Voices Movement emerged as 'a web of self-help groups offering assistance to troubled voice-hearers' [13, p. 6]. In England, there are now over 180 hearing voices groups held in a range of settings, including mental health services, inpatient units, and prisons. Over the past 20 years, hearing voices groups have been set up throughout Europe, North America, Australia, and New Zealand, with 'emerging initiatives in Latin America, Africa, and Asia' [12, p. S285]. The 'main tenet of the Hearing Voices Movement is the notion that hearing voices is a meaningful human experience [12, p. S285]. However, within this movement, members have a diversity of explanations (e.g. spiritual, telepathy, psychological) for what voices represent.

References

1. Wilkinson S, Bell V. The representation of agents in auditory verbal hallucinations. Mind Lang. 2016;31:104–26.
2. National Institute for Mental Health in England (NIMHE) and the Care Services Improvement Partnership. 3 Keys to a shared approach in mental health assessment. London: Department of Health; 2008. Available as a free full-text download from the Collaborating Center for Values-based Practice at: http://valuesbasedpractice.org/. More about VBP/Full text downloads/scroll down to 3 Keys).
3. Romme M, Morris M. Introduction. In: Romme M, Escher S, Dillon J, Corstens D, Morris M, editors. Living with voices: 50 stories of recovery. Ross-on-Wye: PCCS Books; 2009. p. 1–6.
4. Johns LC, van Os J. The continuity of psychotic experiences in the general population. Clin Psychol Rev. 2001;21(8):1125–41.
5. Waters F, Allen P, Aleman A, Fernyhough C, Woodward T, Badcock J, Barkus E, Johns L, Varese F, Menon M, Vercammen A, Laroi F. Auditory hallucinations in schizophrenia and non-schizophrenia populations: a review and integrated model of cognitive mechanisms. Schizophr Bull. 2012;38:683–92.
6. Fulford KWM, Dewey S, King M. Values-based involuntary seclusion and treatment: value pluralism and the UJK's mental health act 2007. Ch 60. In: Sadler JZ, van Staden W, KWM F, editors. The Oxford handbook of psychiatric ethics. Oxford: Oxford University Press; 2015.
7. Page G, Kurth T. Delirium on the intensive care unit. Brt Med J. 2014;349: p7265. Available at: https://doi.org/10.1136/bmj.g7265.
8. Girard D, Pandharipande P, Ely E. Delirium in the intensive care unit. Crit Care. 2008;12:1–9.
9. Briere JN. Child Abuse Trauma: Theory and Treatment of the Lasting Effects. London and New York: Sage Publications; 1992.
10. Herman J. Trauma and recovery. London: Pandora; 2001.
11. Colombo A, Benedelow G, Fulford KWM, et al. Evaluating the influence of implicit models of mental disorder on processes of shared decision making within community based multi-disciplinary teams. Soc Sci Med. 2003;56:1557–70.
12. Corstens D, Longden E, McCarthy-Jones S, Waddingham R, Thomas N. Emerging perspectives from the hearing voices movement: implications for research and practice. Schizophr Bull. 2014;40:285–94.
13. James A. Raising our voices: an account of the hearing voices movement. Gloucester: Handsell Publishing; 2001.

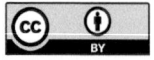

Dharma Therapy: A Buddhist Counselling Approach to Acknowledging and Enhancing Perspectives, Attitudes and Values

35

Sik Hin Hung and Jennifer Yim Shui Wa

35.1 Introduction to the Case

There is suffering, and it is part of life. This is an observation that the Buddha made. In fact, the core of Buddhist teaching is about suffering and the path to end suffering. The Buddha pointed out that the cause of suffering is ignorance, and by eliminating ignorance, suffering can be eliminated. With ignorance, people would develop delusive perspectives, attitudes and value, and, as a result, behave unwisely and bind oneself into all kind of difficulties and sufferings. What the Buddha meant by 'delusive' is the mistaken or dogmatic understanding of reality. The path to eliminate ignorance begins by being aware that there is suffering and developing right view and understanding of realty through the practice of mindfulness and careful attention [1]. The above explanation of the relationship between ignorance and suffering is the core of the Buddhist teaching, the Law of Dependent Origination.

This Buddhist understanding of suffering is the theoretic foundation of Dharma Therapy, a psycho-social intervention that incorporated mindfulness practice and other Buddhist cognitive training to help clients to develop right view and understanding of the stressful situation that they are dealing with. There are a total of seven steps to Dharma Therapy. In the following is a discussion as to how we applied Dharma Therapy to help Mr. Peter Chan to deal with his psychological problems.

S. H. Hung
Centre of Buddhist Studies, University of Hong Kong, Hong Kong, China

J. Y. S. Wa (✉)
Tsz Shan Monastery Buddhist Spiritual Counselling Centre, Hong Kong, China

35.2 Case Narrative

Peter Chan is a 48-year-old Hong Kong Chinese man who was feeling lost and could not find meaning in his life after both parent died one after the other within a year. He is married for over 18 years with no children. Relationship with wife is good and is supportive of each other.

Five years ago, his father was diagnosed to have cancer. The treatment was not effective at all. His father finally gave up all treatments and died half a year later. Unfortunately, his mother blamed herself for not insisting on offering more treatment for her husband. Her guilt drew her into a mental state of depression and eventually jumped to her death. Peter was shocked by her mother's sudden death and felt very sad. He had a contradictory feeling between of not taking good care of his mother, but at the same time, having a feeling of relieve as he didn't know how to deal with his mother's depression. Consequently, his emotion became unstable and developed insomnia. Furthermore, his work as a designer is exerting tremendous pressure on him and he could not concentrate on his work. Eventually, he was diagnosed to have anxiety and panic disorder by his psychiatrist who also gave him 6 months sick leave.

During his sick leave, Peter seek help from a Buddhist counselling center and reported that he had the following problems: whenever he smelt burning incense, raw meat in the market and rotten things, his heartbeat accelerated, felt stuffy and tightness in his chest and panted with heavy sweat. At the same time, he was very anxious and afraid that other people would take notice of his problem. As a result, he wanted to run away and hide from crowded places. He had similar emotional experience before when he was laughed at by some colleagues during a presentation at work. His mind went blank, not until his hands started shaking continuously that he regained consciousness. At that moment, he found himself hidden somewhere in a corner of the room holding his own shaking hand.

After these emotional episodes, Peter noticed that he could no longer control his thought even though he tried. He used to be rational and have a strong willpower to control everything. However, his anxiety and panic attack made him felt helpless and annoyed. He was afraid that his illness would become uncontrollable and could not be cured. Nevertheless, he expected the problem to be resolved with the hope that his life would go back to normal soon.

35.3 Values Arising

During the counselling sessions, the counsellor followed the seven steps of Dharma Therapy [2]:

1. Introduction and preparation session.
2. Become aware of the suffering and unsatisfactory conditions of the current situation.
3. Develop a desire to be liberated from the suffering.

4. Question and investigate the cause of suffering.
5. Observe and learn by paying careful attention to suffering and the cause of suffering.
6. Developing insight and wisdom as to how to bring an end to suffering and the cause of suffering.
7. With insight and wisdom, take the necessary steps to bring an end to suffering.

During the introduction and preparation session, the counsellor explained to Peter that she is only a facilitator to guide and support him on the path to recovery; it is his own motivation and effort that will eventually heal and transform him. Buddhism is a religion that takes the view that we are all responsible for our own thought and behaviour. Other people can only help and educate you to become aware of the problem and causes of the problem. To facilitate the arising of awareness, mindfulness was introduced to Peter to help him build a spiritual oasis where there would be peace and clarity. This is important because the client must first need to acknowledge and learn to live with the present situations, however painful, before he/she can transform or move on to other more satisfactory conditions.

In the second step of the therapy, the therapist guided Peter to become more aware of the unsatisfactoriness of the situations that he is in so that he could develop a stronger commitment to the therapy. At the same time, she helped him to classify the external issues and emotional sufferings that he was facing into two groups: those that he has no choice but has to accept and those that he has an option to change and modify.

During this explorative step, Peter revealed that he felt powerless in face of his parent's death, however, being a man and a successful person, he believed that he should be in charge of his life and be on top of his emotions. But he can't. His depression and anxiety were too much for him to handle. So he had to seek help form the psychiatrist and the counsellor. Furthermore, he felt that being a son, he should have taken care of the well-being of his parent out of filial piety. Now that they have both died tragically, and he felt a sense of shame and guilt; it is a failure on his part because he could not manage his family and live up to the classical value of: "in order to govern the country, one needs to first manage his family; in order to manage his family, he needs to first improve himself" [3].

In the third step of the therapy, Peter was guided by the counsellor to see that there are causes and conditions to his pain and suffering, and with these causes and conditions, pain and suffering would bound to arise. However, there are some pain and suffering that needs not continue. Those are the emotional sufferings that arise due to the subjective perspectives, attitudes and values that Peter held on the tragic deaths of his parent. If Peter can change or update those perspectives, attitudes and values in a more wholesome way, those emotional sufferings could be eliminated. It was necessary for Peter to understand that suffering is dependently originated and will cease to be when causes and conditions stop to be and vice versa as according to the Law of Dependent Origination. Therefore, it was possible for him to escape from the suffering that he was experiencing if he aspires to change the causes and conditions that give rise to his suffering. However, at this stage of the therapy, it is not necessary for Peter to challenge or question those perspectives, attitudes and values because he may not be ready to alter his believe system yet.

The therapist also recommended that Peter should be more compassionate towards himself and accept the fact that he is only an ordinary person. Having compassion towards himself would allow Peter to see that it is normal and reasonable to have painful emotions while experiencing these tragic events. Moreover, being an imperfect world, there will always be imperfection, and we should not expect that everything that we do to be perfect and just right. In Peter case, allowing himself to justifiably live with the pain and suffering was very healing.

Step four of the Dharma Therapy is to help Peter to develop a better understanding of the importance of his mind, more precisely, his thought, perspectives, attitudes and values, and how his thought, perspectives, attitudes and values are correlated to the suffering that he is experiencing. In order for a person to be able to observe the working of his own mind, the practice of mindfulness and meditation is important. By now, Peter had been practicing mindfulness for several weeks, he was instructed to investigate, pay careful attention to and become aware of what is happening in his mind: his thought, perspectives, attitudes and values, and how these mental factors influence his emotions, in order to develop the insight and wisdom that are necessary to bring about the transformation of his suffering.

Step five of the therapy was to help Peter solidify the knowledge and wisdom that he gained from observing the working of his mind. He needed to re-examine which are the facts and events that he needed to accept, for example his parent death, and which are the subjective thought, perspectives, attitudes and values that he can change or update with a more wholesome angle, for example a man should always be on top of his emotions. He was guided to use the Buddhist concept of a person, the five aggregates: form, sensation, perception and thought, volition and consciousness, as a framework to help him develop a better understanding of the working of his mind and, particularly, the relationship between his thoughts, values, emotions and panic distress. The following is an example showing how the mindful process can help him develop a better understanding of the working of his mind in order to be able to deal with his anxiety and panic distress skilfully.

Peter's perceptions, thoughts and values that give rise to his sufferings:

- Death could come so sudden, it is so horrible.
- Embarrassing experience at work: Being laughed at by colleague while he was performing poorly during an introduction of a picture that he created.
- Feeling weak and helpless due to strong emotions such as anxiety and panic attacks.
- Fearing that things will get out of control and he will become useless.

Corresponding volitions that arose due to his perceptions, thoughts and values:

- I want to fight and reject anxiety and other emotions.
- I want to escape from the fact that my parents have passed away, as well as the complex emotions and fears of death.

- Excessive self-protection and defence against dislikes.
- I want to resume and maintain "I am rational and calm," "Life is controllable".
- Eliminate emotions such as anxiety.
- Pursue to get everything back to "normal" and "controllable".

Finally, in Peter's mind and consciousness, he sees that:

- I am the one who is experiencing all sufferings because of parents' death;
- I deserved the suffering because I have not taken care of my parents: self-blaming and grief;
- I felt shameful because my emotional reaction affects my performance at work;
- I should be rational and able but I am losing control of life.

Through the intervention process, Peter understood that a person is made up of five aggregates: form, sensation, perception, volition/mental formation and consciousness. They are interdependent on each other. He also understood that perceptions and thoughts are not facts (Thought rumination); he should be mindful and prevent thoughts from falling into criticism and repetition; he should also examine the excessive attachment to self-identity.

In step six of the therapy, Peter was guided to further examine the context and assumption of the thought, perspectives, attitudes and values that he hold. With a better understanding of the context and assumption behind the thought, perspectives, attitudes and values, he can decide either to hold on to those thought, perspectives, attitudes and values or update/drop them all together. For example, he was suggested to see that his perspective: a man should always be on top of his emotions was built on the context that man should always be strong. However, such a perspective is only culturally based and it is, in many respects, emotionally unwholesome. Therefore, it is perfectly fine for him to feel distress while facing the tragic deaths of his parent.

In step seven, with the updated thoughts, perspectives, attitudes and value, Peter was advised to apply them into his daily life to bring about a transformation. Actually, the transformation just happened slowly without much effort as Peter developed a better understand of the thoughts, perspectives, attitudes and values that he hold. All these transformations happen as a result of the deeper and more wholesome comprehension of the original problem as seen from the perspective of the Dharma, that is all phenomena arise from causes and conditions, and when causes and conditions changes, those phenomena will cease to be or changes accordingly. This also applies to the suffering that Peter was experiencing.

For the end of the Therapy, Mr. Chan was able to resume his lives both in work and daily life. He was able to manage his anxiety and work stress. He also stops taking medication as the psychiatrist also found that he no longer needs the medication.

More importantly, he continues to practice meditation daily which helps him to maintain a mindful and clear mind. Cognitively, he now accepts that life is impermanence. He is now more comfortable with himself while acknowledging that his parents have passed away, something that is beyond his control. He has now learned to enjoy the present moment especially the time with his wife. The evaluation feedback and assessment also showed that his stress, anxiety, depression level have decreased, and his well-being increased after 14 sessions of Dharma Therapy.

35.4 Conclusion

Dharma Therapy was very effective in helping Peter to alleviate the suffering that he experienced as a result of the death of his parent. Through the building of the spiritual oasis, Peter was able to regain some control and clarity of his mind, and as a result, he was guided to become mindful of the content and working of his mind. Through the evaluation of the thoughts, perspectives, attitudes and values that he hold, he was able to let go of old attachments and develop new wholesome perspectives, attitudes and values. With these new perspectives, attitudes and values, Peter developed a more wholesome and healthy way of life.

Building on the Buddhist teaching of the Law of Dependent Origination, Dharma Therapy does seem to be able to help client to effectively deal with their psychological problems. This effectiveness hinges on whether the client is able to develop comprehension and insight of the cause and conditions that lead to suffering. Once the client makes sense of the interaction among his mind contents, action and consciousness, he would be able to manage his feelings and emotions more skilfully and improve overall mental health.

Like other mindfulness intervention, a Dharma Therapy counsellor's own mindfulness and/or meditation practice is very importance to the successful implementation of the intervention.

Acknowledgements This article is based on a real case story which has been anonymized, and we are very grateful that the client agrees to give us the permission to publish his story as a case study. Dharma Therapy is now being used by all the compassionate counsellors of the Tsz Shan Monastery Buddhist Spiritual Counselling Centre to help to alleviate sufferings of their clients.

35.5 Guide to Further Sources

For further information please refer to the following links:

(a) A Randomized Controlled Trial of Awareness Training Program (ATP), a Group-Based Mahayana Buddhist Intervention. https://link.springer.com/article/10.1007/s12671-018-1082-1
(b) Repetitive Religious Chanting Modulates the Late-Stage Brain Response to Fear- and Stress-Provoking Pictures. https://www.frontiersin.org/articles/10.3389/fpsyg.2016.02055/full
(c) Entrainment of chaotic activities in brain and heart during MBSR mindfulness training. https://www.sciencedirect.com/science/article/pii/S0304394016300015

For Dharma therapy being used in an intervention program with mindfulness as one of its key components, please see:

Kwee MGT (Ed.). New horizons in Buddhist psychology: relational Buddhism for collaborative practitioners. Chagrin Falls, OH: Tao Institute Publications; 2010. p. 353–72.

References

1. Bodhi BT. The connected discourses of the Buddha: a new translation of the Sanyutta Nikaya. Boston: Massm Wisdom Publications; 2000.
2. Sik. Dharma therapy: an intervention program with mindfulness as one of its key components [Internet]. HKU Scholars Hub: Home. Tao Institute Publications; 1970 [cited 2019 Dec 6]. http://hub.hku.hk/handle/10722/128225.
3. Confucius. The Book of Rites. Da Xue. James L, translator. The United States: Createspace Independent Publishing Platform; 1885.

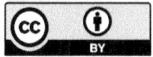

Dangerous Liaisons: Science, Tradition, and Qur'anic Healing in the Dakhla Oasis of Egypt

36

Mohammed Abouelleil Rashed and Werdie Van Staden

36.1 Introduction

The Dakhla oasis is one of six depressions in the Western desert of Egypt. It lies in relative physical isolation from the rest of the country, where the population coalesces around the Nile Valley as it has since the beginning of civilisation in Egypt. The oasis has a General Hospital that covers standard medical specialties except for psychiatry: there are no mental health services in Dakhla. The first port of call for most cases of social, physical, and mental health difficulties are the healers of Dakhla, who play a crucial role in managing the wellbeing of the community. They see everything from marital discord to chronic back pain; from impotence to psychosis; from major depression to bizarre behaviour; and from conflicts at work to schizophrenia.

Whatever the nature of the complaint, the common premise underlying all consultations is the suspicion of spirit (*jinn*) presence or possession and/or evil-doing (sorcery) responsible for the problem. Thus, diverse and seemingly unrelated problems are considered and dealt with within the same practical and moral framework. The healer seeks to detect this evil (e.g. the spirit) and, through a range of interventions, to dispel it. From there, the hope is to restore personal function and social harmony.

M. A. Rashed
Department of Philosophy, Birkbeck College, University of London, London, UK

Department of Philosophy, King's College London, London, UK

W. Van Staden (✉)
Centre for Ethics and Philosophy of Health Sciences, University of Pretoria, Pretoria, South Africa
e-mail: cwvanstaden@icon.co.za

© The Author(s) 2021
D. Stoyanov et al. (eds.), *International Perspectives in Values-Based Mental Health Practice*, https://doi.org/10.1007/978-3-030-47852-0_36

313

In this Chapter, through an ethnographic encounter with a prominent Qur'anic healer in the Dakhla oasis, we demonstrate the interplay of personal and cultural values on the healer's practice. On one hand, the healer is keen to preserve and continue traditional healing practices; on the other, he is keen to innovate and to develop his practices in line with his understanding of scientific concepts and procedures. We conclude by considering the implications of this for the proposed development of mental health services in communities such as the Dakhla oasis, where local healers manage the mental health of the community.

36.1.1 Meeting Sheikh Rayyes

I met Sheikh Rayyes in the course of an ethnographic study carried out during 2009 and 2010 in the Dakhla oasis. He works as a Qur'anic healer in the largest village of the oasis and is among the most famous and sought-after healers in the region. Just over 5 ft tall, with a penetrating gaze, a shaved head, and six digits on both feet and hands, he cuts a striking figure. Due to a congenital anomaly in his legs that was later operated upon at a hospital in Cairo, he walks with a noticeable limp. The operations left him with life-long chronic pain for which he self-administers an intravenous opiate painkiller daily.

Being in the presence of Sheikh Rayyes is unnerving, not least due to the intensity with which he converses with you. He lives in a three-storey building that he shares with his two brothers and their families as well as his wife and four children. In our meetings, we would congregate in his private room, which is also where he receives his many seekers among the possessed, ill, and unfortunate. The room is painted a bright blue and the walls are adorned with various Islamic items: verses inscribed in graceful calligraphy, several calendars with photos of the Prophet's mosque in Medina and the Ka'aba in Mecca, a photo of Al-Aqsa mosque in Jerusalem, and several certificates indicating prizes the Sheikh had won in religious chanting and singing (inshad). In this room I spent many hours with Sheikh Rayyes. I would visit him around 9 in the evening and would stay just short of the call for the dawn prayer. We would converse about possession, sorcery, and the community, and I would observe him at work with those who seek his help.

Sheikh Rayyes, like the majority of healers in Dakhla, practices Qur'anic healing. The main task before a Qur'anic healer is to utilise the divine blessings (baraka) and power of the word of God, the Qur'an, to dispel or contain the evil that has entered in the form of the jinni. The aim is to resolve the mental, physical, or social problems that have resulted from this. Healers do so in two main ways: through the recitation (incantation) of verses (ruqya) that are thought to embody certain powers, and by preparing amulets and holy water that can be used by the person thought to be influenced by the spirit. As Sheikh Rayyes put it, "every verse, every word, every letter in the Book possesses immense baraka."

Transferring the baraka, and therefore the healing power, inherent in the word of God to amulets and holy water is a laborious process. In order to prepare holy water, Sheikh Rayyes fills a large bowl then twirls the index finger of his right hand in the water while rapidly reading and repeating verses and invocations. This process lasts about 20 min. Next, he writes the required verses on plain white paper using ink distilled from the ground mixture of several herbs: za'faran, white musk, gazelle's blood, and rose water. Gazelle's blood, a herb, gives the ink an intense red colour. The paper is then placed in the bowl and the ink gradually dissolves in the water. He then transfers the holy water to several bottles, ready to be used for treatment, for protecting oneself from harm, or for general wellbeing.

36.1.2 Treating Fat'hi

Fat'hi was a young man who consulted Sheikh Rayyes in my presence. He had been harassed by a male jinni for 4 months. It started one evening after he had closed his shop and returned to his mud-brick dwelling. He had been living there alone after his mother's death two years before. As he entered the house, he felt there was someone there. He washed, prayed and went to bed, while trying to ignore this unsettling feeling. The same feeling recurred day after day, always in his house, and 2 weeks later he heard his name called. This progressed from a simple call to what he described as "noise and lots of talk". Initially, this was restricted to the house, but then it carried through with him while at work as well. In the beginning he would go for late night walks and return home only to sleep; he tried to live with it and to ignore it. But when the spirit followed him and spoke to him throughout the day, he found it impossible to work and for the few days leading to the consultation with Sheikh Rayyes he had not been able to open his shop. He had not sought any help during these months, and it was only because he could not afford to keep his shop shut, he explained, that he knew he had to do something about the problem.

On hearing this account, Sheikh Rayyes asked a number of diagnostic questions to ascertain the possibility of spirit interference. He informed him that he was right, that it was probably a jinni interfering with him. The Sheikh then moved closer to Fat'hi and in a powerful voice began reading the verses of the ruqya. These are specific verses from the Qur'an that are used to detect and dispel influences of the spirit world, and are also utilised for general healing and well-being. During this procedure Fat'hi had his eyes closed and was motionless in his chair. Sheikh Rayyes completed the verses, which took about 20 min, and after a short moment of silence asked him how he felt. Fat'hi said he felt calm and it was evident in his features that this was the case. Sheikh Rayyes then resumed further invocations and, upon completion, advised Fat'hi to spend more time observing religious practice: he should pray regularly in the mosque, read the Qur'an on a daily basis both in the morning and before going to bed, and invoke God's name throughout the day. He then gave him two bottles of holy water and asked him to sprinkle it over his body and around the house.

36.1.3 Sheikh Rayyes Innovates

Several weeks after this consultation on one of my regular visits to Sheikh Rayyes, I found him more excited than usual. His face drew the expression of someone who had come upon something significant. He told me that he had conceived a new, modern treatment for spirit influence that could help people like Fat'hi. He said:

> You know how many of the jinn, when they speak through a possessed person, say they are lodged inside the person's body? And do you remember how some of them say they are in the blood or mixed with the blood? Now what if we dissolve the verses into distilled water from the pharmacy and then inject the patient with this holy water? This way the baraka will target the jinn in the blood directly and will be more effective. What do you think?

Immediately and prior to any reflection, I was alarmed by this suggestion. My main concern was that it might not be safe to inject water in which several herbs had been dissolved, not knowing, for instance, the potential for allergic reactions or the impact of residue on arteries and veins; it was a risky practice. When I pointed this out to the Sheikh he thought about it for a moment and said: "No problem then. I don't have to prepare the water this way, I can just read the Qur'an over it".

36.2 Values Arising

From a mental health perspective in the context of the Dakhla oasis, Sheikh Rayyes is consulted for and manages a range of mental health conditions. The case of Fat'hi is a clear example. In pursuing his practice, Sheikh Rayyes is keen to continue his tradition. Qur'anic healing has its roots in pre-Islamic 'magico-religious' remedies including incantation to the many gods in the Arabian Peninsula. Prophet Muhammad had adopted these incantations and purified them of illegitimate polytheistic elements. Sheikh Rayyes is part of this tradition. Additionally, Sheikh Rayyes values innovation. During our meetings, I found his mind to be active, always looking for ways to improve his practice. For example, in order to maximise the *baraka* of the verses, he would sometimes prepare amulets by writing the Qur'anic verses in separate letters, a method he borrowed from sorcerers who prepare talismans and amulets in this way in order to increase their power. His suggestion to inject holy water into a vein is another attempt at innovation, which in this case resulted in a potentially dangerous practice.

What inspired Sheikh Rayyes' to arrive at this idea? We can reasonably surmise that this had something to do with the fact that he self-administers an intravenous opiate on a daily basis, and so is accustomed to the power injected substances can have on one's mental and physical state. He might also have been inspired by my presence, which in my capacity as a medical doctor led to many discussions on mental health practice and psychotropic medication. Overlying this is a serious worry about society's tendency to perceive Qur'anic healers as charlatans or as engaged in backward, unscientific practices. Sheikh Rayyes was aware of these accusations, which can be heard in the coffee shops of Dakhla, and are voiced in various media by doctors, intellectuals, and orthodox religious figures. Accordingly, he was anxious to validate and modernise his practice, and the obvious way to do so was to borrow from the prestige of 'science' and 'medicine' by emulating what he thought of as scientific concepts and practices.

36.3 The Influences of Culture

How does 'science' have this legitimating value for Sheikh Rayyes and the community more broadly? To answer this question, we need to understand the various attitudes to science in the context of the challenges of modernity to more traditional concepts and practices.

This challenge can be heard in the Egyptian Media and is voiced by intellectuals and prominent psychiatrists, all of whom share a tendency to portray the 'supernatural' beliefs upheld by rural and low-income Egyptians as backwards and a sign of ignorance. Consider, for example, Galal Nasr, a prominent journalist and writer in *Al-Ahram weekly*: 'our [the Egyptians] very capacity for reasoning seems to have disintegrated, while our infatuation with myth and the unseen world seems to be on the rise… We have so many schools and universities, and yet here we are entering the twenty-first century with a firm belief in ghosts. We are infatuated with *jinn*, beholden to the darkness of the irrational, and hungry for fables' (15–21 March 2007). The negative portrayal of rural and low-income Egyptians' beliefs is part of the official discourse on modernisation with its emphasis on the value of education and national development: rural and low-income Egyptians are lacking in the first and therefore a hindrance to the second, so the discourse goes.

With this background in place, attitudes concerning science are ambivalent to say the least. On one hand, we find arguments that science is just one part of the package of 'westernisation', a package that many in the community feel the need to resist in that it brings with it 'corrupt' lifestyle and family values. On the other hand, there are attempts to partake in the prestige of science by emulating its procedures and borrowing its discourse, often in a superficial manner. For example, you find every now and again attempts to justify a problematic procedure (e.g. culling the pigs in the wake of swine flu) or a questionable discovery (a machine that cures HIV) by citing 'science' as a grand justificatory category.

The suggestion offered by Sheikh Rayyes can be understood within this web of attitudes as an attempt to partake in scientific method and concepts.

36.4 Conclusions

The development of mental health services in communities such as the Dakhla Oasis requires the cooperation of the community and, crucially, the cooperation of local healers. Healers like Sheikh Rayyes manage the mental health of the community and are almost always the first port of call for a wide range of problems. In order to be able to enlist the cooperation of local healers, it is necessary to understand the values they are keen to promote and the cultural influences on their thought and practice. As we saw in the case study discussed in this chapter, the interplay between traditional practices and scientific concepts and methods, in the context of ambivalent cultural discourses around science and Qur'anic healing, resulted in a potentially dangerous innovation. By understanding these processes through ethnography, it becomes possible for future cooperation between traditional healers and mental health services to lead innovation in a more positive direction.

Acknowledgements Ethical approval for the study on which this case is based was obtained from University College London Research Ethics Committee (UCL Ethics Project ID Number: 1521/001). Approval to conduct research in Egypt was obtained from CAPMAS—the Central Agency for Public Mobilisation and Statistics—through the head of security, Mr. Mohammed Zayed, on 12 May 2009. We are grateful to both for their support.

We are also very grateful to Sheikh Rayyes and others for sharing their stories and for their hospitality.

36.5   Guide to Further Sources

The ethnography reported on in this chapter was carried out by the first author during 2009 and 2010. Excerpts and other material are available here: https://kanzaman.wordpress.com/?s=dakhla.

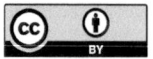

Know Thyself: Jane Discovers the Value of Her Depression

37

Tamara Kayali Browne

37.1 Introduction

Western culture tends to view depression more often than not as something to be avoided and eradicated. (Of course, Western culture is not the only one that views depression in this way, but it is worth remembering that there are other cultures that view it differently. For example, Kleinman [1] notes that dramatic expressions of grief and depression are valued in the Kaluli society of Papua New Guinea. In Shi-ite Muslim Iranian culture, depression is associated with "living justly in an unjust world" and as such, part of a religious experience. Buddhists consider pleasure-seeking as the source of suffering. For them, the state of pleasure-denial, which could be construed as mild depression, is the path to enlightenment. The term "Western culture" in this chapter functions only as a loose term to distinguish itself from other cultures such as these that value depression very differently.) Yet there are individuals who have been through the journey of depression, diagnosis and treatment who challenge this view. Another cultural value—gaining insight and self-discovery—can actually arise from the journey into and out of depression.

Jane's story that follows elucidates such a journey and what can be gained from examining the path that led one towards depression. The story is taken from my qualitative study of 37 women in the UK who were diagnosed with and treated for depression (see Guide to Further Sources). The study examined issues of the self in depression, asking participants for their views on, for example, whether depression/its treatment challenged their sense of authenticity or their views of their future with depression.

T. K. Browne (✉)
School of Medicine, Deakin University, Geelong, VIC, Australia

© The Author(s) 2021
D. Stoyanov et al. (eds.), *International Perspectives in Values-Based Mental Health Practice*, https://doi.org/10.1007/978-3-030-47852-0_37

37.2   Case Narrative: Jane's Story

Jane (not her real name) is a white, middle-class woman who works as a children's social worker. She has a husband and children and was first diagnosed with depression when she was a university student aged about 17, and suffered from it for most of her degree. The event that sparked this first episode of depression was the break-up of a serious romantic relationship—a break-up that left her suicidal. She sought medical help but felt that the support of her friends and seeking solace in religion were the most important factors in helping her out of that first episode.

Since then, she has suffered from bouts of depression throughout her life and has been treated with both medication and talking therapy. The talking therapy prompted her to examine how her early childhood contributed to her sense of self. Her mother left her when she was 1 year old and her father left when she was five. She was then raised by her aunt and her grandparents. She met her mother in her thirties but after a couple of years her mother did not wish to remain in contact.

She describes herself as having been a nervous and withdrawn child, but did not realize the full impact that her childhood traumas and losses had on her until she began talking therapy. As she describes:

> *[...] looking back, a lot of it has got to do with attachment and loss and the denigration of not being worth anything comes to the fact of that early period I would say [...]*
>
> *Me: So how does it help to know why it's happened?*
>
> *I think because before a lot of the reasons I'd put defenses up were to protect myself from other people getting near me in case the same thing happened again. So understanding why they are there and what has happened enables me to bit by bit break that down because there is a reason for it.*

Through her talking therapy, Jane came to understand herself better—something which she believes has been crucial to helping her understand her depression. By learning the reasons behind it, she felt armed with the ability to overcome it.

This is not to say that she does not believe biological factors played any role in her depression. She pondered whether the events that happened to her initiated certain neural pathways, or whether the neural pathways preceded her life events. She thinks her mother may have suffered from depression and therefore wonders whether there is an element of inheritance in her depression. However, she also states, "What I am certain about is because of what has happened in my life I have ended up being depressed."

When I asked Jane in which state she feels authentic, she was unsure, but said that she hopes it is the therapy that has contributed to her authentic self and not the medication. Her reason for this is apparent in the way she speaks about therapy:

> *I would hope that it is the therapy that has made me the real me and given me my confidence and self-esteem and self-worth and all of that. I don't think tablets can do that for you. They can enable you to switch off so that you're not so concerned about things but they can't enable... Well I don't think they can, and they certainly haven't in my case – enabled me to build up those parts of my life, parts of me that I denigrate all the time.*

Me: So if you had to choose one particular form of help, what would you pick?
I would pick therapy. I would pick therapy [...] I think you can use medication to kind of take you out of [a depressive state] a bit so you can cope with the therapy. But I think long-term I think it has to be therapy.

Finally, I asked:

If, in theory, there was a button that you could press that would get rid of depression from your life forever, would you press it?
That is a big question. I suppose in one sense I'd have to say yes because it's not a very pleasant thing to go through and I wouldn't like to see anybody else go through it, particularly my family. In another sense I would have to say it's taught me an awful lot about myself, and I think part of that is because of the therapy that I've had. If I'd have just been on medication I think my answer to that would have just been yeah. But having had the therapy, I think I've learnt an awful lot about myself. I'm much more self-aware and certainly with some of the children that I work with at school, can see things in a different kind of light with greater understanding and respect and empathy. So for that reason I would say no [...]

37.3   Values Arising

Jane's story demonstrates the value of examining the individual's life context, as this proved key for Jane in helping her to understand her depression and, as a result, the tools to be able to overcome it. It was learning the meaning and significance of her past and the context in which her depression arose that was crucial to her improvement. She is careful not to negate the possible role that one's biology might play in depression's aetiology, but whether she had biological factors which predisposed her to depression that was triggered by life events, or whether it was the life events which set in motion certain biological processes, she is not sure. However, she is certain that the life events she experienced were key factors in her depression. Without understanding her own life, she could not overcome depression. In this way, Jane demonstrates the values that society places on gaining insight in order to better understand oneself.

It is also apparent from Jane's story that she does not simply value mental well-being, or mental well-being by any means, but achieving it via learning and insight. This is emphasised by the fact that the insight she gained from therapy was so valuable that she would not choose to be rid of depression forever with the press of a button, despite the suffering involved, due to the opportunity it provides to learn about oneself. While medication, she feels, has its role, it cannot replace the role of therapy, which she sees as helping one understand oneself and the reasons behind one's depression. Jane's story thus also demonstrates two values that can sometimes be seen to be in opposition—the value placed on seeking medical help and taking medication, but also the value in eventually being free of medication.

37.4 The Influences of Culture

The value that Jane places on self-growth through knowledge and insight is reflected in the value placed on it in Western culture. Here, I draw on Ryff's definition of self-growth, which is to "develop one's potential, to grow and expand as a person" ([2], p. 1071). It is not that other cultures do not also value self-growth, but this definition of self-growth has its roots in both the Enlightenment and the Romantic tradition [3]. For instance, the idea that the self could be shaped in whatever direction one desires was popular during the Enlightenment [4, 5]. In addition, the idea that the self must battle against external forces in order to express itself comes from the Romantics [3], as is the view of commitments "from marriage and work to political and religious involvement—as enhancements of the sense of individual well-being rather than as moral imperatives" ([6], p. 47). We can see this nuance reflected in Jane's story, in which she struggled against the influences of her childhood, and drew on religion, work and therapy to enhance her self-growth and well-being. Yet this self-growth, which in Jane's case can only be achieved by examining the context of her depression, contrasts with the widespread culture within biological psychiatry that currently focuses on symptoms rather than their context. Jane's story shows what we may potentially lose with such a focus. In Jane's story, the value placed on gaining insight in broader Western culture won out over an aspect of Western biological psychiatric culture, but this is not the case with everyone.

This clash of "a culture within a culture" of sorts manifests itself in other aspects of Jane's story. Western culture values science and medicine, and the status and legitimacy of the medical profession grant a similar level of legitimacy to the medical approach to depression. However, Western culture also values independence and self-efficacy, as well as "the natural"—all of which can be challenged when one feels dependent on medication (something "unnatural" which one ingests) to achieve or maintain mental well-being. These two values can sometimes be in opposition, as the status given to the medical approach may cause the individual to feel that they must remain on medication for depression indefinitely (especially if this is what their doctor advises) yet there is simultaneously a pull in the other direction coming from a society which also values the ability to function independently of what can be viewed as a chemical "crutch."

Finally, the way depression is often portrayed in society—as something uncontrovertibly negative that one should be rid of—contrasts with the view of some such as Jane who do not view it in such black and white terms. Despite their suffering, they also found value in their journey through depression and recovery. By understanding how and why they became depressed, they could make sense of why they are the way they are. In turn, this insight enabled a self-growth that they felt could not have been achieved through medication alone, or without having been depressed (as this had prompted the need for therapy in the first place). Jane's story thus shows how understanding the context of the individual's depression, rather than relying on symptomatology alone, can be crucial for their recovery.

37.5   Conclusions

Jane's story exemplifies a number of values which manifest in Western culture—some of which are in tension and others not. Depression tends to be portrayed in straightforwardly negative terms—as an illness to be banished. Further, the focus of medical texts such as the *Diagnostic and Statistical Manual of Mental Disorders* is on symptomatology. In contrast, Jane's portrayal of depression is not as black and white. Although it is, in her words, "not a very pleasant thing to go through," the insights she gained from talking therapy were crucial to her self-growth. However, she would not have gained them had she not experienced depression, or had she taken medication alone. Self-growth through insight is also valued by society, but Jane recounts that this would not have been possible for her without understanding her past and how it led her to where she is. It is a testament to the value that can be gained from the journey through depression and recovery if one looks beyond the manifestation and alleviation of the individual's symptoms to the context in which their depression arose.

Acknowledgements   Sincere thanks to all the participants who so generously gave their time to share their experiences for the study from which this case is drawn. Thank you to Dr. Furhan Iqbal for not only assisting with recruitment of participants for the study, but also for providing invaluable support and insightful debate. Thanks also to the Arnold Gerstenberg fund for their financial support for the study.

37.6   Guide to Further Sources

The case presented in this chapter is drawn from unpublished interview material from a study I conducted at the University of Cambridge. Further findings from this study have also been published as a book and two papers:

- Browne TK. Depression and the self: meaning, control and authenticity. Cambridge: Cambridge University Press; 2018 (http://www.cambridge.org/9781316503478).
- Kayali T, Iqbal F. Making sense of melancholy: sub-categorisation and the perceived risk of future depression. Health, Risk & Society. 2012;14(2):171–89.
- Kayali T, Iqbal F. Depression as unhomelike being-in-the-world? Phenomenology's challenge to our understanding of illness. Medicine, Health Care and Philosophy. 2013;16(1):31–9.

References

1. Kleinman A, Good B. Introduction to culture and depression. In: LeVine RA, editor. Psychological anthropology: a reader on self in culture. Chichester: Wiley-Blackwell; 2010. p. 112–8.

2. Ryff CD. Happiness is everything, or is it? Explorations on the meaning of psychological well-being. J Pers Soc Psychol. 1989;57(6):1069–81.
3. Christopher JC. Situating psychological well-being: exploring the cultural roots of its theory and research. J Couns Dev. 1999;77:141–52.
4. Taylor C. The moral topography of the self. In: Messer SB, Saas LS, Woolfolk RL, editors. Hermeneutics and psychological theory: interpretive perspectives on personality, psychotherapy, and psychopathology. Rutgers symposia on applied psychology, vol. 2. Piscataway, NJ: Rutgers University Press; 1988. p. 298–320.
5. Taylor C. Sources of the self: the making of the modern identity. Cambridge: Cambridge University Press; 1989.
6. Bellah RN, Madsen R, Sullivan WM, Swidler A, Tipton SM. Habit of the heart: individualism and commitment in American life. New York, San Francisco: Harper & Row; 1985.

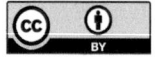

Case Studies in the Culture of Professional Football Players and Mental Welfare and Wellbeing

38

Michael Bennett

38.1 Introduction

There is growing concern about mental health and well-being in football (soccer) and in many other areas of the increasingly competitive world of top-level sport. Statistics abound but there has been little attempt to understand the values (positive and negative) held by the players themselves in relation to their sport and how these interact with those of the clubs by which they are employed to and the impact on their mental health.

This chapter draws on the findings from a series of in-depth interviews I carried out with 12 professional football players about their experience and interpretation of mental health. The study was informed by my own experience as a professional player. It has also been guided by two sources that (as I discuss further below) I have found helpful in understanding and working through the issues highlighted by the study. The first is the ([1], p. 32) 'front stage/backstage' distinction [1], the distinction between what is performed out there, as it were, on the front stage of our lives and the personal meanings and values we embrace in the backstage. The second main guide for the study is the ([2], p. 4). Understood through Du Bois' work, the study explores the veils used by professional players to transcend their experience of being objectified—of being subject to gendered, racialised and other forms of dehumanisation—and denied a legitimate lived experience, an authentic heard voice.

The extracts that follow describe in the words of the players themselves one of four emerging themes from the interviews, called by one of the interviewees *Snowing Balling of Self*. In work of this kind, it is clearly impossible to divorce the

M. Bennett (✉)
The Professional Footballers Association, Manchester, UK

University of East Anglia, Norwich, UK

D. Stoyanov et al. (eds.), *International Perspectives in Values-Based Mental Health Practice*, https://doi.org/10.1007/978-3-030-47852-0_38

way the findings are understood from one's own values. Hence, before describing players' experiences of 'the snow ball effect', I will outline my own values and how these have been shaped by the culture of professional football.

38.2   My Cultural Values

As an ex-professional football, now an academic researcher and Director of Player Welfare at the Professional Footballers Association, I have become aware of the complexity of the different values I carry from my personal life as a black man, a married man, a Christian man and a therapist. I am also aware that these are the cultural values that have been taken from me in the world of football, described by Rhoden [3] as the values that reduce black men in sport to a property.

I am aware further of the reflective insights my counselling and my Christianity give me about my cultural and spiritual values, beyond that which is fixed by being a man, by being black and by working in the professional context of sport. In sport, feelings are denied and one has a single identity, as a *player*, a commodity with decreasing value because of one's age and the loss of body functions [4]. In looking beyond the physical, my spiritual and other cultural values have become crucial to my work and the work that I enjoy. These values and cultures are rarely exposed in the professional setting of football as they are taken to denote vulnerability and weakness. In these cultural encounters, I hold onto my own 'mask', as the ([5], p. 11). I want the dignity of this mask and not to feel that I have to hold a 'mask' to be accepted. I am aware of my spiritual mask, of my veil, in terms of how I see beyond the culture in the room and the values that individuals bring to the room.

The culture of sport, the culture that takes away your values and your individuality, that requires you to give up your values and individuality in order to be accepted, has been an important part of my liberation, to be accepted for who I am as opposed to who I was in the football world. This is where I find the work of ([2], p. 4) helpful. His concept of 'veils' helps me to transcend the professional culture of sport and see and understand how people give meaning to their world. This is important to me. It enables me to observe and evaluate and to see beyond my maleness to engage as a person with a distinct individual identity.

These are the cultural values that have taken my individuality from me in the world of football, the cultural values that can reduce men in sport to a property. I see similar values in the research world in which there is a culture of being accepted if you are academic and bright; and I see similar values in the world of mental health, the values of being seen as normal or abnormal. I position my own values as the search for equality, for equity and for being heard as Michael, not Mickey, a player once owned by a club and told what to do and when to do it. I see the values of research and academic institutions where you told not how to play but to write, how to be heard. In this I seek guidance from the values, Mandela [6] in seeing beyond the racial demands that lead to anger in me, I use the culture of my life in the church, one that is based on seeing beneath the stereotype.

38.3   The Snow Ball Effect and Its Components

As noted above, the concept of the 'Snow Ball effect' was named as such by one of the interviewees in my study. I will call the player in question 'Billy'. I describe the Snow Ball effect in Billy's own words below. The Snow Ball effect was also one of four major themes that emerged from the interviews as a whole using a method of qualitative analysis, Smith [7] This method of analysis defines 'super-ordinate themes' (the snow ball effect being one of these) and their respective sub-elements (called 'clustered subsidiary themes'). The quotes that follow illustrate in the words of the players themselves, first the superordinate theme of the Snow Ball effect, and then four of its 'clustered subsidiary themes'. These are summarised diagrammatically in the Fig. 38.1.

38.3.1   The Snow Ball Effect

Billy—*I likened it to a snowball effect, I started at CM and did well and the snowball grew, your then bought by a premier league club for £2 million and your snowball grows again and you're playing in the premier league and you get sold to another premier league club for £4 million you win the league cup and get called up to the National team and your snowball is a giant and I'm invincible and I'm untouchable and nothing can happen to me and I'm so confident and my ego's huge and then it comes crashing down were I have this traffic accident. A lot of time goes by with memory loss and I'm trying to get back onto my feet my balance and coordination is slowly rebuilding.*

38.3.1.1   Learning to Deal With and Deny Pressure
Michael—*So, my first loan spell at division 2 club was a fantastic time and probably my favourite time down there I was 17 and not long out of school I moved down there with RM and JO and spent most of year in a hotel and looking back on it, it was quite tough. Just getting first team football was quite important and learning to deal with and deny the pressures of fighting to pay the mortgages and people learning to pay their rent was quite interesting.*

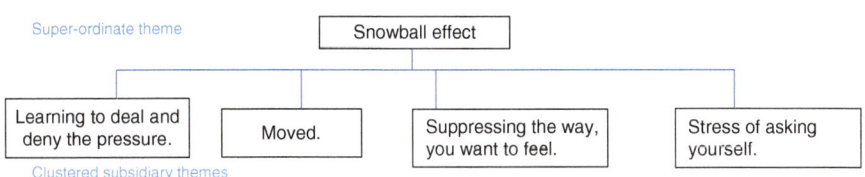

Fig. 38.1 Elements of the 'Snowball effect'

38.3.1.2 Moved

Holly—*In SG the time I was out there was when I encountered my first mental health issues. For me it was like several life stresses all came at one time and I developed some sort of anxiety and depression for around 8–10 months.*

38.3.1.3 Suppressing the Way You Want to Feel

Mark—*Well I made sure I didn't cry because of the way banter was in football and the kind of player I was. I was kind of looked at as a tough player so you 'hold back' and your 'pushing down your feeling basically' your "suppressing the way you want to feel" I didn't go to speak to anyone, I just remember sitting there watching games thinking I wish I wasn't injured and I wish I wasn't here. 'There was no one to reach out to', 'there was no one there', 'there was nothing'.*

38.3.1.4 Stress of Asking Yourself

Charlie—*So yes, it's a lot of pressure, and emotional pressure and the stress of asking yourself did I do good at this did I do good at that ...... it's constantly on your mind. I was always that person who over thought stuff. Did I do good here, or, should I do this and that better?*

38.4 The Culture and Values of Football

These narratives reveal an emerging value and culture co-existing inside the coldness of the culture of sport, a detachment and a failure to recognise its damaging impact on players. Their ego is eroded as they attempt to rebuild themselves in isolation. They learn to be in and part of a culture in which they develop an approach of 'learning to deny and deal with pressure'. Their profession as footballers is one in which they show their feelings in phrases such as 'developed some sort of anxiety and depression'. Such phrases are not a reflection of a clinical culture of 'self-diagnosis'. They reflect a culture in which they use the 'clinical term' in inverted commas to represent feelings that are denied.

Such narratives are readily understood in terms of Goffman's back-stage challenges that are never revealed or made visible [1]. They are also part of what Mandela (2005) would have recognised as contributing to the players' developing internal philosophy of liberation that will enable them to see a world beyond the control of the professional game. The impact of a culture of denial, and of the feeling you have no power, is further revealed in the narrative 'suppressing the way you want to feel' and the 'stress of asking yourself'. These suggest that the three-dimensional character of the professional footballer—its physical essence, its cultural essence and its internal philosophical essence—is rendered unimportant.

38.5 Conclusions

My research has been focused on three moments: the denial of the body as a lived experience, the denial of the culture of a sport that objectifies the body and the internal processes professional players use to get beyond the ([5], p. 4) mask and beyond

Du Bois' ([2], p. 4) veil. As a qualitative study, it seeks the reality of the professional footballer's lived and interpreted experience of stress, denial, moving and transition. Summed up as the snowball effect of the profession, these experiences reflect unrevealed values embedded in the culture of the sport.

As a former player, I am not detached from these experiences. Indeed, I find in my position as a researcher that I am once again trying to co-exist and to conform, this time to the dimensional pressures of the culture of research. I am at risk of ceasing to be an advocate for the lived experiences of professional players but constrained by the research conventions of reliability and validity. In this research, I risk forsaking the sense of myself, everything that I once exchanged for the commodity status of being a professional footballer. Once again, I find myself falling into a dimension, the internal philosophical dimension, in which my cultural identity and the values that support empowerment are invisible. Research and professional football share this cultural void, a void in which the processes of value and cultural denial lead to a delusion about what is value and culture to me.

Acknowledgements There are currently new initiatives in hand aimed at addressing the mental health issues with which this chapter is concerned. My hope is that the experiences of the players reported in this chapter will endorse the importance of these initiatives and provide insights that may contribute to their success.

References

1. Goffman E. The presentation of self in everyday life. London: Penguin Book; 1956.
2. Du Bios WD. The souls of the black folk. Oxford, New York: Oxford University Press; 1903.
3. Rhoden WC. Forty million Dollar slaves: the rise, fall, and redemption of the black athlete. New York: Crown Hardcover; 2007.
4. Hawkins BJ. The new plantation: black athletes, college sports, and predominantly white NCAA institutions. New York: Palgrave MacMillan Press; 2010.
5. Fanon F. Black skin, white mask. London: Pluto Press; 1967.
6. Mandel N. The long walk home. The autobiography. Great Britain: Little, Brown; 1995.
7. Smith JA. Beyond the divide between cognition and discourse: using interpretive phenomenological analysis in health psychology. Psychol Health. 1996;11:261–71.

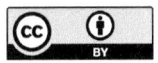

Taryn Knox

39.1 Introduction

Although gay people still face discrimination, being gay has become increasingly accepted in the modern western world. In turn, sexual orientation change efforts (SOCE)—methods used to alter an individual's sexuality, predominantly from homosexual to heterosexual—are largely considered ethically unacceptable. But what if an individual wants SOCE and gives truly informed consent? This question raises a number of conflicting values. A central and unavoidable issue is how these conflicts of values should be resolved. This chapter focuses on whether the conflicts can be resolved by considering whether there are some values that, according to VBP, should not be taken into account.

The chapter explores this issue primarily through the story of 'Matthias' and his therapist 'Kirk' (not their real names). The adapted narrative describes Matthias, a gay man who questions his sexuality and is considering having SOCE. The story is extensively adapted from a case study reported by Andrew Kirby [1]. The overarching question posed by the case study is whether Matthias should have conversion therapy. This question makes explicit the cultural and other values underpinning the issues in a situation of this kind. However, this chapter focuses on which values are relevant for the purposes of decision-making in VBP.

Two notes on terminology. Firstly, the chapter uses the phrase 'SOCE' rather than the more widely known phrase 'conversion therapy'. While the two refer to the same thing, the chapter uses SOCE. This is because the word 'therapy' in 'conversion therapy' signifies that being gay is a disease or illness in need of therapeutic intervention. In contrast, SOCE remains neutral on this issue. Secondly, in the literature, the term *heterosexism* refers to prejudiced institutions and structures, and

T. Knox (✉)
Bioethics Centre, University of Otago, Dunedin, New Zealand

D. Stoyanov et al. (eds.), *International Perspectives in Values-Based Mental Health Practice*, https://doi.org/10.1007/978-3-030-47852-0_39

the term *homophobia* to prejudiced personal attitudes (rather than, as the term suggests, fear) [2]. I use homophobia as shorthand for both homophobic and heterosexual values. In the second part of this chapter, it is suggested that there may be values that do not align with homosexuality, yet are not prejudiced.

39.2   Case Narrative

Matthias (not his real name) is a confident, attractive gay man in his mid-thirties who was raised in a conservative Christian home. He recalls having always been attracted to men rather than women and 'came out' to his parents in his early twenties. Despite some sadness that he had disappointed his parents by being gay, he has generally felt loved and supported by his family. After several short-term relationships, Matthias settled into a happy long-term relationship of 10 years with another man. Matthias enjoys an accomplished career and has a close circle of friends both in and out of the gay community. On entering therapy Matthias described a conflict between his homosexuality and a desire to have children of his own. This, combined with his Christian faith that does not support same-sex attraction, created an underlying gnawing angst that often made him question his gay identity and lifestyle [1].

Over a period of time, Matthias explored these issues with a therapist, Kirk (not his real name), who took a gay-affirmative perspective. While Matthias gained insight into how formative influences contribute to his core belief system and values, Matthias was unresponsive to the gay-affirmative approach. Matthias brings up the topic of SOCE, and asks Kirk whether he thinks it would be a good idea for himself (Matthias) to try it.

Kirk is somewhat taken aback, as he is himself gay and believes that Matthias could lead a happy and fulfilling life as a gay man. Kirk knows that SOCE is available in the city in which Matthias lives. Kirk is not focused on the issue of whether SOCE should be banned, but is more troubled by whether Matthias, in particular, should have SOCE. He also wonders whether he has an obligation to refer Matthias to someone who practices SOCE, even though he (Kirk) is personally offended by the practice.

After doing some research, Kirk finds that SOCE is not currently effective, and in many cases, it is harmful [2, 3]. However, Kirk also reads that recent advances in neuroscience mean that in the near future, there may be SOCE that is both effective and safe [3]. If so, would his intuition that Matthias should not have SOCE still stand up to scrutiny? The issue of consent also crosses Kirk's mind. He knows that many instances of SOCE are either forced or coercive, and holds that any SOCE that is not truly consensual is unacceptable. Yet, Kirk thinks that Matthias may give his truly informed consent to SOCE. If SOCE were safe and effective, and if Matthias gave genuine informed consent, should Matthias have SOCE? And what should Kirk do if Matthias were to ask him to refer him to someone who practices SOCE? Night after night Kirk lies in bed considering these questions.

Kirk is not the only one suffering sleepless nights. Matthias also spends many long nights agonising over whether he should have SOCE. Matthias recognises that his values (his beliefs and desires) are somewhat conflicting. On the one hand, Matthias identifies as gay and is open to gay-affirmation therapy. He definitely values authenticity i.e. being true to his gay self. Matthias also has a deeply loving and respectful relationship with his partner Lachlan. It would be impossible to have SOCE and stay in a relationship with Lachlan. These points make Matthias think that he should not have SOCE. On the other hand, family is very important to Matthias. Not only does he want to have children of his own, he has continuing fears of disappointing his parents. Matthias acknowledges that his religious values are a strong factor causing his uneasiness about his sexuality, as his Christianity has become increasingly important to him.

Matthias recognises the conflict between, on the one hand, his identity as a gay man and wanting to stay in a relationship with Lachlan (which provide reasons not to have SOCE), and on the other hand his desire to have children of his own, please his family and retain his faith (which point in favour of SOCE). He racks his mind to come up with a way in which the conflict could be avoided. Matthias knows that a gay man can have children of his own. But what he really wants is to have the biological children of both himself and his partner, and it is currently impossible to have the biological children of both Lachlan and himself. The divergence between Matthias' desire to have children and his sexuality remains. Matthias also knows that there are gay-friendly churches in his city—that Christianity is compatible with homosexuality. However, Matthias does not entirely approve of these gay-friendly churches, and maintains that his personal Christianity is incompatible with homosexuality. If Matthias could accept that he can have his own biological children (though not children that are biologically related to both himself and Lachlan) and if he could accept a gay-friendly iteration of Christianity, then there would be no need for him to have SOCE. But Matthias cannot accept either of these things, and concludes that he holds values that are intractably incompatible. His sleepless nights continue.

While tossing and turning the following night, Matthias begins to think about how others may be impacted by his decision to have—or not have—SOCE. He knows that Lachlan would be devastated if he decided to go ahead with SOCE. But to what extent should Lachlan's perspective have an effect on Matthias' decision whether or not to have SOCE? Should he decline SOCE just to keep Lachlan happy? Matthias knows that some of his gay friends would be very angry with him if he were to have SOCE. They would say that doing so would diminish and disempower the already vulnerable gay community [2, 4]. Matthias is sympathetic to this argument to some degree, but wonders whether the needs of the gay community should override his individual desire to have SOCE (if this is indeed what he decides he wants).

Just before drifting into a fitful sleep, Matthias begins to think about Kirk, his therapist. Matthias knows that Kirk is gay, and that he is a strong believer in gay-affirmative therapy. Matthias has developed a meaningful relationship with Kirk, and worries about how Kirk would respond if he (Matthias) were to go ahead with SOCE. But once again, should Matthias do what is right for him or that which is right for others?

Matthias takes the courageous step to discuss some of these issues with Kirk. Kirk mentions that Matthias' gnawing angst concerning his sexuality is not really his own view, but may stem from an internalisation of homophobic sentiment in society. Kirk and Matthias discuss that rather than Matthias having SOCE, society ought to be changing the dubious social norms [2]. Together, Matthias and Kirk explore whether Matthias has had negative experiences relating to his sexuality in family, social, educational or vocational contexts, and has incorporated this anti-gay sentiment into his own belief systems. Matthias denies that his views are caused by an internalisation of external anti-gay sentiment—he maintains that they are truly his own views, and that his desire for SOCE are based on his genuine values. (Without relating it to Matthias, Kirk worries that if he were to refer Matthias to someone practicing SOCE, then he might even be compared to a doctor who gives his or her patient in an abusive relationship Valium, rather than dealing with the underlying problem.)

Matthias then points out that New Zealand—the country in which he lives—is relatively gay-friendly, while recognising that gay people in New Zealand undoubtedly experience some stigmatisation. Matthias goes on to say that it is not the case that he has internalised homophobic views, but it may be the case that he has internalised gay-friendly views. That is, he wonders whether the predominantly gay-friendly values of New Zealand society have actively discouraged him from having SOCE. Does he really want SOCE, but is worried about the social consequences of doing so? Will his gay friends be angry with him? Will he be accused of setting the gay-rights movement back 20 years?

Should Matthias have SOCE? If asked, is Kirk obliged to refer Matthias to someone who practices SOCE? The latter part of this chapter interrogates the conflict of cultural values using the insights of Fulford's 'Values-Based Practice' (VBP).

39.3 Commentary

Matthias's values—his needs, preferences, strengths and aspirations—are of fundamental importance (principle four). Some of Matthias's internal values conflict. He identifies as gay and wants to stay in his relationship with Luke. Yet, he also wants biological children of his own and his personal Christianity is incompatible with being gay. Given the importance of informed consent in health care (here, 'health care' is interpreted broadly to include SOCE), it is clear that SOCE should only be given to Matthias if, after balancing his internal conflicting values, he gives his genuine and informed consent. If Matthias refuses to give consent, the issue largely dissolves. Matthias will not have SOCE, which would align with the values of Kirk, Lachlan and the gay community. The difficulty arises if Matthias decides he does want SOCE, as there is a conflict of values between himself and others.

Rather than focusing on the internal conflict between some of Matthias's values, this commentary focuses on a specific external conflict—the conflict between Matthias's religious values (which support SOCE) and the values of a gay-friendly society (which suggest that having SOCE is not compatible with mutual respect for gay people). Other external conflicts, such as the conflict between Matthias's desire for SOCE and the values of his therapist (Kirk) and partner (Lachlan), are not directly considered.

The chapter considers it to be possible that Matthias's views are not internalised homophobic norms, but does not directly consider whether Matthias has, in fact, internalised anti-gay sentiment in society (see, for example, Cruz in [3]). This is because, even if Matthias's views are internalised anti-gay norms, many choices are 'profoundly influenced by social pressures ... but we wouldn't normally conclude that people are therefore non-autonomous [have not given genuine consent]' [3]. Hence, determining whether or not Matthias has internalised social norms does not necessarily change whether SOCE ought to be available to him. In short, the chapter proceeds on the basis that Matthias' views are not internalised homophobic norms, and even if they were internalised, it does not automatically mean that he should not have SOCE.

Diversity of values plays an integral role in VBP. VBP is clear that, in addition to Matthias's values, the values of other parties involved also need to be considered (principle five). Moreover, decisions are not made by determining the right outcome but by a process that balances multiple legitimately different perspectives. The word 'legitimately' plays two roles. Firstly, it emphasises that having differing values is not a bad thing. Secondly, it hints that there are some perspectives or values that are illegitimate. According to VBP, legitimate values are those that are consistent with mutual respect. Fulford gives the example of racism: racism is incompatible with respect for differences, and so racist values are precluded from VBP. Fulford also considers sexist, homophobic, classist, ageist and ableist values, along with values that are prejudiced towards religion, culture and language, to be incompatible with mutual respect [5].

Pickering (chapter 33, "Covert treatment in a cross-cultural setting") critiques VBP on the basis that the scope of legitimate values differences is the same as the scope of values differences, i.e. that there is no way of distinguishing between legitimate and illegitimate values. But VBP does provide a method for distinguishing between the two, namely, whether the values are compatible with mutual respect. Nonetheless, Fulford does not provide a justification for having mutual respect as the necessary and sufficient condition of a legitimate value. And why 'mutual respect' as opposed to simply 'respect'? Let's put these problems aside, and directly consider the case study in question.

Two problems develop regarding Matthias's situation. Firstly, homophobic values and values that are prejudiced towards religion are not consistent with mutual respect, and in turn are not VBP-able, i.e., cannot be accounted for in the decision-making process. Matthias's desire to have SOCE appears to be a homophobic value, and so is beyond the pale of VBP. It is not a legitimately different perspective and cannot be accounted for in the decision-making process. Given principle four (the patient-perspective principle), this seems very odd. Surely Matthias's values, including his religious values, ought to play a central role when making decisions that primarily, although not solely, impact him. Moreover, all VBP case studies concern the conflicts of values between the various stakeholders, rather than conflicting values held by an individual such as Matt. This suggests that Fulford did not intend VBP to have anything to say about such private decisions.

Secondly, the list of values that are not VBP-able may themselves conflict. For example, female genital mutilation (FGM) may not be compatible with respect for women, but not allowing FGM may be incompatible with respect for cultural values [6]. A comparable paradox arises in Matthias's case. Matthias's values that lead him to consider SOCE could be homophobic, and so incompatible with mutual respect for the gay community and, in turn, not VBP-able. Yet, limiting Matthias's religious freedom (by not allowing him to have SOCE, or not allowing Matthias's religious values to be factored into VBP) is also incompatible with mutual respect. Hence, values that limit religious freedom are not VBP-able, which suggests Matthias's religious values need to be accounted for in VBP.

A potential way of avoiding this paradox is to show that one or both of those values are consistent with mutual respect, and so can be factored into the decision-making process. Carrying out violent anti-gay hate crime is clearly inconsistent with mutual respect. However, Matthias's desire to have SOCE might be compatible with mutual respect if, for example, he thought that while he does not want to be gay, it is fine for other people to be gay. In the same vein, it might be inconsistent with mutual respect of religious groups to ban SOCE. However, taking a more moderate approach, such as requiring Matthias to enter into discussion about the acceptability of SOCE, is likely to be consistent with mutual respect.

VBP might deem all values that might loosely be considered homophobic (and racist, sexist, classist, ablest values and values that are prejudiced towards religion, culture and language) to be inconsistent with mutual respect and therefore not VBP-able. For example, one can imagine that Matthias' parents had dreams of being grandparents. This is most easily achieved if Matthias is straight. The desire for grandchildren could be considered a homophobic value, although it is only homophobic in a benign way. That is, taken on its own, it is only very minimally prejudiced. If all values that are incompatible with mutual respect in a benign way are beyond the pale of VBP, then VBP would become very difficult to operationalise. Hence, it is likely that Fulford did not intend 'values incompatible with mutual respect' to have such a broad reach.

Principles six and seven require those practising VBP to look deeply at the exact values involved. Based on this, when considering whether a perspective is compatible with mutual respect, it appears that VPB requires us to consider the precise value or perspective involved. It would be easy to blithely label Matthias's desire to have SOCE as homophobic. However, VBP requires more, namely, to consider whether Matthias's particular view is consistent with mutual respect. Matthias's view—while he does not want to be gay, it is fine for other people to be gay—is, at least arguably, consistent with mutual respect.

Of course, some people may consider Matthias's view to be incompatible with mutual respect, i.e. to be homophobic. They might point out that as the gay community has faced much oppression and stigmatisation in the recent past (and still faces this discrimination to some degree), Matthias's desire for SOCE is not just a simple choice between, say, vanilla and chocolate ice-cream. Put bluntly, they would say that Matthias's desire to have SOCE is a loaded choice—it is a choice that, despite Matthias's intention, expresses to society that being gay is wrong or sinful. Thus, they would say, Matthias's religious values (which support SOCE) are incompatible with mutual respect and therefore not VBP-able.

But is Matthias's desire for SOCE really a loaded decision? Perhaps it is closer to a simple choice than first appears. In an ideal society—a society entirely free of homophobia and heterosexism [2]—choosing to have SOCE would be a 'simple' choice, akin to choosing between ice-cream flavours. It would not be a loaded choice. That is, there is no oppression or stigmatisation in an ideal society, and so opting to have SOCE would not perpetuate oppression or stigma. New Zealand, where Matthias lives, is not an ideal society. Sexual injustice undoubtedly exists. This means that Matthias's desire to have SOCE is not entirely a simple choice. However, New Zealand is a relatively gay-friendly community. The gay community is not as persecuted as it once was. As being gay is becoming increasingly acceptable, perhaps Matthias's desire to have SOCE is becoming closer to a simple preference. If so, then Matthias's desire to have SOCE is more likely to be compatible with mutual respect, and hence, his religious values (which support his desire for SOCE) are VBP-able.

39.4 Conclusions

Many readers from the modern Western world might have the intuition that SOCE is unacceptable. This chapter has challenged that intuition by considering the diversity of values involved in considering whether safe, effective and consensual SOCE would be acceptable for someone in Matthias's position.

In VBP, the legitimate values (those that are compatible with mutual respect) of everyone involved must be considered in the decision-making process. The chapter has suggested that only some homophobic values are incompatible with mutual respect. It is possible Matthias's position—he thinks it is okay for people to be gay, but does not want to be gay himself—to be compatible with mutual respect. This is especially so in a relatively gay-friendly society such as New Zealand, as an individual's decision to have SOCE is less likely to express the view that it is not okay to be gay.

It is possible that VBP will come to the conclusion that safe and effective SOCE should be available to Matthias, should he decide this is what he wants. Some might consider this to be a shortfall of VBP. However, recall Matthias's concern that he really does want SOCE but has internalised the predominantly gay-friendly views of New Zealand society. VBP provides space to consider this position. In turn, VBP can help to come to a decision that does not ensure the well-being of the gay population at the expense of people like Matthias.

Many questions concerning this case remain unanswered. Is it really the case that Matthias's desire for SOCE is not based on internalised anti-gay sentiments? To what extent should the perspectives of Lachlan, Kirk and the gay community influence Matthias's decision about whether SOCE is right for him? What impact would Matthias having SOCE have on the gay community—would it turn 'Queer villages into ghost towns' [4]? Would Kirk (Matthias's therapist) have an obligation to refer Matthias to someone who practices safe and effective SOCE? It is unlikely to be the case that VBP can definitively answer all these questions. Nevertheless, we should not forget that the power of VBP lies in its recognition of all mutually respectful values.

Acknowledgements Thanks to Andrew Kirby for the use of his very rich case narrative.

39.5   Guide to Further Sources

National LGBTQ Task Force. https://www.thetaskforce.org/

Stuff. 2018. "I thought I was a freak": one man's experience with gay conversion therapy. Stuff. 2018. https://www.stuff.co.nz/national/health/105368961/i-thought-i-was-a-freak-one-mans-experience-with-gay-conversion-therapy

Human Rights Watch. 2017 "Have You Considered Your Parents' Happiness?" | Conversion Therapy Against LGBT People in China. https://www.hrw.org/report/2017/11/15/have-you-considered-your-parents-happiness/conversion-therapy-against-lgbt-people

BBC. 2017. China "gay conversion": accounts of shocks and pills. https://www.bbc.com/news/world-europe-41996322

References

1. Kirby A. Gay-affirmative therapy and emerging integrative solutions. N Z J Counsell. 2008;28(2):37.
2. Delmas C, Aas S. Sexual reorientation in ideal and non-ideal theory. J Polit Philos. 2018;26(4):463–85.
3. Earp BD, Sandberg A, Savulescu J. Brave new love: the threat of high-tech "conversion" therapy and the bio-oppression of sexual minorities. AJOB Neurosci. 2014;5(1):4–12.
4. Behrmann J, Ravitsky V. Turning queer villages into ghost towns: a community perspective on conversion therapies. AJOB Neurosci. 2014;5(1):14–6.
5. Fulford KWM. Values-based practice: fulford's dangerous idea. J Eval Clin Pract. 2013;19(3):537–46.

6. Kingma E, Banner N. Liberating practice from philosophy – a critical examination of values-based practice and its underpinnings. In: Loughlin M, editor. Debates in values-based practice: arguments for and against. Cambridge: Cambridge University Press; 2014. p. 37–49. (Values-based practice). https://www.cambridge.org/core/books/debates-in-valuesbased-practice/liberating-practice-from-philosophy-a-critical-examination-of-valuesbased-practice-and-its-under pinnings/8C609F0E1E8FEBCE38E0E0B437BBFC99.

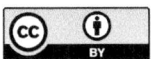

Values, Meanings, Hermeneutics and Mental Health

40

Michael TH Wong

40.1 Introduction

Mary (not her real name), the woman whose story is described below, was seen at the Neuropsychiatry Clinic of the Queen Mary Hospital in Hong Kong. This is the only tertiary referral centre for neuropsychiatric disorders serving the whole of the Hong Kong. She had agreed to the referral by her psychiatrist because her involuntary movements were not responding to treatment. Her story is based on that of a real person but her name and other identifying details have been changed to protect confidentiality.

Mary's story illustrates some of the ways in which values (notably cultural in origin) influence the experience, expression, interpretation and treatment of bodily symptoms; and how these in turn interact with the management of mental health issues related to underlying and unaddressed psychosocial and spiritual values. I will first present her story in the form of a medical case history and then offer a brief hermeneutic analysis of her story as a narrative in which there is a complex interplay between values, culture, meanings and mental health. Finally, I will return to Mary's story to show how the medical assessment and hermeneutic understanding together guided the way her problems were managed and the outcomes of her story.

40.2 Mary's Neuropsychiatric History

Mary was a 46 year-old married clerk who had been depressed on and off for a decade and probably with a brief episode of psychotic breakdown. She was referred to the Neuropsychiatry Clinic for assessment of persistent abnormal movements

M. TH. Wong (✉)
Department of Psychiatry, Li Ka Shing Faculty of Medicine, The University of Hong Kong, Hong Kong, China
e-mail: mthwong@hku.hk

© The Author(s) 2021 341
D. Stoyanov et al. (eds.), *International Perspectives in Values-Based Mental Health Practice*, https://doi.org/10.1007/978-3-030-47852-0_40

apparently arising as side effects of the medication she had been prescribed for her mood disorder with psychotic symptoms.

She had seen two private psychiatrists over a period of about 7 years. The first had prescribed a number of antidepressants and antipsychotics (including risperidone). Over a 5-year period on this regime she had shown no obvious improvement and indeed had developed muscle twitching and tremor. A neurological assessment including various scans revealed no abnormal findings. The neurologist concluded that she had 'tardive dyskinesia' and 'dystonia' affecting the muscles of her face and her right upper limb. These are forms of movement disorder known to occur as side effects particularly of antipsychotic medications such as risperidone. The second private psychiatrist thus stopped Mary's risperidone and switched her to a different antidepressant and an anti-anxiety agent, diazepam. These changes had been made 2 years previously but she had continued to be anxious and depressed and there had been no improvement in her involuntary movements.

In her background, there was no family history of mental illness or movement disorders. Her birth was uneventful and her early milestones were normal. As a child she had been generally well apart from a tendency to falls that she developed around the age of 6. A paediatrician advised that this was due to the fact that her legs were of slightly unequal length. The difference however was only noticeable through measurement and no treatment was indicated. She had no other medical or psychiatric history other than as an adult developing episodes of dizziness, tremor and anxiety after skipping meals in order to finish her work on time. These were compatible with hypoglycaemia (low blood sugar) and she had never had any form of eating disorder.

Her childhood was generally happy apart from an episode of serious sexual assault when she was just 13 years old. What happened was that she was attacked by a stranger on her way home from school who dragged her into a road side bush, pulled her trousers off, and tried to have sex with her. Fortunately, a passer-by realised what was happening and chased the man away. Mary meantime ran home and did not tell anyone what had happened.

Mary was average at school and managed to enrol in a university where she successfully completed a diploma in English. She went on to get work as a clerk and to get married. There were however on-going stresses both at work and in her marriage. As to her work, she had been employed in clerical roles since leaving university but found work very stressful. This was not because of the workload but because of never-ending problems dealing with difficult colleagues.

The stresses in her marriage on the other hand were sexual and psychosocial in nature. She had been married for 17 years by the time she was seen in the Clinic but the marriage had never been consummated. The difficulties seemed to arise from the fact that before they married she had told her then husband-to-be that she had had sex in a previous relationship. She had decided to make this confession because she believed at the time that as they were both practicing Christians she had to be honest with her future husband. The result was that when they attempted sexual intimacy on the first night of their marriage Mary had experienced dyspareunia (pain on intercourse) and her husband had given up because he did not want to hurt her.

After this experience they started to sleep in separate rooms. Mary regretted her confession. She stopped attending church with her husband and they slowly drifted apart. They considered divorce but decided against that because it was against their religion. Mary had suggested they might see a marriage guidance counsellor but her husband had repeatedly rejected this idea. Importantly, Mary had not spoken of her marital difficulties with either her neurologist or psychiatrist because they had not asked her about her sexual history.

She described herself as sentimental and an introvert, not good at dealing with stress and a person who preferred to avoid confrontation at all cost. She enjoyed music, drawing and cinema.

Physical examination in the Neuropsychiatry Clinic revealed physiological tremor of both hands but no involuntary movements suggesting dyskinesia or dystonia. She only had one brief startle like movement during the 2-h assessment and that happened when she was performing Mini Mental State Examination (MMSE). She said that was what she was told as her movement disorder. There was no localising or lateralising sign. She was anxious and depressed. She was not suicidal. Her speech was spontaneous and coherent. Thought form and content was normal. No perceptual disturbance was elicited. She scored 28/30 for MMSE as she was very nervous during this assessment, managing only one out of three items for 3-min recall. She did very well on other items otherwise. Her insight and judgement were good: she was fully aware of her longstanding anxiety and depression but was puzzled and frustrated about her involuntary movements which had been diagnosed as tardive dyskinesia and dystonia secondary to the use of Risperidone.

40.3 Hermeneutic Analysis

The relevance of hermeneutic analysis is that one of the key issues of the patient-psychiatrist interaction is how to address the tension between the subjective and the objective, and between explanation and understanding. The former focuses on cause and effect and is empiricist. The latter is concerned with significance and is meaning-based.

In essence, the patient-psychiatrist interaction involves how to correlate between or bring together the subjective (experience, expression and understanding of symptoms from a first-person perspective) and the objective (observation, organization and explanation of symptoms from the third-person perspective) with the aim to find a formulation that makes sense to both parties leading to a management plan that can achieve remission of symptoms, rehabilitation of functions and recovery of health and well-being.

There are two key challenges. One is that of multiple discourses in psychiatry—biological, psychological, social and spiritual. How does a psychiatrist help patients make sense of the relationship between these different discourses? How can and should a psychiatrist promote dialogues between these different discourses in order that patients can have a whole person discourse rather than a fragmented or incoherent one? The other one is that mental health and ill health are experienced and expressed by a person within a cultural context. How can we facilitate these different culturally contextualized voices to be heard and understood properly between patients and psychiatrists especially in this day and age of cultural plurality and diversity?

The discipline of psychiatry has not done well with respect to these challenges. There has been an unfortunate swing of psychiatry between "brainlessness" (*neglecting* neurobiology) and "mindlessness" (*over-focusing* on neurosciences) at different phases of her development [1]. There is in addition an ongoing ambivalence or negligence of the relevance of culture religion and spirituality to psychiatry [2, 3].

Schleiermacher's nineteenth-century notion of the "hermeneutic circle" showed us that the process of interpretation is an open if not never-ending pursuit, oscillating between the understanding of the whole and the analysis of the part of whatever we are to study. Dilthey's categories of "explanation" (*Erklären*) and "understanding" (*Verstehen*) indicate that understanding and meaning do not arise automatically from demonstrating correlation or causal relations. Heidegger added a metaphysical dimension to our understanding of hermeneutics turning hermeneutics as epistemology into hermeneutics as ontology, arguing that interpreting and understanding are essential features of being human. After Heidegger, Gadamer pushed the argument further, stating that we all have different backgrounds and presuppositions— "prejudice," which is a fact of life that we all need to acknowledge and use as a starting point to achieve optimal mutual understanding. Gadamer called this process of achieving mutual understanding between individuals with different backgrounds and presuppositions a "fusion of horizons," a term that Ricoeur took up when in dialogue with him [4].

Ricoeur in his book, *The Conflict of Interpretations* [5], proposed a crucial step—that of "explaining in order to understand" or as he put it "to explain more in order to understand better" to address the perpetual dialectic between explanation and understanding. His article "Creativity and Language" in *The Philosophy of Paul Ricoeur* [6] develops this step into the process of dialogue between "ordinary" everyday language ("first discourse") and "scientific" or "specialist" languages ("second discourse") and, which in turn has been further expanded to a "third discourse," proposed but never worked out by Ricoeur himself, to bridge the human and the natural sciences, the subjective and the objective, explanation and understanding [4, 7].

This "third discourse" has been formulated subsequently as a multi-layered discourse that is comprehensible to both patients and psychiatrists, not only symptoms but also behaviour and function, correlates biopsychosocial [8] and spiritual dimensions, not reducing them to any particular or single perspective, to explain but *not* to explain away, to understand and search for meaning and significance, explain more in order to understand better, and thus achieving a *therapeutic hermeneutic circle*. It is in this sense a "whole person discourse" in which patients and psychiatrists *explicitly* and *consciously* using ordinary everyday language and "specialist" languages together to express their experience, in a *correlative* but *non-reductive* way that promotes both explanation and understanding [4].

40.4 Hermeneutic Understanding and the Outcomes of Mary's Illness Experience

With this hermeneutic perspective outlined above, Mary's presenting narrative can be summarized as follows:

I am not happy (ordinary discourse) because I had a severe depression and a psychotic breakdown and developed involuntary movements which are the side effects of the antipsychotic medications prescribed to me (biological/neuroscientific discourse). I had a breakdown because of the stress at work and the fact that my marriage was not getting anywhere (psychosocial). My marriage is not even con-summated because I told my husband that I had premarital sex which is against our Christian faith (religious/theological discourse). I kind of understand that he is a very religious and traditional man and would find that as sinful and guilty (cultural and ethical) but I thought his love for me can help him overcome that but apparently has not. Now I have to get support from my friends instead (psychosocial) and I wish one day I could make sense of all these with my faith which says truth, good-ness and beauty and faith, hope and love will prevail and that I can still be happy healthy and feeling fulfilled even if all these problems never go away (spiritual/religious/theological).

And the hermeneutic analysis can be as below:

Mary presents with a neurobiological problem and expects a pharmacological solution. The psychiatrist clarifies signs and symptoms and advices her that her original neuropsychiatric problem is more or less gone and the so-called persistent involuntary movement is now to do with something else—hypoglycemia which needs to be addressed via a lifestyle adjustment (don't refrain from eating for too long). That relieves her from her neurobiological focus and allows her to discuss her other longstanding and outstanding issues—stress at work, nonconsummation of marriage and ongoing estrangement with her husband. This facilitates, motivates and empowers her to engage with other discourses—ethical/philosophical (is pre-marital sex right? Should I have lied?) values/cultural (is this simply Christian values or Chinese morality?) and religious/spiritual/theological (now that damages have been done and cannot be undone, how do I achieve meaning, health, happiness and fulfillment again through my faith?)

The outcome of Mary's assessment in the Neuropsychiatry Clinic reflected in part the findings of the medical assessment and in part the deeper understanding of the values and cultural influences on her narrative provided by the hermeneutic understanding as just outlined. The values and cultural factors involved are described further here.

Thus, drawing on her medical assessment, Mary was advised that the neuropsy-chiatric assessment had found no ongoing evidence of tardive dyskinesia or dysto-nia. Indeed, these movement disorders were in remission now after the cessation of the antipsychotic (risperidone). Her persistent tremor and exaggerated startled responses were very likely to be part and parcel of her anxiety and depression. She was receptive to this medical reformulation and agreed to try a higher dose of her antidepressant. Drawing however on hermeneutic understanding, she was also advised to seek help from a Christian therapist with experience in marital and sexual counselling to address the non-consummation of her marriage and on-going psychosexual, relationship and communication problems with her husband.

With this two-pronged medical-plus-hermeneutic approach Mary's anxiety and depressed mood improved. Drawing on the medical side, she managed to see her so called movement disorder more clearly—in place of persistent tardive dyskinesia or dystonia she understood her tremor as being related to anxiety, and its occasional worsening and associated startle response to be a result of episodic hypoglycaemia due to missing meals. She thus started to take regular small meals to prevent hypoglycaemic attacks and found that helped to minimise her anxiety and depression in general and the episodic startle attacks in particular.

Drawing on the spiritual side of her understanding Mary made contact with one of her Christian friends and started to attend an all-women bible study group. She found the fellowship helped her overcome her social isolation and regain her confidence. She became motivated to re-examine her Christian faith and to address her marital and sexual issues from a religious perspective. Her husband seemed to be pleased that she had started to reconnect with her Christian faith. He began talking to her again and on one occasion put his arm around her shoulder to express his care and encouragement, although he withdrew immediately when Mary tried to reciprocate with intimate gestures. Following this incident and drawing on her newfound confidence, Mary brought up the issue of getting help from a Christian marital and sex therapist again. We do not know how this is going to work out yet. But at least her husband said he would consider the idea rather than as he had in the past rejecting it out of hand.

40.5   Hermeneutics Values and Culture

The hermeneutic analysis above suggests a complex interplay between values (her own and those of other people), culture, meanings and mental health.

First, The relationship between behaviour, function and symptoms. Her neurologist interpreted Mary's symptoms as tardive dyskinesia and dystonia and that diagnosis stayed with her despite the change of the nature of her physical signs. She continued to use the same diagnostic labels to describe her own experience and perception. This seems to have been the case for her previous psychiatrists too. One way to understand this is that the diagnostic label given by an expert neurologist has an impact on the capacity of both Mary and her psychiatrists to perceive otherwise. Valuing expert opinions over one's own appears to have influenced the way she interpreted her symptoms which in turn determined how she behaved as a patient and functioned as a wife and at work.

Second, the role of multiple discourses—biological, psychological, social and cultural/religious/spiritual. For Mary, the biological discourse—that she had movement disorders and a sexual dysfunction—played a dominant role in her own personal narrative. The dominance of this discourse had steered her away from her psychosocial and spiritual discourses: yet these were more relevant to her ongoing stresses and associated psychosexual issues both at a personal and marital level. The reformulation of her highly focused biological discourse into a broader and comprehensive multi-layered correlative and non-reductive one freed her up to review her psychosocial and religious discourses resulting in a re-invigoration in her self-esteem, religious life and marital relationship.

Third, the influence of each of these particular discourses on one's meaning and values system. The particular juxtaposition of different types of discourse in a person reflects one's educational, professional, ethnic, cultural, religious and spiritual backgrounds. The capacity to assemble a relevant multi-layered correlative and non-reductive personal narrative that does not impoverish one's lived experience is not straightforward. In the case of Mary, her interaction with her neurologist, her psychiatrists, her husband and her Christian friends had both positive and negative influences on her capacity and readiness in sorting out how different values systems were affecting her.

Fourth, the increasing relevance of these values as our society is becoming more multi-cultural. The Hong Kong into which Mary was born is predominantly Chinese. The influence of Chinese culture on her roles as an individual, as a wife and as an employee at work is significant. There is an expectation for her as a woman to be submissive and passive and this clearly influenced the way she behaved as a wife, as an employee and as a patient. The value placed on politeness and modesty made her unforthcoming about her sexual and marital issues. The value of social acceptance made her focus on her bodily symptoms rather than her mental health problems (these being still heavily stigmatized) [9]. The cultural influences are further evident in that Mary was brought up in Hong Kong while it was still under British rule. This gave her access to and preference for Western Medicine rather than Traditional Chinese Medicine. The professional and expert status of medical doctors is highly respected, and this further exaggerated the power imbalance in the doctor-patient relationship towards the authoritarian medical side of the dyad. The westernized culture also allowed exposure to the Christian faith that had a significant influence not only on Mary but also her husband, on their sexuality, marriage and relationship. The perceived guilt and sense of sinfulness associated with premarital sex affected Mary's emotional life and that of her husband that it led to non-consummation of their marriage.

Fifth, hermeneutics facilitates values-based practice and improves clinical outcomes. Values-based practice (VBP) is a skills-based approach to working more effectively with complex and conflicting values related to diagnosis and treatment that are not only affected by moral values of patients or ethical and professional codes of psychiatrists but also personal preferences, desires, wishes and expectations of both. VBP is not straightforward and involves beginning with an awareness of values, clarity of where values are in the reasoning process and improving knowledge of values, followed by using communication to resolve value conflicts, starting with patients' values, resolving conflicts in values by balancing different values rather than by a pre-prescribed rule and making decisions in partnership with patients, and finally achieving the right outcome by good process and by applying the above principles of VBP and not by an outcome based on previously laid down regulations or rules [10]. This whole process requires from both patients and psychiatrists starting from the beginning to the end non-stop attention to presuppositions, assumptions, beliefs, habits, preferences, biases and prejudices, constant dialogue, clarification and negotiation as well as repeated reflections, revision, reformulation and decision. All these tasks are facilitated by hermeneutics which acknowledges the plurality and diversity of narratives, polysemy in words, surplus of meaning and conflict of interpretations of any discourse. The notion of hermeneutics that "to explain more in order to understand better" provides an approach that emphasizes the importance of ongoing dialogue between evidence-based practice and values-based practice and promotes the partnership between patients and psychiatrists in achieving personalization of care and improving clinical outcome.

40.6 Conclusions

The experience and expression of mental ill health involve a complex interplay of values and culture that goes beyond the familiar biopsychosocial formulation. Psychiatry has been limited by her tendency to swing between the extremes of "brainlessness" (neglecting neurobiology) and "mindlessness" (over-focusing on neurosciences) as well as her ongoing ambivalence and negligence of culture religion and spirituality. This results in sub-optimal explanation and understanding of the clinical needs of patients. Hermeneutic commentary that analyses clinical history as a multi-layered personal narrative and formulates intervention and management in a correlative and non-reductive manner provides a whole person and personalized approach that facilitates values-based practice (VBP) and improves clinical outcome.

Acknowledgements My sincere thanks to Dr Jocelyn Dunphy-Blomfield, colleague and mentor, for introducing me to hermeneutics and arranging me to meet with Paul Ricoeur, her friend and teacher, to discuss how the dialectic between explanation and understanding really works.

40.7 Guide to Further Source

Wong MTH. Ricoeur and the Third Discourse of the Person: From Philosophy and Neuroscience to Psychiatry and Theology. London: Lexington Books; 2019.

References

1. Eisenberg L. Mindlessness and brainlessness in psychiatry. Br J Psychiatry. 1986;14:497–508.
2. Wong MTH. Theological anthropology as informed by the changeux-ricoeur dialogue on science, philosophy & religion. In: Verheyden J, Hettema TL, Vandecasteele P, editors. Paul ricoeur: poetics and religion. Leuven: Uitgeverij Peeters; 2011. p. 519–29.
3. Royal Australian & New Zealand College of Psychiatrists. RANZCP position statement 96. The relevance of religion & spirituality to psychiatric practice. Section of history philosophy & ethics of psychiatry. Melbourne, VIC: RANZCP; 2018.

4. Wong MTH. Ricoeur and the third discourse of the person: from philosophy and neuroscience to psychiatry and theology. London: Lexington Books; 2019.

5. Ricoeur P. In: Ihde D, editor. The conflict of interpretations: essays in hermeneutics. Evanston: Northwestern University Press; 1974.

6. Ricoeur P. Creativity in language: word polysemy, metaphor. In: Reagan C, Stewart D, editors. The philosophy of Paul Ricoeur: an anthology of his work. Boston, MA: Beacon Press; 1978. p. 120–33.

7. Changeux J-P, Ricoeur P. What makes us think? A neuroscientist and a philosopher argue about ethics, human nature, and the brain. Debevoise MB translator. Princeton, NJ: Princeton University Press; 2000.

8. Engel GL. The need for a new medical model: a challenge for biomedical medicine. Science. 1977;196:129–36.

9. Fan R, Guo R, Wong M. Psychiatric ethics & confucianism. In: Sadler JZ, Fulford B, van Staden CW, editors. Oxford handbook of psychiatric ethics. Oxford: Oxford University Press; 2015. p. 603–15.

10. Woodbridge-Dodd K. Values-based practice in mental health and psychiatry. Curr Opin Psychiatry. 2012;25:508–12.

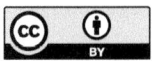

Disha: Building Bridges-Removing Barriers: Where Excluded and Privileged Young Adults Meet

41

Sadhana Natu

41.1 Introduction

'Disha' which means Direction is a Speak Out and Peer Support Group started in 1992 in a Pune City College in India for students, which I facilitate. Against the backdrop of globalization in India in 1991, I thought that such a group was the need of the hour. It is a gender-just, non-discriminating, humane platform that allows dialogue, debate and dissent. It also creates a space for friendships, bonding and nurture. The commonalities and differences help to embrace 'multiple realities' which in turn help to look at life, issues and conflicts in a new light [1]. The group is managed by student coordinators and those who participate range from urban poor to those who come from various states in India and various countries. There are first- and second-generation learners as well as well-to-do students, the group is truly inclusive. This aspect is both a challenge and the strength of the group. The Model that we follow is Peer Support, Peer Learning, Feminist Counselling and Empathetic Listening. What works is that they can validate, challenge as well as view their experiences against the backdrop multiple realities and gain a sense of proportion [2].

I am describing these vignettes which are outcomes of discussions on a couple of topics that are areas of concern for the students in order to narrate the effectiveness of listening to and learning from diversities, which is the catalyst for change in the Speak Out and Peer Support Group. The sheer multiplicity of voices enables the

S. Natu (✉)
Department of Psychology, Modern College, Ganeshkhind, Savitribai Phule Pune University, Pune, India

Women's Studies, Pune University, Pune, India

Psychology, Pune University, Pune, India

National and international Journals of Psychology, Pune University, Pune, India

Disha Peer Support and Speak Out Group, Pune University, Pune, India students to hole their own singular experience under a lens. I have chosen two topics that bring out this diversity and multiplicity beautifully.

41.2 Vignettes of the Discussion on Loneliness in Disha

The students who hailed from rural areas and poorer backgrounds confessed that they felt isolated and alienated from both their surroundings and classmates due to the cultural differences and lifestyle in the city. They were trying their best to adjust and assimilate and wanted to feel that they 'belonged'. The middle and upper middle-class students spoke more about personal loneliness, feeling disconnected, cut off, alone if their friends or families did not listen or respond to them, as against the social loneliness of their other classmates. The students from other states and countries spoke about a deep sense of 'being an outsider' who had difficulties with local language, culture, practices and hence felt bereft at times. The solutions that were put forth were that they should try to speak out as they had done in the group, ask for help and the local students should take the initiative in reaching out to those who were new to both the city and life away from homes. The discussion foregrounded the existence of multiple realities and contexts and underscored the need to build bridges in order to bond across this sea of contrasts.

41.3 Vignettes of the Discussion on Meanings of Freedom in Disha

A student hailing from a rural area said that studying in a College in a city gave her the freedom to dress in a way of her choice, talk to boys, take in the sights in the city and enjoy the entertainment that the city had to offer. She also had the freedom to pursue her academic dreams. All of this was non-existent while she was studying in a school and junior college in her village. Another student from a neighbouring state expressed that staying 'away from home' he could avail of a lot of freedoms! Take decisions about food and clothes choices, choose friends, entertainment, hobbies. He was monitored constantly by his parents through calls on the cell phone; nevertheless, he was happy with his 'limited freedoms'. The discussion also included their views about gender differences in rationing out freedom. The restrictions, demands and accountability were more applicable to the female students. The male students had more freedom compared to the females. One student felt that Disha was a 'safe place', and she felt truly free in this group. Free enough to talk about her sexuality. She said that she was gender fluid and called herself queer. She had no support from her parents and family, but with her peers in Disha who discussed their concerns so openly, she wanted to share this part of her life. Another girl spoke about the caste discrimination she faced, both subtle and direct. She said that all freedoms come with responsibilities, the constitutional responsibility to treat your fellow beings as equals! The group responded with maturity and solidarity towards all the issues raised vis-a-vis freedom: caste, sexuality, gender, rural-urban divide and more. The wonderful part of the discussion was that the coordinators, while summing up, exhorted the group to analyse and understand the differences and similarities amongst each other as young adults and not homogenize the group. This artificial homogenization takes away the inherent inequalities that existed within the group. A good way ahead was to acknowledge them, accept them and to work actively towards removing discrimination and bigotry and try to achieve true psychological freedom and security for individuals and groups. The fact that this discussion took place on 14 August, the eve of Indian Independence Day made it more meaningful and poignant. The session ended with a chorus recital of Gurudev Rabindranath Tagore's epic poem 'Where the Mind is without Fear' from the Geetanjali.

41.4 Alumnus Disha Coordinator Profile

I am a Role Model too!

For the rest of the college, I did not exist. Why? I am dark, I come from a poor background, do not wear fancy clothes and I am certainly not attractive! It does not amount to much that I topped the college every year, am sincere, kind- hearted. That does not matter. You must have 'attitude' and you must impress, and you must be able to speak English. The only place where what I said mattered, where I mattered was Disha! It is a platform for the intellect, the mind and emotions. Nobody judges you. Your background does not matter. In fact, after I did my Master's in Social Work overcoming all odds, I have been invited several times to interact with the present members and hailed as a role model of sorts!

When I embarked on an MSW course I had a tough time emotionally, mentally and financially. I was really depressed. But thank God, I could not afford the fees of a professional- I survived! My friends from Disha and my MSW course and my mentor helped to come to grips with the situation and to deal with my problems. This journey has made me stronger and happier than I ever was. I share my story with a younger group in Disha every year [1].

41.5 Disha Coordinator Profile 1

Hansa*, 24 years (*name changed) is from a Scheduled Caste family. She comes from a family of five members. They live in a <u>basti</u> (slum settlement) for 30 years. Her father works in leather repair and her mother is a domestic worker. Both are daily wage earners. She has done her Graduation in Psychology and Post- graduation in Social Science. She went the 'Learn and Earn' way. Her family said "For how long will you study? If you get further education, it will only help your in laws, how is it of any use to us". They wanted her to work in a Call Centre and earn lots of money and support her family. They could not fathom why she wanted to continue her education.

Meanwhile, in the classroom and College she felt isolated and abandoned. "The homogeneity with so-called friends felt fake and forced". "Though I did not glorify or capitalize on my hardships, the reality check was too much for my classmates, when I spoke about my family and home".

In the Disha, Peer Support Group, students of different backgrounds—caste, class, and gender, nationalities came together and interacted on an equal footing. A space was created for discussion and not a debate (debate and discussion have a crucial difference—debate has a 'winner'; discussion is more about laying out views—hence dissensual). It has been about sharing commonalities, dreams, love, attraction and friendships. She got involved in analysis and finding solutions and felt empowered. Leading the group as a Coordinator helped her in resolving her own problems too. She learnt how to look at life dispassionately. Others looked up to her and this helped to build her self-esteem. Her subaltern life experiences became her lode star instead of 'something to hide'.

41.6 Disha Coordinator Profile 2

Manoj*, 22 years (name changed) came from a well to do family, was self- assured and articulate. He was interested in academics, theatre and ambitious. His role as Disha Coordinator and interactions with a diverse group made him examine his own lived reality more deeply. He realized that a lot of the other students had financial problems, they lived in crowded spaces and could not afford to entertain or enjoy college life. Some of the sessions on myriad topics such as sexuality, aspirations and love etc. made him realize that he had a lot of autonomy and very little struggle in his life. He also learnt to care for others and connect with those who needed help and moral support. All this was new for him. He realized that but for Disha, their lives would not have intersected at all since college students hang out with PLU (people like us, their own type). This experience was both challenging and rewarding for him. It gave him a sense of proportion and an opportunity to connect with an entire world which was not like his own. It helped him in resolving his personal problems and endowed him with a deep sense of social responsibility. He marveled at the way in which some of his classmates whose life was full of struggle were happy with so little! This motivated him to factor struggle into his life goals. He is now a budding social entrepreneur, who is not merely working for profit.

Both these Coordinators remark very often that the bonds that they forged in Disha are qualitatively different from their other friendships, since this platform allowed people to bare their souls and act real, these bonds are special.

41.7 Values Arising in the Discussion and from the Profiles

In both the discussions, the reader must pay attention to the values of plurality and inclusion. The life experiences must be understood in the context of the backgrounds of the students. When compared with each other the impact of caste, class, gender, region, nation on lived reality becomes clear and just like the participants, the readers will realize that intersectionality plays a huge role in day-to-day living and decision-making and is at the core of mental health. Loneliness and isolation are otherwise viewed through a very narrow lens of individualism, but with many contexts, the subtle differences between different categories become clear. It is these differences in turn, which offer entry points and solutions. That there are many freedoms and that it is not absolute is a revelation in the discussion. This is a learning experience for many. The conflicting value systems between the classes of privileged and underprivileged are also comprehended in Disha discussions. Negotiations, strategies that are deployed change according to class and location and though we speak of universal values, multicultural contexts define, challenge and reconstitute values. Disha offers this large canvas to the students.

The three profiles offer the readers a bird's eye view of the processes of validation and interrogation that are deployed in Disha. In every session and every topic that comes up for discussion, both the coordinators as well as participants question the issues and the conflicts that arise because of their own location. Questioning privilege and entitlement, engaging with disadvantage and struggle create a churning of ideas as well as action. Mainstream spaces in Psychology seldom do this. Coordinators from different backgrounds are selected carefully for representing all kinds of voices and to connect the privileged and the excluded and marginalized. Many myths are busted, stereotypes about caste, religion, nationality, race, gender, sexualities are discussed and questioned. Students learn to make an informed choice based on facts and lived experiences that they hear and share rather than forming opinions based on biases and prejudices. The coordinators play a crucial role in this endeavour and empower others and become empowered and inclusive too.

41.8   The Influences of Culture on This Story

Pune City is a mini-metro, close to the metropolis Mumbai. Its academic institutions are full of a rich diversity and hence Disha operates within a rich, multicultural context. It caters to both local and global netizen students. This is the exciting and formidable part of running a Speak Out and Peer Support Group for the last 27 years. The understanding of culture here is hence neither homogeneous nor narrow. These young adults, post-millennials are connected to the world through the Internet and social media and are also deeply rooted in the multicultural Indian context. The students from countries as diverse as Mauritius, Uganda, Sri Lanka, Afghanistan, Uzbekistan who are studying with the Indian students and who participate in Disha bring in their own cultural complexities. It is these different strands, with some commonalities and a lot of differences that are constantly challenged, interrogated and unpacked to yield rich insights about psycho-social issues, individual, interpersonal, cross-cultural problems and experiences. In the last few years, the challenges that young adults in India are facing have multiplied. India has the highest suicide rates in the world with maximum number of young people on the brink, worse it may soon turn out to be the biggest killer in the country [3]. So apart from dealing with distress, Disha helps to mitigate and ameliorate the mental health of many students on the campus in a non-clinical, non-judgemental, non-hierarchical and non-threatening fashion and this is the raison d'etre of the group.

41.9 Conclusions

Disha Peer Support and Speak Out Group offers 'safe space' to students who represent a multilayered and multicontextual diversity. It brings in the complexities of various locations which help to tease out and unpack several psycho-social issues that a typical clinical, counselling or therapeutic setting does not. It challenges the student coordinators as well as the faculty members who are facilitators, since there are no ready-made thumb rules. The peer learning and cross-cultural learning are huge. Disha also helps to shine a light on contextual and intersectionality-related social realities that are key to offering solutions for mental health issues and out of the box practices where students are peer counsellors, with facilitative (and not directive, performative) roles. It draws out principles such as validation and reflexivity and creates an enabling ethos for the lives of the privileged and the excluded to intersect and inform each other's lived reality. In the process, all those who participate in these sessions which revolve around current concerns that change every month and year, go back enriched and armed with life skills. Disha also creates an organic synergy that is beyond the synthetic 'feel good', more humane, earthy, multihued and syncretic. There is a Counselling Cell that is run in the institution, where a lot of self-referral is done as well as referral by staff members. But this is only for critical cases. Primacy is given to Disha, where students themselves are 'healers' and mentors. While faculty members who are facilitators do train Disha coordinators, in the meetings (sessions) their role is more of observers and they make interventions, only when necessary. The transactions in the sessions are multilingual, with translations and hand holding (language specific) which allows all voices to be heard.

Acknowledgements Students have presented the Disha model and learnings at local, national and international conferences. Dr Sadhana Natu has also presented several Disha learnings in national and international conferences. This chapter is based on the collective learnings of many. Students have also written three articles based on their experiential learning and contribution to Disha in local language journals and newspapers.

41.10 Guides to Further Sources

https://www.moderncollegegk.org/psychology-dep.php

References

1. Natu S. College mental health: the Disha experience, vol. 365–66. Pune: Medico Friends Circle Bulletin; 2015. p. 10–3.
2. Natu S. Youth and Mental Health: Urban, Rural and Fringe Realities, Conference Proceedings. Pune: Siddhivinayak College; 2015. ISBN 978 81 9314440 4.
3. Patel V, et al. Suicide mortality in India: a nationally representative survey. Lancet. 2012;379:2343–51.

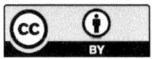

Online Counseling "The World Without a Label"

Lejla Kuralić-Ćišić, Meliha Bijedić, Irma Dobrinjic,
Nermina Kravić, Aida Duraković, and Dajana Stajić

42

42.1 Introduction

In post-war Bosnia and Herzegovina, there has been a noticeable increase in the number of people, especially young people, who face behavioral and emotional problems. The problems are wide ranging: they run from anxiety, depression, and withdrawal, through social problems, attention problems, difficulties thinking, somatic problems without clear medical causes, and even to problems of rule violation, aggressive behaviors, various types of addiction, learning disabilities, and more severe psychiatric illnesses and disorders.

Often the problems begin with a person having difficulties in the social environment in which they live. The prevalence of young people with emotional and behavioral disorders ranges from 13% to 22% of the total population in our Bosnia and Herzegovina [1]. This is a clear indication that many young people are in need of assistance and counseling. The problems are amplified by people fearing that they will become labeled if they decide to engage with one of the regular mental health

---

NOTE: The authors are all team members of the online counselling organisation "The World without a Label"; Tuzla 75000, Bosnia and Herzegovina.

L. Kuralić-Ćišić (✉) · M. Bijedić · I. Dobrinjic · A. Duraković
Department of Behavioural Disorder, Faculty of Special Education and Rehabilitation,
University of Tuzla, Tuzla, Bosnia and Herzegovina
e-mail: lejlamar@gmail.com

N. Kravić
Department of Child and Adolescent Psychiatry, Psychiatric Institution of Tuzla,
Tuzla, Bosnia and Herzegovina

D. Stajić
Department of Psychotherapy, Non-governmental Organization "Amica Educa",
Tuzla, Bosnia and Herzegovina

© The Author(s) 2021
D. Stoyanov et al. (eds.), *International Perspectives in Values-Based Mental
Health Practice*, https://doi.org/10.1007/978-3-030-47852-0_42

institutions. Young people in particular assume (perhaps not unreasonably) that by attending an institution they will get "stuck" with a label. The result is that, hesitating, their problems get worse.

This is where we found in our work an ally in the virtual world. Given the fact that we now live to a large extent in a virtual world, in which all of our needs are satisfied through the basics of online communication, we recognized the need for adopting a similar approach in establishing new and improved access to mental health services for children, young people, and adults. We changed our approach to access and moved to allowing our users to get the help they needed (whether socio-educational, psychological, or psychiatric) through their computers, laptops, and phones, and from different parts of the country or indeed the world, and all without going near a clinic.

The online platform we developed with our partners (see Acknowledgments) offers a "World Without a Label." It is the first counseling center of its kind in Bosnia and Herzegovina, and it is also a platform for the future in the wider world. It brings together in one place experts in behavioral, psychological, and psychiatric problems. Its approach is both evidence-based and values-based: it was created, on the one hand, on the basis of long-term preparations and research into the effectiveness of virtual interventions consistent with strategies for promoting and preserving young people's health in general; and on the other hand, on the basis of careful assessments of the needs of the people—especially the young people—that the program is intended to serve. The result is an online platform that offers specialist counseling for young people (including with their parents' permission, underage children) and for adults. An online counseling service is also available to parents who want to support their children in overcoming life difficulties. The approaches offered are socio-pedagogic, psychotherapeutic, and psychiatric, including behavior modification treatments with primary and secondary prevention.

The platform lives up to its name—it is a "World Without a Label"—in that all treatments are delivered in the virtual environment through Skype's online platform. Those who need help are required to visit the site "onlinesavjetovaliste.com" and fill out the form. After the application has been sent, the multidisciplinary team makes a real-time triage of the problem and sends the patient to an appropriate online expert. The intervention is again done through Skype and is completely anonymous.

The story that follows illustrates how the program works to provide a world without a label, allowing clients to access help without fear of prejudices against mental health, by providing an expert service within a virtual environment and with full confidence anonymity.

The boy concerned (who is clearly above-average computer literate) refuses face-to-face therapy (at least in the first instance) but then engages successfully with our innovative online service.

The anonymity of online counseling services gives users a sense of control, and users simply open up because there is no possibility of first contact.

42.2   Adnan's Narrative

Adnan was a young teenager, born in 2002, who first attended our Child and Adolescent Clinic accompanied by one of his parents. The concern was that he had been showing behavioral problems—extremely poor social interaction with peers; and spending most of his free time on his computer playing video games. He came reluctantly and only at the urging of his parents.

Adnan was an only child living in a complete family with both his parents. He attended the local elementary school, was in the final grade, and an excellent student. At school, he had very little communication with peers and no best friend. In the early years of his schooling he was occasionally mistreated and bullied. He later responded to this bullying physically—he bullied the bullies back and after that they stopped mistreating him for good. But subsequently he expected only the worst from other people and constantly thought he was being attacked by others for no reason. Most of the time he was a very calm child though always ready for self-defense. Since preschool, he had spent a lot of time on his computer mostly playing war-related video games. He had always been fascinated by the war itself, by the arts of killing, and he dreamt about being a professional soldier when he grew up. When he was 7 years old, he started following internet sites for military training.

Adnan's mother had a history of psychiatric illness: she had been treated in the Day Hospital of a local psychiatric clinic where in group psychotherapy she recalled her own war-related rape trauma; she experienced this in her early 20s, where soldiers of the opposing army systematically raped their captives. Adnan's father was a former member of their national army and he himself suffered many war traumas. Adnans's parents met after the war. They knew all about each other's war-related traumas but they never talked about them in front of their son.

Our formulation was that unconscious transgenerational transmission of the parents' war trauma (see below) had led to a specific formation of Adnan's personality traits reflecting his lack of confidence and fascination with war. The boy refused group therapy but engaged well with your on-line programme.

42.3   The Transgenerational Transmission of War Trauma

War trauma is in many ways specific: it causes destruction, death, and wounding of a large number of people; it has occurred from the enemy's hand; and it leaves feelings of helplessness, loss of trust in others, and a sense of humiliation. Hate, prejudice, and negative feelings are among the well-recognized common reactions to war trauma. Less well recognized is "transgenerational trauma transmission" where the victim transmits trauma to their children with the result of keeping it alive for the generations to come.

Importantly, trauma of this kind may be transmitted unconsciously and even where, as in Adnan's story, the original victims try to avoid passing on their trauma by not talking about it in front of their children. We have seen this following the war in Bosnia and Herzegovina in the 1990s when systematic rape of Bosnian women was for the first time in history characterized as a war crime. It is believed that more than 20,000 women were raped in the war in Bosnia and more than a thousand children were born afterward origin [2, 3]. Such children are born into a world that may lack the basic prerequisite for normal mental development, the availability of a primary object (mother) to become a good content of the child's personality, or what Winikot has called a "good enough mother" [4]. The processes involved in this are in part but importantly unconscious. For example, work on facial mirroring has shown interactions that, organized through constant regulation and experiences of mutually coordinated and synchronized responses, form the basis for the affective development of the child [5, 6].

What picture then could the child who was born out of rape get from their mother's eyes? How could a mother laugh or look forward to giving birth to that child knowing how she became pregnant? And how will her feelings affect her child's emotional development? The result is trauma which becomes transgenerationally transmitted influencing the formation of identity and self-image of children [7].

42.4 Beyond Direct Transmission to the Generations to Come

We seek to tell the story of children now in their 20s who were born as "war-time children of rape" in an attempt to publicize and acknowledge the existence of these so-called "invisible children," or Bosnian war children.

Such unspoken secrets have the effect of creating messages within the environment in which the Bosnian war child is growing up, messages affecting his or her sense of inadequacy, of feeling guilt about the emotional state of the mother who was raped, and a sense of disgust because rape is stigmatized in society and its origin does not belong anywhere. These messages are not confined even to those directly affected but (as with our story above of Adnan) may spread indirectly to the children of those affected. The result is a process of transgenerational trauma that becomes self-sustaining spreading to the children of the victims of war and from them to the next generation, to the children of these "invisible" children themselves.

Silence and closeness with their attendant guilt and shame keep these children, now young people, imprisoned in their personal worlds without as they see it hope of exist. Paradoxically, society's acknowledgment that such children exist, and are in and around us all these years, often brings massive disbelief and sometimes outright rejection. It does not surprise us, precisely because of this, the need for online privacy counseling. Such a service offers a safe space for acknowledgment bringing with it not rejection but support and understanding. That is why simply writing about these children and their stories can be helpful. Acknowledging what happened, difficult as it is, could make an important contribution to healing and treatment for both sides, for our "invisible war-time children" and for the society in which they are growing up to have children of their own.

42.5 Conclusions

Our story of Adnan has illustrated that in addition to all the well-known pathogenic circumstances in which people live in post-war Bosnia and Herzegovina are the "invisible children" born after war-time rape. For these children and their parents, support is very much needed and professionals have an obligation to respond to their needs. Appropriate responses require an interactive multidisciplinary team approach focused on recognizing that socio-emotional health depends on identifying the effects of trans-generational transmission of trauma and seeking help for it in a safe environment.

This is what our online counseling center "A World without a label" aims provide. We believe it has great potential to contribute to solving the post-war mental health problems of young people (also children and adults) and to create the motivational patterns that support changing risky behaviors and persisting in implementing those changes. As counselors, we offer the opportunity for our young people to address their problems with a professional team but without the fear of being labeled or judged in any way. The service in addition is able to offer a duration of treatment that is limited not by the limitations of available resources but only by the intensity and duration of the difficulty presented by the young person and their own needs and vulnerability. Our hope is that as we gain experience of the program, it will lead to development of a number of similar online mental health counseling centers in Bosnia and Herzegovina and elsewhere.

Acknowledgments We would like to thank the parents of the child for their cooperation on the case and the Faculty of Education and Rehabilitation and University and Clinical Center, Department of Psychiatry, Tuzla.

42.6 Guide to Further Sources

The websites below provide an overview and insight into just some of the materials we used to disseminate activities.

https://www.facebook.com/svijetbezetikete/

https://www.youtube.com/watch?v=4fKl8flGFKI

https://www.youtube.com/watch?v=9FUQbynGHXU

https://www.klix.ba/lifestyle/zdravlje/bih-dobila-prvo-online-savjetovaliste-za-pomoc-osobama-s-psiholoskim-problemima/180507126

1 also be good if you have any web links to materials illustrating the work of the center.

References

1. Stevanović D, Kuralić-Ćišić L. Creativity development and prevention of behavioral disorders. Lukavac: INDA; 2017.
2. Bećirbašić B, Šečić D. Invisible casualties of war. In: Bryant-Jefferies R, editor. Counselling victims of warfare: person-centred dialogues. London: CRC Press; 2005.

3. Volkan VD. Blood lines, From ethnic pride to ethnic terror. New York: Farrar, Straus, Giroux; 1997.
4. Winnicott DW. Transitional objects and transitional phenomena. In: Winnicott DW, editor. Playing and reality, 1951. Harmondsworth: Pelican; 1971.
5. Thomas EAC, Malone TW. On the dynamics of two- person interactions. Psychol Rev. 1979;86:331–60.
6. Tronick E. Infant's communicative intent. In: Stark B, editor. Language behavior in infancy and early childhood. Holland: Elsevier; 1981. p. 5–16.
7. Stern D. The interpersonal world of the infant: a view from psychoanalysis and development psychology. New York, NY: Basic Books; 1985. (1985) and (1998). ISBN 978-0-465-03403-1 https://en.wikipedia.org/wiki/The_Interpersonal_World_of_the_Infant.

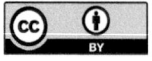

Part VI

Reflections

The Realpolitik of Values-Based Practice: An Introduction to Part VI, Reflections

43

Bill Fulford

In this final Part of the book, we present three chapters reflecting on aspects of the challenges experienced by their authors in implementing values-based approaches in their respective contexts. This is the realpolitik of values-based practice. The challenges as we will see are real and really difficult. They are likely to be in some respects greater still for implementing a culturally enriched form of values-based practice—for one thing, a culturally enriched form of values-based practice necessarily involves an extended range and complexity of operative values. Though in this connection, we should not lose sight of the fact that, as many chapters in earlier Parts of the book have shown, engaging with cultural values brings with it many resources as well as challenges.

As Table 43.1 indicates, the three chapters in this Part fall naturally under three shared values identified by a group of us in the course of one of the writing development workshops we ran in connection with the book. The workshops are described further in our concluding chapter 47, "Co-writing Values: What We Did and Why We Did It". The shared values we adopted were adapted from a framework of similar shared values developed by NIMHE[1] to support its work of policy

---

[1] NIMHE, the National Institute for Mental Health, England, was a policy implementation body set up by the UK government around the turn of the century. The derivation of the NIMHE Values Framework including its origins in expertise by experience as well as expertise by training is described in chapter 47.

Authors
The editors with input from the contributors to Part VI

B. Fulford (✉)
St Catherine's College, University of Oxford, Oxford, UK
e-mail: kwmf@kwmfulford.com

© The Author(s) 2021   367
D. Stoyanov et al. (eds.), *International Perspectives in Values-Based Mental Health Practice*, https://doi.org/10.1007/978-3-030-47852-0_43

Table 43.1 Annotated table of contents for Part VI, Reflections

implementation. Dubbed the '3 Rs' of values-based practice, these are respectively, **R**aising Awareness, **R**ecognition and **R**espect.

In the remainder of this chapter, we will first summarise the experiences of implementation described by contributors to this Part. As will be seen, the three chapters together provide powerful insights into the challenges of what it means to 'do' values-based practice for real. We will then contextualise these challenges within the framework of the '3 Rs' as this plays out across the book as a whole.

43.1   The Three Projects

First in line is a project illustrating the first of the '3 Rs', Raising Awareness of values.

43.1.1   R for Raising Awareness

As noted in chapter 1, "Surprised by Values: An Introduction to Values-Based Practice and the Use of Personal Narratives in This Book", raising awareness of values is the first and foundational skills area of values-based practice. Raising awareness turned out to be crucial in a project run by Kim Woodbridge-Dodd and Evette Hutchinson on which they reflect in chapter 44, "Reflections on the Impact of Mental Health Ward Staff Training in Race Equality and Values-Based Practice".

Kim and Evette's reflections on their project are presented in the form of a dialogue. In this dialogue, they look back on their experiences of first running and then evaluating the impact of a training project for front-line mental health ward staff that combined race equality with values-based practice. Kim (who is white) initiated, designed and organised the training and evaluation. She also delivered the values-based practice training. She is a nurse herself and was the operational manager of the staff completing the training. Evette (who is black) was external to the organisation and was invited to evaluate the programme. The project was funded and commissioned by an implementation arm of central government, the Care Services Improvement Partnership (CSIP). The ward was high achieving. The staff had recently gained a rare 'excellent' rating in a national assessment.

What stands out from Kim and Evette's vantage point of hindsight is the extent to which their early expectations of the training differed from what happened in practice, and how this was linked to their own cultural positioning in the project, respectively, as a white person (Kim) and a black person (Evette). In their dialogue, Kim and Evette candidly share their narratives of working through the difficulties and issues the training raised, such as the realisation that the white staff were finding the race equality training very challenging, and the black ward staff responses revealing their distress in relation to racism and dismissive attitudes or outright denial from their white colleagues. We come back below to the nature of these difficulties and the issues raised. As we will see, they provide a powerful illustration of the challenges of raising awareness of values in values-based practice.

43.1.2   R for Recognition

Chapter 45, "Connecting Patients, Practitioners and Regulators in Supporting Positive Experiences and Processes of Shared Decision-Making: A Case Study in Co-production" then follows with a project illustrating the second 'R' of values-based practice, Recognition. 'Recognition' in this context means recognising that (consistently with the Two-Feet principle of values-based practice, see chapter 1, "Surprised by Values: An Introduction to Values-Based Practice and the Use of Personal Narratives in This Book"), values come into all areas of health care including diagnostic assessment.

In chapte 45, Fiona Browne, Steven Bettles, Stacey Clift and Tim Walker describe their project. The authors of the chapter represent one of these constituencies—they are all health service regulators in the General Osteopathic Council (or GOsC, the regulator for osteopaths in the UK[2]). As a regulator, the GOsC might seem to some a perhaps surprising champion of values-based practice. 'Surprising' because regulation is widely regarded by practitioners as offering mainly a safety net against bad

---

[2] The GOsC is embedded in the statutory regulatory environment of health care in the UK. It is in turn overseen by the Professional Standards Authority, which reports on the performance of ten health and care professional regulators in the UK including the General Medical Council, the General Dental Council and others.

practice. In this respect, regulation has sometimes had the unintended consequence of acting as a barrier to good practice. In mental health, notably, regulation is often blamed for producing a risk-averse culture that is inimical to recovery: this is reflected in Waldo Roeg's story (chapter 32, "Discovering Myself, a Journey of Rediscovery"), for example, where he notes that a more enlightened attitude to risk management was an important factor in his own recovery.

It is particularly encouraging therefore that it is as senior regulators that the authors of this chapter should have been active in driving their whole programme of supporting positive practice along values-based lines. As they describe, this involved exploring what matters to patients in an osteopathic consultation. But consistently with the inclusive approach to values of values-based practice, it also involved exploring what matters to osteopaths. It was in this regard a genuine *co*-production. And reflecting the Recognition 'R' of values-based practice, what mattered to all stakeholders turned out to include not only how treatment was delivered but also how problems were assessed diagnostically. Again, we return below to the outcomes of the project and the challenges these present for implementation.

43.1.3 R for Respect

The third 'R' of values-based practice, Respect, directly reflects its premise. 'R' for Respect stands for the premise of values-based practice in 'mutual respect for differences of values' (see chapter 1, "Surprised by Values: An Introduction to Values-Based Practice and the Use of Personal Narratives in This Book"). The importance of an underpinning premise of Respect particularly when cultural values are in play, is powerfully illustrated in this Part by Colin King, Simon Clarke, Steven Gillard and Bill Fulford's chapter 46, "Beyond the Color Bar: Sharing Narratives in Order to Promote a Clearer Understanding of Mental Health Issues Across Cultural and Racial Boundaries".

The narrative of this chapter is developed from Colin King' and his colleagues' very different perspectives on working together over a number of years on various projects aimed at improving inter-ethnic and cross-racial understanding in mental health. The stakes are high: in the UK (as in a number of other countries) young black men are many times more likely to be treated psychiatrically on an involuntary basis than their white counterparts; and there are indications that this may reflect cultural rather than medical factors—epidemiological studies for example show that the rates of disproportionate treatment follow administrative boundaries [1].

Small wonder then that as Kim Woodbridge-Dodd and Evette Hutchinson found in their combined race equality and values-based training programme (chapter 44, "Reflections on the Impact of Mental Health Ward Staff Training in Race Equality and Values-Based Practice"), the values issues raised are deeply conflicting. We had similar experiences of conflicting values in our writing workshops developing the book (described in our concluding chapter 47, "Co-writing Values: What We Did and Why We Did It"). And conflicting perspectives is exactly what Colin (who is black) and his colleagues (who are white) experienced. *So* conflicting indeed were their perspectives that without a shared commitment to the mutual respect underpinning values-based practice, their working relationship would surely have broken down long ago.

That their relationship has not broken down, that, as we describe further below, their project continues to make progress towards getting 'beyond the colour bar', shows the power of the premise of Respect underpinning values-based practice particularly where, as in this instance, it is cultural values that are in conflict.

43.2 The 3 Rs

That all three projects turned out to be in different ways difficult, indicates, if indication were needed, that values-based practice itself is difficult. Raising awareness of values is difficult; Recognition of the role of values in all areas including diagnosis is difficult: above all, Respect for differences of values is difficult.

43.2.1 R for Raising Awareness

The difficulty of the first R of values-based practice, Raising awareness of values, is well shown by Kim and Evette's shared learning from their programme combining race equality with values-based training. Their programme indeed captures much that is important about the role of cultural values in mental health. The ward culture enabled staff to engage with culturally compatible values such as the autonomy of service users (including their rights in relation to having choices), and in achieving improved mental health through narratives of recovery. It was these values that had led to the ward staff's coveted 'excellent' rating for their work with service users. But when it came to working across racial boundaries, discriminatory values soon came into play. With hindsight, this might have been anticipated. Ward culture after all is not free from wider societal cultural norms, beliefs and assumptions. In contrast to the wider society, however, the playing out of values in behaviours within the ward environment can be more open to scrutiny and observation, particularly, as in this instance, in training.

A further important point from Kim and Evette's reflections is about self-awareness. Kim and Evette's willingness to move beyond the theory of values-based practice and to expect it of their own behaviour, both at the time of the project and when reflecting back, enabled considerable learning from the experience. Perhaps as Kim and Evette surmise, earlier engagement in values-based practice and ways of understanding racism could have supported staff on the race equality training to achieve more equal and respectful ways of working together. Black and white staff members certainly believed that there would be benefit from continuing forums of the values-based kind in which the differences between them and their white colleagues could be explored in a safe space that supported mutual understanding and resolution.

We noted in chapter 1 (and again in chapter 15, "Vectors of Best Practice: An Introduction to Part III, Practice") our own failure of self-awareness in values-based practice as reflected in the unacknowledged values of individualism that had driven its development to date. This as we emphasised continued despite the philosopher Sridhar Venkatapuram's early observations to this effect [2].

There is a sense in which this whole book is about remedying that failure of self-awareness by focusing on the importance of cultural values at least in mental health (for of course they are important across the board). The importance of cultural values is clearly flagged in the exemplars given in Part I. Then again, many of the new theoretical resources highlighted in Part II are resources for raising awareness of cultural values: aesthetics, phenomenology and topic-focused resources such as feminist philosophy are all highly sensitive to cultural values; and African philosophy offers a range of resources for working with cultural values that have no direct counterparts in Western thought and practice.

Raised awareness of values was important too in the aspects of values-based practice covered in Part III. The different values represented by the 'extended multidisciplinary team' of values-based practice, these in turn providing a resource for the values-based concept of 'person-values-centred care', reflected the cultures of the different professions making up the multidisciplinary team. In Part IV, the examples included from the wider values tool kit were all 'tools' for working specifically with cultural values (trans-cultural ethics, anthropology, and reinforcing the message about the resources of African thought and practice, the use of indabas in policy making). Part V, training, was in a sense all about training for raised awareness of values. The first skills area is explicitly about 'raised awareness' but knowledge, reasoning, and communication skills, all contribute in values-based practice to the task of raising awareness. Notice again in this Part the importance of new resources for raising awareness available to a culturally enriched form of values-based practice: Michael Bennet's methodology (chapter 38, "Case Studies in the Culture of Professional Football Players and Mental Welfare and Wellbeing"), for example, combining expertise by experience with social science methods, Dharma therapy from Buddhism (chapter 35, "Dharma Therapy: A Buddhist Counselling Approach to Acknowledging and Enhancing Perspectives, Attitudes and Values") and the Disha project in India (chapter 41, "Disha: Building Bridges-Removing Barriers: Where Excluded and Privileged Young Adults Meet").

43.2.2   R for Recognition

The importance of the new resources available to a culturally enriched form of values-based practice is further evident in respect of its second 'R', Recognition— Recognition of the role of values alongside evidence in all areas of health care including diagnosis.

The importance of cultural values in diagnostic assessment in mental health is again evident in three chapters in Part I (chapters 3, "Antonella: 'A Stranger in the Family'—A Case Study of Eating Disorders Across Cultures", 4, "The Role of Culture, Values and Trauma in Shaping Abnormal Bodily Experience in Migrants" and 5, "Premorbid Personality and Expatriation as Possible Risk Factors for Brief Psychotic Disorder: A Case Report from Post-Soviet Bulgaria"). In each case, their exemplar narratives took us directly to the importance of these diagnostic cultural values. Diagnostic values were similarly evident in Part IV (chapters 25, "A Cross-Cultural Values-Based Approach to the Diagnosis and Treatment of Dissociative (Conversion) Disorders", 26, "Treatment of Social Anxiety Disorder or Neuroenhancement of Socially Accepted Modesty? The Case of Ms. Suzuki", 27, "Nontraditional Religion, Hyper-Religiosity, and Psychopathology: The Story of Ivan from Bulgaria" and 28, "Journey into Genes: Cultural Values and the (Near) Future of Genetic Counselling in Mental Health") covering the three principles defining the relationship between values and evidence in values-based practice in its role of linking science with people. The further links in the chain of connections linking science with people, to which we pointed in the introduction to that Part (chapter 24, "Linking Science with People: An Introduction to Part IV, Science"), running as it does from research through regulation to clinical guidelines, are all about cultural values. The selection of research topics is guided by cultural values. Research itself is driven by a strong set of cultural values (to which Steven Gillard points in his contribution to chapter 46, "Beyond the Color Bar: Sharing Narratives in Order to Promote a Clearer Understanding of Mental Health Issues Across Cultural and Racial Boundaries"). Regulation reflects the cultural values of the wider society (such as being risk-averse). The values of the wider society are also reflected in clinical guidelines to the extent that these are constructed by combining evidence with health economic values.

It is thus particularly apposite that chapter 45, "Connecting Patients, Practitioners and Regulators in Supporting Positive Experiences and Processes of Shared Decision-Making: A Case Study in Co-production" should be by a health professional regulator, the General Osteopathic Council, regulation being itself a key link in the chain connecting science with people. As its authors describe, there were many difficulties in developing their project: the values of stakeholders were difficult to characterise, requiring a number of workshops using different methodologies. There will, as they anticipate, be further difficulties to come in evaluating the project. But they have led the way nonetheless in getting tangible results. Building on their foundational work on the values of the key stakeholders in osteopathic care, the General Osteopathic Council has produced a series of innovative resources to help osteopaths deliver care that is consistent with their own values while at the same time more effectively meeting the needs of their patients. Following their lead, similar developments are under way with other UK regulators (such as the General Dental Council); and the focus of the programme as a whole on positive practice is supported by the Professional Standards Authority (see the Guide to Further Information in chapter 45).

It is also apposite that chapter 45, in representing the 'R for Recognition' of values-based practice, should be about osteopathy. It might be thought that osteopathy being (primarily[3]) about bodily health, its processes of diagnostic assessment would be value free. To the contrary, as the story in chapter 45 illustrates, and as the resources produced by the programme make clear, the vectors of best practice in osteopathy no less than in mental health include diagnostic values. The example of osteopathy is the more striking as an instance of 'R for Recognition' because, as chapter 45 describes, with one exception, osteopaths start with enviably high patient satisfaction ratings. The exception is patients being less confident they have a sufficient say in how they are treated. In this respect, therefore, osteopathic patients share with service users in mental health a sense of loss of autonomy, suggestive of paternalistic practice. In mental health, moreover, as Waldo Roeg's story (chapter 32, "Discovering Myself, a Journey of Rediscovery") shows, restoring a sense of control is a first and often key step towards recovery. If therefor as chapter 45 shows, diagnostic values are important to restoring a sense of control in a discipline with such high overall patient ratings as osteopathy, they will hardly be any less important in mental health.

43.2.3　R for Respect

Like 'R for Recognition', the third 'R' of values-based practice, 'R for Respect', is widely represented throughout this book. Values-based practice as we have several times indicated is premised on mutual respect for differences of values. As a premise therefor, we should not be surprised to find that 'R for Respect' is pervasive. But the premise comes most decisively into its own in the outputs of values-based practice in balanced decision-making. Without mutual respect, the dissensus on which the distinctive balancing processes of values-based practice directly depend (see chapter 1, "Surprised by Values: An Introduction to Values-Based Practice and the Use of Personal Narratives in This Book") would simply not be possible.

---

[3] Osteopaths frequently see people whose bodily problems reflect psychological causes (such as stress-induced muscle tension) and most adopt a holistic biopsychosocial approach to assessment.

The three chapters on balanced decision-making included in Part III (Practice) illustrate the dependence of dissensus on mutual respect for differences specifically of *cultural* values. This is well illustrated by Guilherme (G) Messas and Maria Julia (MJFR) Soares (chapter 19, "Alcohol Use Disorder in a Culture that Normalizes the Consumption of Alcoholic Beverages: The Conflicts for Decision-Making") exploration of the role of cultural values in the context of treating alcohol use disorder in a culture that normalises alcohol consumption. In this context, cultural values are at the heart of the conflicts for decision-making they describe; and as their case narrative so vividly illustrates, resolving (or at any rate managing) these conflicts requires a capacity for dissensus; it requires, that is to say, a capacity for respecting what is important for the patient in question while at the same time not abandoning the clinician's own values of evidence-based interventions.

Other chapters in Part III provide important illustrations of the resources for Respect opened up by engaging with cultural values. Drozdstoy Stoyanov and Bill Fulford's chapter 20, "Living at the Edge of Compromise: Balkan Pluralism as a Resource for Balanced Decision-Making" and Werdie van Staden's chapter 21, ""Thinking Too Much": A Clash of Legitimate Values in Clinical Practice Calls for an Indaba Guided by African Values-Based Practice", both take us to the heart of the matter with the resources they respectively offer for managing pluralism. The essential pluralism of values-based practice as we noted in chapter 1, leaves it vulnerable to what the political philosopher Isaiah Berlin identified as the 'challenge of pluralism'. This challenge arises from what Berlin took to be the fact that people generally default to monism: they want definite answers not balanced judgements. Berlin's challenge of pluralism, furthermore, is no merely theoretical challenge. To the contrary, it crops up in many areas of practice. It was evident in the UK for example in the difficulties experienced in implementing values-based practice in relation to involuntary psychiatric treatment [3] and to diagnostic assessment [4]. The example of Balkan pluralism (chapter 20, "Living at the Edge of Compromise: Balkan Pluralism as a Resource for Balanced Decision-Making") thus gives hope that the default to monism is, as Stoyanov and Fulford indicate, a learned not innate feature of human behaviour and hence one that in principle can be unlearned. Werdie van Staden's chapter (chapter 21, ""Thinking Too Much": A Clash of Legitimate Values in Clinical Practice Calls for an Indaba Guided by African Values-Based Practice") complements this conclusion by illustrating the use of the African indaba as a powerful process through which the required learning demonstrably takes place.

All of which, coming back to chapter 46, "Beyond the Color Bar: Sharing Narratives in Order to Promote a Clearer Understanding of Mental Health Issues Across Cultural and Racial Boundaries", speaks to the importance of the experience of Colin King and his colleagues of the power of mutual respect in supporting dissensus. As noted above (and as described more fully in chapter 46) without mutual respect their project would have been pulled apart by the highly conflicting perspectives that as a racially mixed group they brought to it. As it is, however, they are making progress towards their aim of getting 'beyond the colour bar' and establishing co-production between people of different colours (black and white) in mental health.

The progress of the group, as their chapter describes, is partly by way of deeper theory, partly by way of practical outputs. As to theory, Colin King, drawing on the novel sociological and literary work on race of the turn-of-the-century Black American writer, WEB Du Bois [5], and others, has introduced the concept of pre-production as a necessary prerequisite for genuine co-production. As to practice, Colin King (who is black) and Simon Clarke (who is white), working through their roles as joint leads of the Network for Whiteness and Race Equality in the Collaborating Centre for Values-based Practice in Oxford, have run a number of innovative sessions raising awareness of the cultural values in play in mental health. A further indication of the innovative nature of this programme is that working in collaboration with Michael Bennet (chapter 38, "Case Studies in the Culture of Professional Football Players and Mental Welfare and Wellbeing"), its outputs build in part on coaching models used in professional football.

43.3 Conclusions

That values-based practice is difficult is the message of the three chapters in this Part. Reflecting on their experiences of implementing values-based practice in their respective programmes, the experiences of the authors of the three chapters illustrate the difficulties presented by values-based practice, in raising awareness of values, in recognising the role of values in all areas of health care including diagnosis, and in maintaining the mutual respect by which values-based practice is underpinned.

These themes, as we have seen, reflected across the book as a whole, indicate the extent both of the additional challenges raised by and of the additional resources available from a values-based practice that is enriched by engaging with cultural values. All of which is good news for mental health. As a number of chapters in the book indicate, recovery in mental health depends critically on the three Rs of Raising awareness, Recognition and Respect.

References

1. Weich S, McBride O, Twigg L, Keown P, Cyhlarova E, Crepaz-Keay D, Parsons H, Scott J, Bhui K. Variation in compulsory psychiatric inpatient admission in England: a cross-sectional, multilevel analysis. Health Serv Deliv Res. 2014;2(49):90.
2. Venkatapuram S. Values-based practice and global health. Chapter 11. In: Loughlin M, editor. Debates in values-based practice: arguments for and against. Cambridge: Cambridge University Press; 2014.

3. Fulford KWM, Dewey S, King M. Values-based involuntary seclusion and treatment: value pluralism and the UK's Mental Health Act 2007. Ch 60. In: Sadler JZ, van Staden W, Fulford KWM, editors. The Oxford handbook of psychiatric ethics. Oxford: Oxford University Press; 2015.
4. Fulford KWM, Duhig L, Hankin J, Hicks J, Keeble J. Values-based assessment in mental health: the 3 keys to a shared approach between service users and service providers. Ch 73. In: Sadler JZ, van Staden W, Fulford KWM, editors. The Oxford handbook of psychiatric ethics. Oxford: Oxford University Press; 2015.
5. Du Bois WD. The souls of the black folk. Oxford: Oxford University Press; 1903.

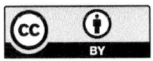

Reflections on the Impact of Mental Health Ward Staff Training in Race Equality and Values-Based Practice

44

Kim Woodbridge-Dodd and Evette A. Hunkins-Hutchinson

44.1 Introduction

In 2008, following implementation of the UK's 2006 Equality Act, before the UK's Equality Act 2010, the authors undertook a project to evaluate the impact of combining race equality with values-based practice training for staff on an acute inpatient mental health ward. The aim of the project was to see whether training in values-based practice would help staff to embed race equality practice into their work.

One author (Kim) was the operational manager for the ward; the other author (Evette) was the external evaluator for the project. The project was initially scoped out by Kim and three senior ward colleagues (all three were nurses). A steering group was set up comprising of Kim, ward colleagues, the race equality trainer, and Evette. This formed the core membership, with others, such as the regional Delivering Race Equality lead, and an additional qualified nurse from the ward, joining on occasion. The race equality training sessions were run by a national lead in race equality training who was involved in initial discussions about the delivery of both elements of the training, race equality, and values-based practice. They were also aware of the evaluation element but took no part in the evaluation other than to contribute feedback on their experience of running the race equality sessions.

Thirty-four core staff members were offered the training: the mix was 7 men and 27 women; 21 were white, 11 black, and 2 were of mixed heritage. Most were registered mental health nurses and held posts with different levels of responsibility.

K. Woodbridge-Dodd (✉)
Faculty of Health, Education and Society, University of Northampton,
Northampton, Northamptonshire, UK

E. A. Hunkins-Hutchinson
Faculty of Arts, Humanities and Cultures, University of Leeds, Leeds, UK

D. Stoyanov et al. (eds.), *International Perspectives in Values-Based Mental Health Practice*, https://doi.org/10.1007/978-3-030-47852-0_44

The staff completed a day-and-a-half race equality training followed by a day-and-a-half values-based practice training. To evaluate impact, participants were invited to attend two focus groups, one immediately after the race equality training and one immediately after the values-based practice session. In addition, staff shared their reflections with the evaluator whilst in practice during a 2-day period following the second focus group. Further details of the training and evaluation can be found in the reference at the end of the chapter (see Guide to Further Sources).

We reflect here on the project from our perspectives, respectively, as operational manager (Kim) and external evaluator (Evette), focusing on, (1) early expectations, (2) initial impressions, (3) evaluation and report on findings, (4) thinking back, and (5) what we would do differently. As will be seen, our reflections in some areas coincide and in others diverge. We conclude with a brief section summarising our shared learning points for the future.

44.2   Early Expectations

Kim

Reflecting on my early expectations for the project, I realise how little I knew about the challenges that race equality training could pose for all staff, black, white and all people of colour. At that time, we, the staff of the acute inpatient ward, were feeling very positive. We had just received a rating of 'Excellent' from the Care Quality Commission (the standards regulator for the UK's National Health Service), an award that very few services receive.

This rating endorsed all the dedicated work of staff in improving the experience of people using our ward. We held frequent discussions with our service users to understand what their issues were, if any, and their recommendations for improvements. There was active service user presence on the ward in the form of an independent service user advocate and routine visits by a community faith representative. Training had been completed by staff on the 'recovery approach' to mental health care (see chapter "Living at the Edge of Compromise: Balkan Pluralism as a Resource for Balanced Decision-Making") delivered by a service user jointly with a staff member. The physical environment had also been transformed as a result of an 'Enhancing the Healing Environment' project in collaboration with a UK NGO, the Kings Fund.

At the time of the training programme there had been an increasing national focus on Black and Minority Ethnic (BME) equality in mental health. This had been prompted by several reports highlighting the lack of understanding within services of the needs of BME service users. The UK's Equality Act had also recently come into effect requiring public bodies to implement race (and other aspects of) equality in their services. All this meant that as Operational Manager responsible for the ward I wanted to build on our success by supporting the staff to feel confident delivering race equality in their everyday work. My expectation was that this would be a natural extension of our earlier work responding to service user feedback. In previous jobs I had encountered very

defensive reactions from healthcare staff when service users questioned the established ward culture. Here by contrast staff had embraced such challenges and my expectation was that they would respond similarly to delivering race equality.

Hence my excitement when we secured funding from the UK Department of Health. Rather than just sending out a covering memo about the new corporate 'Equality policy', with instructions that it must be implemented, we now had the opportunity to provide staff with a comfortable space (the training took place in a hotel with refreshments) and time to think through what racism was and how it could be addressed on the ward.

Again, I did not anticipate any difficulties. In addition to my earlier experience of staff members' positive attitude to change, I knew them all well—my office was just off the ward area and I spent much of my time either on the ward or nearby. Yet as described further below, a key learning point for me was my surprise at just how difficult for staff the training in this area proved to be.

Evette

Since 'Empire Windrush' docked at Southampton race and equality has been a challenge for both the new-comers (British West Indians) and the host community. Both these communities were diverse in every sense, such as dress, food, and culture. Many came to work in the NHS. However, many became service users within the mental health services through compulsory admissions. With the lack of uptake voluntarily by this community and the over representation of men within all areas of mental health services, these disparities were highlighted in the publication 'Breaking the Circles of Fear', [2] after which came Delivering Race Equality' [3].

When I was approached by Kim to evaluate this project, I knew there would be challenging moments, as race equality training is never straight forward or without its challenges. But given that as Kim has described the organisation was in a good place, although I had more reservations than Kim, I too expected staff to be open to engaging positively with the challenge.

By way of background, I was told that there would be two separate training sessions, one on race equality led by an expert in this field (who was also black), and one on values-based practice led by Kim (who was already well known for her work in this area). I was introduced to members of staff to whom my role within the sessions was explained. As an evaluator I did not take part in any of the conversations or group discussions that developed during the sessions.

The race equality trainer and I were not known to each other or to the organisation. We are all female. We thus reflected the racial but not gender mix of the ward staff. The race training was very informative and as some participants expressed concerns as to the reasons why the training was on race, expressing their concerns that it would have been more helpful if It was on diversity. There clearly was a lack of understanding of what was intended by the training. Staffs' behaviour was very different when Kim (their manager) was present, they were more attentive, less confrontational and more engaging.

44.3 Initial Impressions

Evette

Kim and I met after each session to reflect on the day. This allowed us to work through our own challenges. The sessions aided our focus on the original purpose of the training sessions and my role as evaluator. What I found particularly helpful was that as operational manager, Kim was very open during our discussions, at times expressing frank surprise at the behaviour I observed of some staff members, and this despite having had in some respects a very different experience of the groups from me. For some members of staff this safe space enabled them to express concerns that they had previously kept locked away perhaps even from close friends and family.

Kim

At the time I ran the values-based practice workshops I was aware that there could be challenges as people struggled to work out what the approach meant to them and in their practice. But once staff grasped the basis of values-based practice they were creative in seeing ways to apply it in their work.

In our sessions with ward staff the challenges became harder when the conversation turned to how they worked with each other. Here however my initial impression was that staff found the framework of values-based practice helpful in allowing them to talk about difference. This enabled some very sensitive conversations between white and black staff about their experience of working together. For example, it became apparent that what could be viewed as being abrupt was often due to having to translate what the person wanted to say from their first language to English, and vice versa. There were also what I found painful accounts of black staff being distressed by what appeared as casual comments made on the ward and white staff members having no idea that these comments had been hurtful.

An encouraging finding from our initial feedback was that all staff said they would value a regular forum, run on similar lines, where they could discuss and work through difficult issues. The session had been viewed very positively and it had been good to air some of the concerns staff had about working with each other across racial differences. Without a forum of this kind problems were likely to remain unaddressed, sometimes resulting in negative impact on staff morale and health.

Evette

The race equality training although fairly standard was challenging as it emphasised difference and how one should behave in certain situations, for example if one is being bullied, or verbally abused on account of race.

Many of the staff found some of the issues raised by the training challenging and difficult to discuss, for example issues involving behaviours and diet that were different from the norm. Comments were made such as "why should we have to change—this is our country". Those from overseas on the other hand felt that they had come to a country that they believed they understood (having grown up within a similar educational system). The reality they found was completely different. Black staff felt they were not supported when racially abused verbally or even physically by patients; white staff would blame this on the patients' illness as 'part of their crisis' or claim that black staff 'had a chip on their shoulder'. These are of course old clichés yet still frequently used by staff to undermine or fail to challenge inappropriate behaviours. The result is that such behaviours are all too frequently overlooked, and the victim is made to feel like the perpetrator.

Staff members, black and white, were obviously very effective in their work. The group activities however highlighted failures in their relationship across racial lines, with black staff reporting how they often went home feeling very distressed and fragmented on a personal level. One result was that when it came to activities within the group they chose people from their own background. Debate was lively within same-race groups but flowed less readily when the facilitator mixed the groups up. A noticeable if worrying finding was that the race equality trainer was quite often treated disrespectfully, with suggestions that for example that she was biased or that her facts were incorrect.

Staff also found feedback in the one-to-one interviews challenging. When the transcriptions were handed back for checking I had many comments opening with 'I did not mean...'. White staff in particular would be almost indignant to see their own words in front of them and felt they had to justify them.

The values-based practice session went a lot more smoothly. I noticed the engaged and respectful attitude staff adopted towards the trainer, i.e., Kim, as their own operational manager. Even though some of the ideas of values-based practice were unfamiliar to them they were willing to participate in the exercises without the objections or lack of enthusiasm that had thwarted the Race Equality training. Staff even managed to put some of the values-based practice training straight into practice.

I took the contrast between their reactions to the two kinds of training as showing that staff members were not resistant to change but that change would have to come on their own terms irrespective of the potential benefits for their work and personal environment.

Kim

The first I was aware that there were issues arising was when Evette mentioned that the race equality trainer was having a hard time and that she had received some very negative responses from the participants. I spoke to the trainer who as noted earlier was very experienced and an expert. They confirmed yes there were issues and they agreed to send me their feedback on the training. This feedback indicated that some white staff were not engaged with the training and were being very disruptive. Some of these staff held positions of authority in the team and therefore influenced how others responded during the training. The feedback also noted that some staff members had commented that service user racist incidents on the ward were not taken seriously and that follow-up actions were not always evident.

44.4   Evaluation and Report on Findings

Evette

Four post-training focus groups were held. The groups were smaller than any of the training sessions. During the focus groups staff seem more inclined to raise issues that they had not felt able to raise before perhaps because they were afraid of the response they would receive in the larger group. I remember feeling that some of these debates would have been wonderful in the main sessions as they raised pertinent questions that the larger forum may have found useful. For example, there was much discussion about why the race equality session was focused on race and not on diversity. I noted that white participants were happier to engage in discussions around diversity than they were around race. It was almost as if the staff were intimidated to speak of race in an open and honest way. It is one of those discussion they should not be had in open for fear of saying the wrong thing. A vital opportunity was lost for open and honest dialogue between very diverse people, who as professionals went about the duties with diligence, efficiency and professionalism.

Some staff members felt that diversity rather than race quality was much more relevant to their work. Yet this was flatly contradicted by the sometimes openly disrespectful behaviour I had seen displayed in the training sessions. The atmosphere was sometimes such that I would find myself cringing inwardly at the level of disrespect shown even towards the race equality trainer and at the hostile reaction when she raised issues of race.

Kim

During the time when Evette was running the focus groups, I received concerns from a colleague involved in the project that the independent evaluator (Evette) was biased and reporting the findings in an unfair and negative way on the white staff. I checked with Evette and was reassured that verbatim accounts had been taken and shared with those taking part in the evaluation. My understanding from Evette that each participant had opportunity to double check the accuracy of the transcripts of the comments. Following this Evette submitted her findings and analysis to me and to the project group. This initial report of findings was agreed by the project group and was then used as the basis of a final project report, authored by myself and Evette and also shared with the group, that was for wider stakeholder circulation.

Through this process participants were satisfied the information contained in Evette's data collection was accurate, and the conclusions drawn in final project report were reasonable and fair. This was a journey for me where I could have used my position to override Evette's report to me, or ignored the feelings of the staff, or both to enable a less uncomfortable and more positive account of the training. However, through giving participants the opportunity and time to reflect on their accounts recorded by Evette, and by including participating colleagues in decisions about what was said in the final report, we were able to respect the different perspectives and achieve some difficult learning from the experience. The final project report included the following agreed conclusions:

1. There was a lower than expected level of general knowledge in relation to race equality practice. For example, an understanding of what is meant by the terms race and racism, how the service policy on racism could be implemented in practice.
2. More specifically, there was a lack of awareness/appreciation of the meaning of race as opposed to diversity or ethnicity, and its importance and effects.
3. The difficulty experienced by staff in discussing race, racial harassment and racism in a group with a mix of black and white staff could not be resolved by talking from a professional perspective alone and drew from individual's personal selves (experiences, beliefs, feelings, values).
4. The impact of racial abuse by service users towards staff whilst staff were caring form them was raised. How this should be addressed did not appear to be completely resolved or consistently addressed.

To share the learning from this experience, Evette and I, with the necessary approval, used the final project report as a basis for an article published in Mental Health Practice [1].

44.5 Thinking Back

Kim

Looking back on the project, I wonder how many other service areas I have spent time on with teams that have appeared to be professional, confident, and open to discussion and challenges to their custom and practice, yet where the reality was very different. If I was so unaware of the race issues within my own teams that I knew so well, surely I had been no more aware on other situations.

My concern is that without having the space to directly and personally discuss these issues, they are brushed off with oft-repeated yet contradictory assurances that, yes, we show careful attention to any race equality issues arising, and, no, there are no such issues here.

Evette

Completing the evaluation was not without its challenges for me. As a black woman, I was constantly having to dismiss my own personal feelings about some of the attitudes, misinformation and outright disrespectfulness of some members of staff during the sessions, having to remind myself of my role within the process and my own professionalism, which was to be unbiased and report only the facts.

I felt that although the training in both values-based practice and Race Equality offered staff the opportunity for personal development and growth, not all staff members were receptive to this. The project highlighted not only to myself, the team and trainer that the journey through race training is not without its challenges no matter how many time you are involved, either as a black trainer, evaluator or participant, but each time you learn new ways of dealing with the situation. Values-based practice can be a very influential tool in helping to move this debate forward.

Kim

What I found hardest about the project was the extremely uncomfortable feelings I experienced, that I was somehow letting my staff down—white as well as black—when they had trusted me. I felt white staff had been hurt by being as they saw it unfairly called racist when they worked so hard to make the ward a good and caring place. I realised that black staff had also been hurt by their experiences of racism not having been taken fully seriously and acted on. I had been simply unaware of just how badly their working lives were affected by the racist treatment they experienced, even if this was described as banter or misunderstanding.

I have since learnt a lot about why white people like myself find it difficult to talk about race equality, particularly how 'judged' we can feel when discussing our own behaviour and practices.

Evette

What I find interesting is that whilst no one person was called a racist they, by their own admission, felt that their actions had led others to feel uncomfortable, and as such they themselves acknowledged that their behaviour was racist, but of course they would not call it such.

44.6   What We Would Do Differently

Kim

I would hold the values-based practice session before the race equality session. This would have prepared the ground by encouraging discussion about how we all have a culture within which we are embedded, one of which we are unlikely to be aware, and yet which includes assumptions and beliefs that drive own behaviour. Values based practice brings these implicit cultural values and beliefs to the fore.

Evette

Yes, the race equality training would have benefited from values-based practice. Staff would have already been exposed to the importance of implicit and explicit values and differences of values, and the challenges that diverse groups encounter particularly when people share the same working space, yet do not share or appreciate their different cultural assumptions.

This would have had other benefits: it would have given staff the opportunity to engage with the concept of change; and it would have equipped them to acknowledge, appreciate and open their minds to alternative ways of working. As could be seen from the ward observations, were staff members were actively putting into practice some of the lessons taken from the VBP workshops.

Kim

I agree, I have searched to understand why this project was so difficult, reflecting on my position as a white person, as a values-based practice facilitator, and as a manager. I think there are many ways of understanding the concept of culture, and there are many cultures, (nursing, mental health ward, English), relevant to this experience. I wonder if one consequence of the national health service mental health ward culture is that the focus on professional accountability and the monitoring processes of clinical governance produce a culture where staff can only be seen as good or not good, with no option for a middle ground. As a staff group discussing race equality and racism on the ward, a middle ground is needed, as coming to understand and recognise racism may require some self-reflection, uncomfortable insights and painful awareness raising about ward culture and personal practice.

Evette

I firmly believe no matter how difficult this journey was for all concerned everyone would have learnt something from the experiences.

44.7 Conclusions

We would like to offer the below key learning points from our experience with the Race Equality and values-based practice project.

1. Be aware that being open to challenge and change in one area of healthcare (such as service user involvement) does not automatically lead to being able to be open to other challenges (race equality training). This has significant implications for understanding how cultural change works on wards.
2. The benefit of introducing values-based practice before race equality training workshops.
3. Being aware that white people find it very difficult to talk about racism.
4. Be prepared for your own position in modelling/using values-based practice when events/issues arise during training sessions.
5. Have a respectful and trusting relationship between trainers and evaluators, even if their perspectives differ.
6. Know what you are going to do if people within the evaluation strongly disagree with what you are doing, the findings and believe the trainer and the evaluator are biased.
7. Remember, there are always conflicting values, treat them all with respect.

8. Finally, be careful about what you wish for, the aim of the project was to get staff personally engage with the training rather than just 'ticking the box' for race equality training. They really *did* engage. That is why it so was difficult and painful.

Acknowledgements We would like to thank all the staff that took part in the race equality and values-based practice training. They helped us learn and understand, they were often brave and sensitive when discussing difficult and challenging issues. We would also like to thank Petronella Mwasandube OBE who ran the race equality and Cultural Competence Awareness training. Finally, we are grateful to the Department of Health for funding the project through a small grant and the NHS for giving us permission to complete the study and to publish the findings.

44.8 Guide to Further Sources

44.8.1 Books

White Fragility by Robin DiAngelo published 2018 by Beacon Press. This is helpful if you are interested in understanding why white people sometimes feel very uncomfortable in race equality training. Robin DiAngelo wrote the book following her experiences in America of being a white person running race equality training and the challenging responses of white people.

Also helpful is: *Between camps: nations, cultures and the allure of race.* Paul Gilroy 2000. Penguin Books.

44.8.2 Workbook

Whose Values? A workbook for values-based practice in mental health care by Kim Woodbridge and Bill (K.W.M.) Fulford. Published in 2004, it is available as a download from valuesbasedparctice.org/More about VBP/full text downloads and scroll to training materials. Although produce a few years ago, it provides a simple and practical guide to values-based practice in mental health.

44.8.3 Reports

The House of commons *Enforcing the Equality Act: the law and the role of the Equality and Human Rights Commission.* Tenth Report of Session 2017–2019. Available from https://www.parliament.uk/business/committees/committees-a-z/commons-select/women-and-equalities-committee/inquiries/parliament-2017/enforcing-the-equality-act-17-19/ This gives a recent and interesting overview of policy and issues related to the Equality Acts.

Breaking the Circles of Fear: A review of the relationship between mental health services and African and Caribbean communities https://www.centreformental-health.org.uk/sites/default/files/breaking_the_circles_of_fear.pdf.

Reference

1. Dodd K, Hunkins-Hutchinson E, Fulford W. Race equality training and values-based practice. Ment Health Pract. 2011;15(2):28–32.
2. Department of Health (2005) Delivering race equality in mental health care: An action plan for reform inside and outside services and the government's response to the independent inquiry into the death of David Bennett. Retrieved from http://www.dh.gov.uk/en/Publicationsandstatistics/Publications/PublicationsPolicyAndGuidance/DH_4100773.
3. Sainsbury Centre for Mental Health (2002) Breaking the Circles of Fear: A review of the relationship between mental health services and African and Caribbean communities https://www.centreformentalhealth.org.uk/sites/default/files/breaking_the_circles_of_fear.pdf.

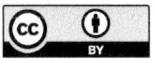

Connecting Patients, Practitioners and Regulators in Supporting Positive Experiences and Processes of Shared Decision-Making: A Case Study in Co-production

Fiona Browne, Steven Bettles, Stacey Clift, and Tim Walker

45.1 Introduction

The aim of the project in osteopathic regulation described in this chapter was to develop resources that could be used by osteopaths and patients to support them to make more explicit what was important to them and to enhance patient agency through shared decision-making. The project, which built in part on a background development programme in values-based osteopathy, ran in two main phases: Phase I focused on increasing understanding of the values of osteopaths, their patients and the regulator; Phase II focused on developing support resources. As will be seen, an understanding of the cultural values of osteopathy proved to be central to both phases of the project though in very different ways. In the first phase, cultural values proved to be relatively simple to elicit and to organise into a shared framework of values (see below), but in the second phase, the framework turned out to be very difficult to apply in practice.

The project was guided by two themes of growing importance across contemporary health service regulation: the need to support good practice as well as preventing bad practice [1, 2]; and the use of more evidence-based approaches [3, 4]. In relation to these themes osteopathy offers a promising area for exemplar projects in that studies have reported very high levels of care, for example with up to 95% overall patient satisfaction in the OPeN study [5] and similarly in a YouGov study [6] using categories derived from the CARE Measure [7]. Within this overall figure, however, items that related to patient empowerment in the context of shared decision making stood out as an area for potential improvement from the perspective of patients. The items included: 'fully understanding your concerns'; 'helping you to take control'; and 'making a plan of action with you' and were suggestive of a potentially paternalistic approach to care by practitioners. Hence the focus of our project on patient empowerment and shared decision-making.

F. Browne (✉) · S. Bettles · S. Clift · T. Walker
General Osteopathic Council, London, UK

© The Author(s) 2021
D. Stoyanov et al. (eds.), *International Perspectives in Values-Based Mental Health Practice*, https://doi.org/10.1007/978-3-030-47852-0_45

The project as a whole is described in detail elsewhere [8]. We focus in this chapter on the insights it provided about the role of cultural values as a bridge between osteopaths, their patients and the regulator. We start with a case narrative illustrating the impact of the cultural values of osteopathy in practice.

45.2   Case Narrative: Jennifer's Story

Jennifer's story is fictitious but based on a composite of cases from everyday osteopathic practice. The story is presented here as it was used in the background development programme in values-based osteopathy on which the project was in part based. It is presented here as it was used in the context of that development programme, that is, in two parts with two brief questions for the reader at the end of the first part, about his or her reactions to that point.

45.2.1   Part 1: Initial Assessment and Treatment

Jennifer is a middle career manager working full-time in a medium sized media business. Her background is in design, but these days she spends most of her time in mainly administrative roles, sitting at a computer plus travelling to consult with business clients. She enjoys her job, but the current economic climate has made it difficult to find new clients and she says there are rumours of redundancies going round the business. She has been in her job for some years so she thinks she is safe, but these days who knows?

She visits an osteopath complaining of headaches and aching across her shoulders and upper back with an occasional pain into her left arm when she's particularly stressed or tired. It has been slowly developing over the last few months. She hasn't seen her doctor for fear of what she might say and because she doesn't want to start on a regime of pill taking.

Otherwise she is in good health with no history of significant illnesses or operations, though she did have a fall from her horse when she was 15 and was badly concussed. They told her she'd had a minor neck injury. She recovered ok and isn't aware of any repercussions from the accident. Her weight is within normal ranges and she claims to eat well, though she has little time for regular exercise, something she used to do a lot of when younger.

She is married with two teenage boys who are both into competitive sport. This involves them in frequent competitions as well as training sessions during the week.

When the osteopath examines her standing and moving, Jennifer looks tense and a little 'ill at ease', but she says she feels comfortable. Her upper thoracic and cervical spinal movements are all a bit less than the osteopath expects for someone her age, and there is considerable hypertonia (tension) in the paraspinal muscles. There is no dizziness on neck movements.

When the osteopath examines her lying supine, Jennifer flinches when he feels round her neck. The osteopath asks her if she has pain, which she denies but then goes quiet. The osteopath senses there is something wrong, but he doesn't know what it is and there is no further discussion about this. The osteopath finds a local area of restricted mobility in C 2–4 and Jennifer tells him that it feels tender particularly on the left side.

The osteopath concludes that her problem is mainly stress related, and that pressures of work and home are maintaining hypertonic tissue, impairing fluid flow in the area and that there are mild inflammatory changes in the soft tissues. He treats using some gentle soft-tissue techniques and joint articulation with the aim of freeing the area and improving fluid exchange.

45.2.2 Questions for the Reader

From either a patient or an osteopath perspective please think about.
1. What was good about the osteopath's approach to helping Jennifer?
2. Were there areas where they showed less than optimal practice?

We will come back to these questions later but for the moment please think about them particularly with issues of patient empowerment and shared decision-making in mind, and how these issues might interact with cultural and other values.

45.2.3 Part 2: First Follow-Up

Jennifer returns for a follow up appointment a few days later. She reports that she felt very sore for 36 hours after treatment but that has now eased and if anything, she feels a little better overall. While she is being examined and given further treatment for her neck, there is an awkward silence and then she says that perhaps she ought to explain that she was sexually abused by a relative when she was a child, which also included threatening her never to say anything to anyone. He had reinforced that message by putting his hands around her throat. Since then she has never felt comfortable lying exposed and she can freak out if someone puts their hands around her neck.

45.3 Understanding Jennifer's Story

Rather than commenting directly on Jennifer's story from our perspective as a regulator, we will explore the issues it raises through materials from our workshops. Being co-produced, these materials reflect the perspectives of us as a regulator, osteopaths and osteopathic patients. We give a brief overview of the project as a whole and then illustrate its outcomes with sample findings from two of the workshops, one from Phase I (eliciting values) and one from Phase II (developing support materials).

45.3.1 The Co-development Workshop Programme

Three development workshops were held between 2014 and 2017. The first two workshops (Phase 1) focused on eliciting values and employed methods adapted by a senior academic in the University College of Osteopathy (formerly the British School of Osteopathy), Stephen Tyreman (see Acknowledgements), from those developed for surgical training by the Collaborating Centre for Values-based Practice in Oxford.

The last workshop (Phase II) focused on developing support resources was run in partnership with another regulator (the General Dental Council). For this workshop, we employed an independent social research organisation, Community Research, working with the team responsible for Phase I. We present here sample materials from the two phases of the project by way of illumination of the issues raised by Jennifer's narrative above.

45.3.2 Phase I Workshop Materials: What Makes a Good Osteopath

The focus in this first phase was on the values by which good practice in osteopathy is defined from the perspectives, respectively, of regulators, osteopaths and their patients. Stephen Tyreman (for the University College of Osteopathy) and Bill Fulford (for the Collaborating Centre) developed and led this phase using interactive exercises adapted, as noted above, from the values-based training materials developed in Oxford) and case studies.

Table 45.1 illustrates the key outcome from one of the interactive exercises in Phase I. Participants were asked to write down three words that they felt described a 'good osteopath'. It was emphasised that they should approach this not as a theoretical or general exercise but from their own particular perspective, whether as an osteopathic patient, an osteopath or other (the latter included regulators). The result was a wide diversity of responses with no obvious or outstanding differences between the three groups. We noted that all three groups agreed that a good osteopath showed a combination of

- **People-focused values**: care/empathy/compassionate/reflective.
- **Task-focused values**: skills/techniques/expertise/knowledge/experience.

This finding was encouraging from a regulatory perspective in that these shared values corresponded with the Osteopathic Practice Standards (core standards of conduct and competence for osteopaths) and other established regulatory standards for health professionals (see Guide to Further Sources, below). They thus provided prima facie validation of the role of these standards in supporting shared decision-making. Applying these findings to the story of Jennifer and others like it, we can see that the shared values illuminated both positive and negative aspects of osteopathic practice. Thus, on the positive side, we could say that the osteopath performed well against task-focused values: they made a technically competent

Table 45.1 Descriptions of a 'good osteopath' from patients, osteopaths and regulators

Patients	Osteopaths	Other (including regulators)
Patient centred (1)	**Effective (1)**	**Expertise (1)**
Efficacy (1)	**Professionalism (1)**	**Knowledgeable (1)**
Accuracy of outcome (1)	**Reflective (1)**	**Clinically sound/competent (1)**
*Identifying and **improving condition** (1)*		**Integrity (1)**
Professionalism (1)		*Trustworthy (1)*
Confidence in their ability (1)		*Good listener (1)*
Communication interaction in identifying needs (1)		*Clear communication of management plan (1)*
	Compassionate (3)	
	Empathy (3)	
Caring (3)	*Care (3)*	*Caring (3)*
Empathic/empathy (3)	*Empathy (3)*	
	Integrity (3)	**Integrity (3)**
Competent (3)		**Competent (3)**

[Note: Bold italic = Task-focused values; Italic = People-focused values; Bold = other values]

osteopathic assessment of the presenting problem and provided appropriate treatment and follow-up for the patient that she found helpful.

On the other hand though, we could say that the osteopath performed less well against people-focused values: the osteopath misread Jennifer's hesitations and silences about being examined. Indeed, the osteopath's whole approach, at least as represented by the language of the case study, reflected a lack of engagement with what was important from the patient's perspective—the language is focused on what the osteopath thought, for example, '*the osteopath concludes that …*'—and there is no suggestion (in the story as presented) of the osteopath taking time or giving Jennifer space to say what was important to her about what was going on.

This mismatch of values goes to the heart of the challenge we had set ourselves as regulators of embedding standards. It could be assumed that despite the osteopath not really exploring what was actually important to the patient at that time, she might well have rated him within that 95% positive satisfaction for the profession as a whole (noted above, [5]). After all, measured against the task-focused values, the osteopath had done well—Jennifer did feel better. But the osteopath did less well measured by the people-focused skills—they missed (or misread or failed to respond to) important signals relevant to empowering Jennifer: in the terms of the CARE Measure items ([7] and see introduction above), the osteopath did not appear to be 'fully understanding (Jennifer's) concerns', or to 'help (her) to take control', and to 'make a plan of action with (her)'.

45.3.3   The Cultural Values of Osteopaths and Jennifer's Story

The origins of these misreadings in the cultural values of osteopaths became clear through the workshop discussions in Phase I. As described further in the sources given below (see Guide to Further Sources), osteopathy is a manual therapy with palpation of tissue quality and mobility being key to patient care. The findings from palpation furthermore can only be interpreted in the light of a full background history. When this is done well, the patient will often feel they have been really listened to—a key component, as many among our participants pointed out, of the high patient satisfaction ratings achieved by osteopaths.

Osteopaths, moreover, tend to undertake a global assessment of a patient's musculoskeletal system rather than just the symptomatic area [9]. Hence, osteopaths will often request that patients undress so as to facilitate a broad osteopathic examination. Osteopathy thus tends to be by its nature an intimate intervention—it involves close physical contact with the patient in varying degrees of undress and so potentially feeling nervous and uncomfortable can be a common patient response. Couple this with the fact that osteopaths often work as sole practitioners in quite isolated practices, and the potential for misunderstanding becomes clear.

45.3.4   A Draft Framework of Values

Based on the above findings about the cultural values guiding osteopathic practice and their prima facie relevance to regulatory standards, and working with our academic partner, Professor Stephen Tyreman, our programme developed the framework of values shown in Fig. 45.1.

Our idea at this stage was that the framework would help to illuminate what was important to patients and practitioners by supporting them to make more explicit the values driving their interaction. Through improved understanding the framework would thus serve as a basis for developing support materials for improving patient agency and shared decision-making. When we came to test this idea, however, with an extended group of participants and additional cases, we found that far from clarifying the values involved, the Framework became a distraction. Participants struggled to map their values onto the Framework and ended up instead debating the merits of the Framework itself. It was at this point that we had the opportunity to partner with the General Dental Council in taking the project to its next phase.

45.3.5   Phase II Workshop Materials: Developing
Support Resources

The General Dental Council had worked successfully with the independent research group, Community Research, who suggested an innovative approach to tackling the challenges of implementing shared decision-making directly. Using an exercise developed by Community Research with the steering group for the project, called

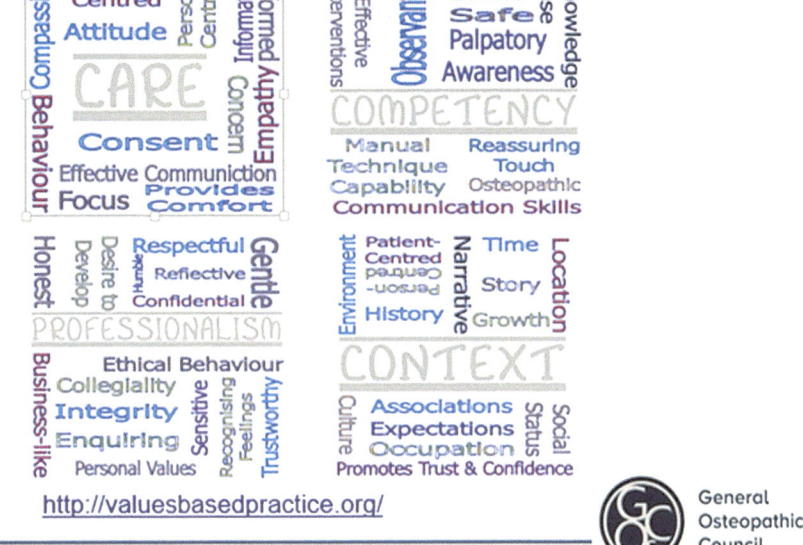

Fig. 45.1 Draft framework of shared values for osteopathic practice (The copyright of this figure is the property of the General Osteopathic Council. It was developed in partnership with Professor Steven Tyreman (see text and Acknowledgements) as part of the Council's programme described in this chapter)

'Fruits, Pests and Roots', this involved participants identifying, respectively, the benefits of and barriers to patient empowerment and a positive consultation, and actions that could be introduced to overcome the barriers. Written on coloured post-it notes, these were then added to a tree diagram as shown in Fig. 45.2.

This exercise was helpful particularly in pointing to the diversity of factors participants identified across the board in relation to shared decision-making. This finding went some way to explaining the gap in our Phase I findings between the relative ease with which we were able to identify key cultural values and the difficulties we experienced when we came to applying them in practice. This in turn suggested that there could be 'no one size fits all' approach to developing support resources for patient empowerment and shared decision-making.

45.3.6   Developing Prototype Support Resources

Taking into account the 'no one-size-fits-all' finding from the workshop programme, the team has developed a series of different tools to support patients and practitioners to prepare for consultations that would enhance patient empowerment and

Fig. 45.2 Fruits, pests and roots exercise from Phase II

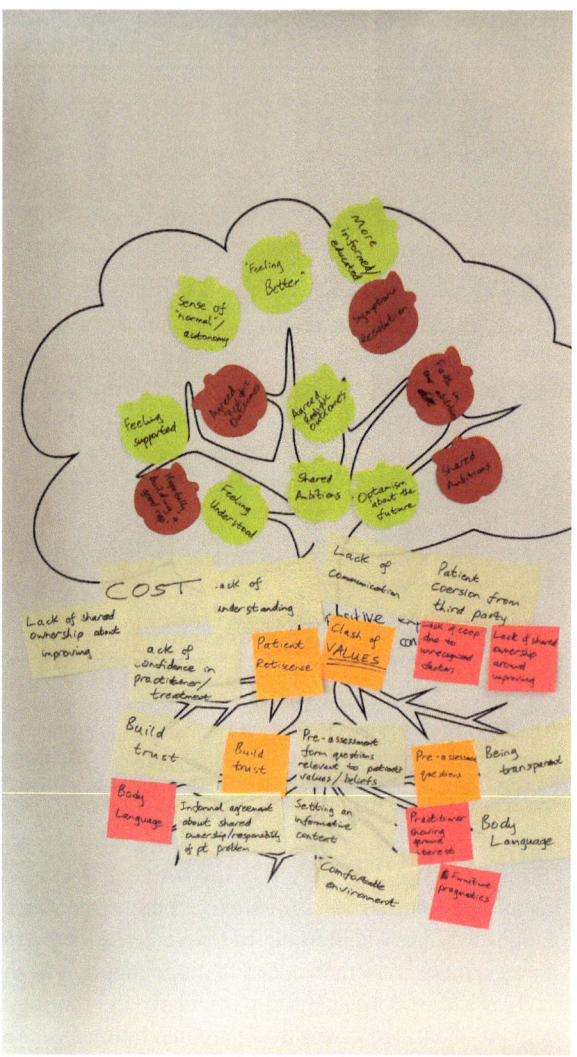

shared decision-making. Reflecting regulatory guidance and recent changes in the law on consent [10], this has included raising awareness of the values (of what is important to) the particular patient concerned [11]. As in Jennifer's story, this is not always self-evident: Jennifer presented with pain and stiffness in her neck, but her response to being examined pointed to underlying concerns that limited her engagement and there was little, if any, evidence of shared decision-making. These resources are listed with links below (see [8] and Guide to Further Sources). As noted earlier, they have been generally well received, at this early stage, and we plan more formal testing of their impact in the next stage of the project.

45.4 Conclusions

In this chapter, we have described a two-phase project that we developed in our role as regulator, aimed at enhancing patient empowerment and shared decision-making in the context of osteopathic clinical care by supporting patients and osteopaths to make more explicit what is important to them in a consultation. The first phase of the project, concerned with eliciting values, showed the potential role of shared values as a bridge between patients, practitioners and regulators. When it came to implementation, however, in the second phase of the project, building on these values proved considerably harder than we had anticipated. What became clear was that a 'no one-size-fits-all' approach would be needed to support implementation. Examples of the range of support resources we are currently developing are provided below in our Guide to Further Sources.

Osteopathy as we have indicated is a promising area for work of this kind given the high levels of patient satisfaction generally achieved by osteopaths. Lower scores, however, for items indicating patient empowerment and shared decision-making are important, as we have also indicated, particularly from a regulatory perspective to the extent that these are reflected in recent changes in the law on consent [10, 11]. Jennifer's story in this chapter shows the importance of cultural values underpinning both positive and negative aspects of osteopathic practice. Insights into these values emerged readily in Phase I of our project. That such insights are, however, not sufficient was made abundantly clear by the difficulties of implementation we encountered in Phase II. These difficulties we believe suggest the need for building further on contemporary moves in health service regulation towards empirically informed approaches to supporting good practice.

Acknowledgements We would like to warmly acknowledge the support and guidance of:

- Harry Cayton, at the time of the project, Chief Executive of the PSA (Professional Standards Authority).
- Professor Stephen Tyreman of the University College of Osteopathy.
- Professor Bill Fulford of the Collaborating Centre for Values Based Practice.
- Mr. Guy Rubin of the General Dental Council.
- Ms. Rebecca Addis and Ms. Kate Waller of Community Research.
- All our patients and practitioners. We are grateful to the General Osteopathic Council and the General Dental Council for funding this project. The General Osteopathic Council employed all the authors at the time of the study but without requiring a grant number.

Sadly, Stephen Tyreman died before the end of the project. This was shortly after being awarded the Institute of Osteopathy President's Medal for 2018. For an appreciation of his work, please see: https://valuesbasedpractice.org/who-are-we-2/list-of-project-partners/list-of-individuals/stephen-tyreman/.

45.5 Guide to Further Sources

45.5.1 The Osteopathic Practice Standards (2019)

These are given here: https://standards.osteopathy.org.uk/.

They are consistent with the corresponding standards for medicine in the UK given in the General Medical Council's publication Good Medical Practice at: https://www.gmc-uk.org/ethical-guidance/ethical-guidance-for-doctors/good-medical-practice.

45.5.2 The Cultural Values of Osteopathy

These are reflected, for example, in the curriculum elements included in the Guidance for Osteopathic Pre-Registration Education (GOPRE) at https://www.osteopathy.org.uk/training-and-registering/becoming-an-osteopath/guidance-osteopathic-pre-registration-education/).

45.5.3 Prototype Resources

As noted in the chapter, we have developed a range of prototype resources to support patient empowerment and shared decision-making in osteopathy by helping patients and practitioners to make more explicit what is important to them in a consultation. These have been well received by practitioners and patients, and in a further phase of the project, we plan to assess their actual impact in practice. For details including links to the on-line resources please see [8].

References

1. Law Commissions. Regulation of Health Care Professionals Regulation of Social Care Professionals in England. Law Commission, Scottish Law Commission and Northern Ireland Law Commission. Report number: LAW COM No 345, SCOT LAW COM No 237, NILC 18, 2014. https://s3-eu-west-2.amazonaws.com/lawcom-prod-storage-11jsxou24uy7q/uploads/2015/03/lc345_regulation_of_healthcare_professionals.pdf. Accessed 21 Dec 2019. Subsequent dialogue in relation to this is an example about this framing of regulation.
2. Tyreman S. Evidence, alternative facts and narrative: a personal reflection on person-centred care and the role of stories in healthcare. Int J Osteopat Med. 2018;28:1–3. https://doi.org/10.1016/j.ijosm.2018.04.005.
3. Professional Standards Authority. Rethinking regulation. 2015. https://www.professionalstandards.org.uk/docs/default-source/publications/thought-paper/rethinking-regulation-2015.pdf. Accessed 21 Dec 2019.
4. McGivern G, Fischer M, Palaima T, Spendlove Z, Thomson O, Waring J. Exploring and explaining the dynamics of osteopathic regulation, professionalism and compliance with standards in practice. Report for the General Osteopathic Council. 2015. http://www.osteopathy.

org.uk/news-and-resources/document-library/research-and-surveys/dynamics-of-effective-regulation-final-report/. Accessed 21 Dec 2019.

5. Leach CM, Mandy A, Hankins M, Bottomley LM, Cross V, Fawkes CA, Fiske A, Moore AP. Patients' expectations of private osteopathic care in the UK: a national survey of patients. BMC Complement Altern Med. 2013;13:122. https://bmccomplementalternmed.biomedcentral.com/articles/10.1186/1472-6882-13-122. Accessed 21 Dec 2019.

6. You Gov *Public Perceptions Study*. Report for the General Osteopathic Council. 2018. https://www.osteopathy.org.uk/news-and-resources/document-library/research-and-surveys/public-perceptions-study/. Accessed 21 Dec 2019.

7. CARE Measure. The Consultation and Relational Empathy (CARE) Measure. http://www.caremeasure.org. Accessed 21 Dec 2019.

8. Browne F, Bettles S, Clift S, Walker T. Connecting patients, practitioners and regulators in supporting positive experiences and processes of shared decision-making: a progress report. J Eval Clin Pract. 2019;25(6):1030–40. https://doi.org/10.1111/jep.13279.

9. Tyreman ST. The concept of function in osteopathy and conventional medicine. PhD thesis, Milton Keynes: Open University; 2001. http://oro.open.ac.uk/59356/. Accessed 14 Jan 2020.

10. Supreme Court. Montgomery (Appellant) v Lanarkshire Health Board (Respondent) (Scotland). UKSC 11, 2015. https://www.supremecourt.uk/cases/uksc-2013-0136.html. Accessed 21 Dec 2019.

11. Herring J, Fulford KWM, Dunn D, Handa A. Elbow room for best practice? Montgomery, patients' values, and balanced decision-making in person-centred care. Med Law Rev. 2017;25(4):582–603. https://doi.org/10.1093/medlaw/fwx029.

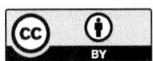

**Beyond the Color Bar: Sharing
Narratives in Order to Promote a Clearer
Understanding of Mental Health Issues
Across Cultural and Racial Boundaries**

46

Colin King, Simon Clarke, Steven Gillard, and Bill Fulford

46.1 Introduction

The 'back story' to this chapter is a long-term collaboration between the authors—one British black man (Colin) and three British white men (Simon, Bill and Steven)—aimed at getting 'beyond the colour bar' towards better understanding of their respective cultural perspectives.

Their four narratives (written independently) reveal their very different perspectives on their experiences to date. As such, it might seem that their collaboration has failed. But as they describe in their co-written commentary, held together as they are by the premise of mutual respect, the differences between them point to new understanding of the factors driving the diagnosis and treatment of mental health issues.

46.2 Colin King's Narrative

I am a black, African, mental health diseased case, one dimensional in terms of the culture of the individuals I associate with. I cannot work in a cultural vacuum with other people who do not declare or wish to look at their dimensions of their world they accept without been attached to an identity based on race [1]. They can only see themselves through me, it is a deceit that goes unchallenged particularly when given the badge of the mental health survivor. I see the deadness of their soul [2]

C. King · S. Clarke
Coordinator of the Whiteness and Race Equality Network, St Catherine's College,
University of Oxford, Oxford, UK

S. Gillard
Social & Community Mental Health, Population Health Research Institute, St George's,
University of London, London, UK

B. Fulford (✉)
Fellow, St Catherine's College, University of Oxford, Oxford, UK

© The Author(s) 2021
D. Stoyanov et al. (eds.), *International Perspectives in Values-Based Mental
Health Practice*, https://doi.org/10.1007/978-3-030-47852-0_46

when they talk and how they act in the cultural contexts in which we give meaning to our relationships, asking for my experiences as the knowledge they need to research me. They rarely exchange their experiences, their heritage, the foundations of who they are, they hide behind the scientific exoneration of detachment. In this culture exists the process of white denial, black emotional expression, white rationality, black feelings of despair and injustice. Culture is a whiteness understanding its whiteness through black experiences of becoming mentally ill. Listening through its theories and models that protect its whiteness, that rationalises what it hears and sees in the culture of the black people it interacts with, so it has no responsibility, it is absent in this cultural space, the space that Rosaldo [3] sees as cultural truths.

Culture has emerged in my experience as an entry into a whiteness that is never visible [4]. It is walking into academic institutes and meeting with white academics who talk in cold tongues, look at you as a mystery and activate indifference to an examination of their white codes, which Ladner [5] sees as old colonial reference points. Race, racialisation and discrimination appear to detach its ability for self-reflection. The culture of whiteness I enter cannot be articulated or evidenced in the contexts in which we meet. My capital remains my mental health diagnosis, my 'schizophrenia', my power is my ability to articulate and express without threatening the culture of whiteness that does not expose itself as a culture. Similar to Littlewood and Lipsedge [6] it is something that happens as the unknown, undetected and absent. I enter a culture in which I am made visible and the other, white men, white women, are invisible. They chose when to become visible, they are not vulnerable to their experiences of their culture being labelled and constructed as a mental disorder. Culture in this process of researching, writing, and discovery of the truth of partnership working, is assumed and never discussed. It's part of a culture of deceit, we meet periodically and enter each other's world, in a meeting room, a café, McDonald's, the National Film Theatre, we have no appreciation or invitation to announce how our external world and values enter us and form the culture in which we work in these contexts. It is the terror of what whiteness can do if discussed [7], the terror of being guilty of a truth that is culturally painful to own.

I live in and through a culture where whiteness gives me inferiority, cultural differentials and self-narcissism, what Fanon [8] refers to as 'negrophobia'. I consequently take part in a culture in which I form distance and an alien response to those who are alien to my world. I talk, drink coffee, listen and then go home waiting for the next meeting interspersed by emails or even a phone call. This is the social distance with the white other, I maintain as a cultural distance in which I avoid contamination. I don't feel part of their culture in which I am defined, rarely do they offer themselves as part of sharing their culture. I rarely enter into their personal social world, what Goffman [9] calls their back stages, unless it is academic, scientific, or research based. Rarely do I see the culture behind what Fanon [8] refers to as the 'white mask'. I am left in a culture of emptiness and failed promises that materialises where I experience cultural inequality, where I am always the black diseased schizophrenic.

46.3   Simon Clarke's Narrative

Our collaboration has given me opportunities to work in a way that is co-operative, that seeks to build bridges between methodologies which are generally seen as being in conflict. I have learnt through coproduction to value processes that facilitate change, that question assumptions about working methods and approaches to Mental Health and well-being. As a white practitioner I have begun to open up, to reflect on how my whiteness informs my view of the world. I have had to come to terms with the fact that my whiteness can impose a view of reality that is not shared by people whose cultural references and norms are different from my own. My learning has come through the experience of facilitating the workshops and seminars that we have run under Colin's leadership, from taking part in the regular meetings we have to review progress and from the work I have done in supporting Colin in editing a book that he is writing about the processes that we are exploring.

The glue that binds our work together is the drive that we all have to improve communication between professionals and service users in terms of assessment and diagnosis in mental health services. We want to promote ways of working that will ensure that all voices in the process are given equal weight, that peoples' lived experiences are valued and understood. For me this has meant being prepared to see how my experiences as a white middle class man are shaped by privileges that are not so readily available to others. I'm reminded of what the musician Archie Shepp said when he was asked about the blues. 'The blues (is what) we have every day as black folks—going to school, going to work, going to play.' (Quoted in a Radio 3 Profile-January 2019) It is hard to be yourself if every day you feel you have to watch yourself or justify yourself just for being you.

This is also about acknowledging the historical contexts that underpin belief systems and being prepared to question, rather than accept things at face value, particularly when that face is a white face speaking from a position of entrenched privilege. Indeed, what I find so refreshing and new about this coproduction project is the fact that Colin has focused our work on bringing together methodologies from across the board so that we can learn from Fanon as well as Foucault, from Freud as well as Du Bois. We can draw water from many different wells.

46.4   Steven Gillard's Narrative

Before I started to work with Colin, Simon and Bill my thinking about mental health research and race was probably something along the lines of 'should do more, could do more'. Actually I think I did do more once, when I was working in the voluntary sector. That was around the time of the 'Engaging and changing' agenda, when there was at least some acknowledgement that it wasn't so much the case that people from BAME communities were 'hard to engage'; rather that mental health services, such as they were, could be really hard to engage with. And in the voluntary sector we had a freedom to try things, to do something a bit different, running 'culturally-specific' versions of the services we provided with our evaluations demonstrating at least a measure of approval from the people we sought to engage.

But we know that, over the years, with this and other policy initiatives not really impacting on the inequalities that plague mental health services, this kind of cosmetic modification of what we habitually do somehow isn't enough. On top of that, having since moved into the big, bad world of clinical academic research, even that reasonably modest approach suddenly becomes difficult, and this in a world where there are no rewards for being difficult. It is a stultifying paradox of academic peer review that asking bold, step-change questions is met with an ingrained scientific risk adversity, with an incremental approach to enquiry grounded in mutual citation the way to go in career development. So we give ourselves a pat on the back for remembering to collect data on ethnicity and performing an underpowered subgroup analysis. After all, 'you can't do everything at once', 'someone else will do the race stuff better'. I've been doing research for nearly 20 years now that places people with lived experience of mental distress at the heart of designing and doing research. Isn't that somehow enough?

I'm guessing that in reading this you have, by now, noticed something about my voice that it has taken me these 20 years to realise. That my first person plural, my 'we', is White. (And my third person plural, my research subjects, are Black, are Other). In effect, I find myself hard-wired to objectify both the mental health system and its academic bedfellow as ubiquitously White, always asking 'how are we going to make things better for them'. Not only does this efface the existing achievements of colleagues of colour who bring far more insight and expertise than I will ever manage; it also fails to acknowledge that the solutions here might not be the exclusive preserve of White clinical academia. Indeed, that the origins of race inequality in mental health might in themselves lie in this tacit refusal to relinquish control over the production of knowledge about mental health; to open up that productive space.

I think that is the main lesson I have learnt—to date—from our 3 years of working together. This is where I think we have attempted to locate our coproduction. It is in the acknowledgement that none of us actually brings anything complete, in and of itself, to this process. There is no 'I' or 'him', or at least not in the sense that we might privilege the first person when we speak of ourselves (and subjugate the third person—each other—as an object of study or treatment). So the bit I think I've managed to do so far, to some extent, as a researcher, lies in not asserting what I think I might know, in being ready and willing to give up control over a research process, to let others do and decide, shape and create, even if I'm convinced it might be done better, done 'properly', my way.

46.5   Bill Fulford's Narrative

'Is a puzzlement!' Reflecting on several years working with Colin and (latterly) Simon and Steven I find my state of mind kin to that of the King of Siam in the Rogers and Hammerstein musical The King and I—and I suspect for much the same reasons.

Colin and I go back to 2004 when we worked on a project exploring concepts of mental disorder for a mental health NGO. I was an advisor to the project. Colin was the successful applicant for the post of Lead Researcher based on his innovative and challenging ideas for how the research should be carried out. The project was at one level a complete success—it produced important findings that were published in a report from the NGO in question. But it also failed in that instead of implementing Colin's ideas it morphed into a very different (and less innovative and challenging) form. Colin's plans involved direct exploration of the 'front stage/back stage' values driving psychiatric diagnosis. But what we actually did was a series of on-line questionnaires. There were at the time good reasons for changing the project in this way (such as the limited extent of our funding). But the effect was de facto *colonisation.*

Over this same period Colin and I worked together separately on his intellectual autobiography. Here I can claim a degree of at least partial insight. I had published a chapter-length version from Colin in a collection on Reconceiving Schizophrenia [10] and encouraged him to develop his ideas into a book. Yet despite being an experienced and several times published author, Colin seemed completely unable to do this. It took a year but I finally realised I was asking him to write in a language (my language) in which what he had to say, simply could not be said.

Thus far is the extent of my insight. I recognise that I failed to get beyond the colour bar in our original research project. I also recognise that I failed again in the first iteration of Colin's intellectual autobiography. Not only that but I recognise that getting beyond the colour bar is important at many levels in mental health. There are, in particular, good reasons (from my own field of values-based practice) to believe that our failure as a culture to get beyond the colour bar lies at the root of the disproportionate use of compulsory psychiatric treatment in young black men. But here my insight fails. It fails with the all-important experience of whiteness. Despite Colin's best efforts over several years the very concept of whiteness remains to me almost entirely opaque.

Such is the nature of partial insight that I can see why this might be so. I can see that my own values of whiteness may be a barrier to self-understanding. I can see too that this may be in part adaptive. My whiteness after all, set besides Colin's blackness, brings with it a tension that may in the end prove to be productive. It would be easy (though to be sure not that easy) for me to disown whiteness for blackness (or for Colin vice versa*). This is indeed how the King of Siam's puzzlement is resolved in the musical. On the King's deathbed his eldest son and now acknowledged heir apparent decrees that the country will move decisively to Western values. But the aims of our project—consistently with the dissensus of values-based practice—admit no such one-sided resolution. So for me for now it remains 'a puzzlement'.*

46.6 Commentary: Mutual Respect of Bust?

Values-based practice is neither black nor white. It is, rather, essentially and irreducibly, plural. It is from the pluralism of values-based practice that its key strengths but also its deepest challenges are derived. Both are evident in these four narratives. As to its strengths, the four narratives show the positive role played by the premise of values-based practice in mutual respect for differences of values. This operates at several levels. First, it is through mutual respect that notwithstanding the highly challenging nature of the differences between them, the group holds together. Colin, drawing on the background experience he brings to the group, writes of 'the dead-ness of their soul … when they talk … asking for my experiences as the knowledge they need to research me. They rarely exchange their experiences … (hiding) behind the scientific exoneration of detachment'.

Colin's experience is thus of being made visible as a Black man by contrast with his white colleagues' elective invisibility. There is a particular irony here. Within the very group that aims to get beyond the colour bar there is a colour bar indeed, the colour bar of whiteness. Yet the holding power of the premise of mutual respect is such that instead of the group breaking apart in the face of 'failed promises', it sur-vives and, indeed, thrives. Colin, working initially with Bill and latterly with Steven, has generated significant research outputs (his work on racism and sport has been recognised with a national award). Working with Simon and Steven, he has set up the very active Whiteness and Race Equality network within the Collaborating Centre for Values-based Practice run by Bill (valuesbasedpractice.org). These tan-gible products of the group's work reflect the premise of mutual respect actively at work. It is easy for those of like mind to collaborate. What is evident here is those of unlike and potentially conflictive minds collaborating to good effect.

One particular output from the Group is a growing awareness of the importance of whiteness as a tacit culture. Steven makes the point in terms of his habitual use of personal pronouns in research: 'my first person plural, my "we," is White. (And my third person plural, my research subjects, are Black, are Other)'. Colin, similarly, though drawing on the work of the mid-twentieth century French West Indian psy-chiatrist and philosopher, Frantz Fanon, writes: 'In this culture (of the Group's meet-ings) exists the process of white denial, black emotional expression, white rationality, black feelings of despair and injustice. Culture is a whiteness … that protects it … that rationalises what it hears and sees in the culture of the black people it interacts with … it has no responsibility, it is absent in this cultural space …'. And again, later … 'Rarely do I see the culture behind what Fanon [9] refers to as the "white mask"'.

Here, then, with this insight into whiteness is progress towards the Group's aim of getting beyond the colour bar. Yet with this comes a sharp reminder of the chal-lenge of pluralism noted in the introduction to values-based practice (chapter 1, "Surprised by Values: An Introduction to Values-Based Practice and the Use of Personal Narratives in this Book"). This is in evidence here. We may identify in principle with Simon's call for us to ' … draw water from many different (method-ological) wells'. But achieving this in practice, as Steven describes, requires break-ing free from a scientific research culture based on peer review that adopts '…an incremental approach to enquiry grounded in mutual citation …'. Peer review and mutual citation have a proven track record as powerful ways of driving scientific advances. But herein lies precisely the challenge for values-based practice. For the very power of peer review and mutual citation is the power of monism not pluralism.

46.7   Conclusions

This chapter has presented four very different perspectives on the experiences of its four authors (one black man and three white men) of working together over a num-ber of years. The shared aim of the group is to bridge their cultural divide (to get 'beyond the colour bar') and thus cone to an understanding of (and thereby remove) the current disparities in mental health provision between black and white.

An emergent finding from their collaboration is the importance of an implicit culture of 'whiteness' as a factor potentially driving inequalities in mental health. That their collaboration has been in this way productive notwithstanding the differences between them reflects the premise of mutual respect at work. This brings with it the challenge of pluralism inherent in values-based practice. The experience of the Group to date suggests that the premise of mutual respect will have a key role to play in overcoming the challenge of pluralism inherent in values-based practice.

46.8 Further Information

For details of the Whiteness and Race Equality Network please go to: valuesbased-practice.org/what do we do/networks—and scroll down the page.

References

1. Small S. Racialised barriers: the black experience in the United States and England in the 1980's. Critical studies in racism and migration. New York: Routledge; 1994.
2. Du Bois WD. The souls of the black folk. Oxford: Oxford University Press; 1903.
3. Rosaldo R. Culture and truth. The remaking of social analysis. London: Routledge; 1988.
4. Dyer J. 1994. https://www.theguardian.com/society/2017/nov/08/jacqui-dyer-race-mental-health-act-black-people-detentions-inequality.
5. Ladner J. The death of white sociology. London: Routledge; 1972.
6. Littlewood R, Lipsedge M. Aliens and alienists: ethnic minorities and psychiatry. London: Penguin Books Ltd; 1982.
7. Hook B. Black looks, race and representation. New York: Routledge; 1991.
8. Fanon F. Black skin, white mask. London: Pluto Press; 1967.
9. Goffman E, Lemert CC, Branaman A. The Goffman reader. Oxford: Blackwell Readers; 1967.
10. King C. They diagnosed me a schizophrenic when I was just a Gemini: the other side of madness (Chapter 2). In: Chung M, Fulford KWM, Graham G, editors. Reconceiving schizophrenia. Oxford: Oxford University Press; 2007. p. 11–28.

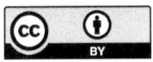

Co-writing Values: What We Did and Why We Did It

Bill Fulford

47.1 Introduction

This book is ambitious. It was ambitious in its original scope and aims. It has been ambitious in implementation. It is ambitious for the future.

In this concluding chapter, we describe the processes we adopted in pursuing our ambitions for the book and take stock of its outcomes. We look first, in Sect. 2, at the challenges that were presented by the co-writing approach that we adopted. Section 3 then describes how we deployed the resources of values-based practice in addressing these challenges. Finally, Sect. 4 reflects on outcomes. We offer no further justification for our ambitious co-writing approach than the range and quality of the contributions to the book. We conclude with a brief reflection on the implications of the book for the future of person-centred care not just in mental health but in health care as a whole.

47.2 What We Did (a)—Finding the Challenges

As we described in our Preface, this book came about as an unintended though welcome consequence of the 'embarrassment of riches' of personal narratives that resulted from our initial call for contributions. Faced with the wide diversity of these contributions, it became immediately clear that as Editors (being, although geographically diverse, all white, male and psychiatrists), we were ill-equipped to represent the book as a whole.

Authors
The Editors with input from all contributors

B. Fulford (✉)
St Catherine's College, University of Oxford, Oxford, UK

D. Stoyanov et al. (eds.), *International Perspectives in Values-Based Mental Health Practice*, https://doi.org/10.1007/978-3-030-47852-0_47

Various options for remedying this were considered at an initial writing workshop convened by the Lead Editor, Drozdstoj Stoyanov, and hosted by one of our contributors, Hasanen Al-Taiar, under the auspices of the Royal College of Psychiatrists in London. It was this workshop that settled on co-writing as a values-based strategy for capturing the full range and diversity of the proposed contributions to the book. A second workshop then took this strategy forward by developing a shared framework of values within which as co-writing contributors we would all work. (The second workshop is described further in Sect. 3.)

47.2.1   First Workshop: Raising Awareness of Values

The first workshop brought together a small group recruited, for practical reasons, locally from among those able to attend but broadly reflecting the range of backgrounds and experiences of contributors to the book as a whole.

The programme for the day started with two exercises routinely used in values-based practice training sessions to raise awareness of values and of differences of values.[1] The aim at the time was to give our contributors an introduction to values-based practice by experiencing it for themselves. But as is so often the way with exercises in values-based practice we got more than we had bargained for! So effective were the exercises in raising awareness of values and (more particularly) of differences of values that a number of (sometimes painful) clashes of values emerged among participants.

The depth of the challenges presented by these clashes of values is illustrated by the sample comments that follow. These reflect the range of comments on one of the dominant themes, Respect and Disagreement. They are partly as made in the first workshop, partly as reprised in the second, and partly as subsequently submitted by way of follow-up.[2] We return to some of the other themes below (see Risks, Resources and Strengths). Although anonymized, the comments are reproduced with the permission of those concerned.

- *Speaker 1—is the resolution that XX* (whose values had upset and offended some participants) *resigns?*
- *Speaker 2—my reaction is the opposite—I agree this has made for an uncomfortable meeting but it is good that things have been said openly so they can be dealt with rather than get sat on.*
- *Speaker 3—if the book as a whole doesn't represent my values I will withdraw but this doesn't mean I agree with everything in every chapter—so its about facing our challenges—not an easy thing to do—but we have to agree to acknowledge differences.*

---

[1] The exercises used were the 'three words' exercise and the 'forced choice' exercise—these are described fully in the sources indicated in the Guide to Further Information at the end of this chapter.

[2] The extracts given here are representative of the comments and views expressed on the theme of Respect and Disagreement in the course of a much longer discussion (continuing in all for over an hour and a half across the two workshops). The numbering of the speakers is solely for purposes of differentiating them and does not reflect the order in which they spoke.

- *Speaker 2—my standards are 'am I proud of my contribution and will my contribution make a difference?'*
- *Speaker 3—there is an important difference between disagreeing and taking offense. We must behave in a way that is consistent with the book so may agree to disagree but so long as we all believe in values-based practice, and in actually doing it, a key part of what we are about is to share and acknowledge differences.*
- *Speaker 2—my desire to say what I want to say may sit alongside things I think are wrong.*
- *Speaker 3—it's not about agreement but about finding that framework of respect within which we may disagree without taking offense.*

Through this and similar discussions, we found the originally planned 'introduction to values-based practice' morphed into a substantive and as it proved particularly intense exercise in values-based practice itself. We took this exercise forward, following the last speaker's suggestion, with the development in the second workshop of a shared framework of values.

47.3   What We Did (b): Facing the Challenges

The second workshop—kindly convened by another of our contributors, David Crepaz-Keay, at the Mental Health Foundation[3]—focused as we have said on establishing a framework of shared values within which we could all agree to work in taking the book forward.

As a key component of values-based practice, such frameworks should be established on a locally agreed basis among those directly concerned (see Table 1.2, chapter 1, "Surprised by Values: An Introduction to Values-Based Practice and the Use of Personal Narratives in this Book"). It was just such a locally agreed framework that the second workshop gave us the opportunity to produce. Led on this occasion by Kim Woodbridge-Dodd and Evette Hunkins-Hutchinson (authors of the reflective chapter 44, "Reflections on the Impact of Mental Health Ward Staff Training in Race Equality and Values-Based Practice"), the group agreed to adopt a modified version of a framework of shared values developed some years ago to support the policy implementation work of NIMHE [1].[4] Those present contributed suggestions for modifying this framework. It was then circulated for comment to the group as a whole. The version finally adopted is given in Fig. 47.1.

---

[3] The Mental Health Foundation is a mental health NGO based in London (see https://www.mentalhealth.org.uk). David, who is the author of chapter 22 "Three Points in Time: How Values and Culture Affected my Life, Madness and the People Around Me" and first author of chapter 28 "Journey into Genes: Cultural Values and the (Near) Future of Genetic Counselling in Mental Health", is the Head of Empowerment and Social Inclusion at MHF.

[4] NIMHE (the National Institutes for Mental Health, England) was a policy implementation body set up by the UK's Department of Health some years ago to support what at the time was an ambitious programme of mental health services reform. NIMHE's first Director, Anthony Sheehan, convened an interdisciplinary group (of which one of us, KWMF, was a member) tasked with producing a Framework of Values to guide its work.

The modified NIMHE Values Framework adopted in developing the book

The work of the editors and authors will be guided by three principles of values-based practice:

1) **Recognition** – as editors and authors we will recognize the role of values in all areas of mental health policy and practice and will aim to reflect this in developing the book.

   We recognize that no judgement can be 'value free' but results from such factors as class, background and culture.

2) **Raising Awareness** – as editors and authors we will be committed to raising awareness of the values involved in different contexts, the role/s they play and their impact on the development of this book.

   Our commitment to raising awareness of values will include recognizing our own values and how these reflect our very different backgrounds and life experiences. It will also include acknowledging the privilege we have of being able to adopt and write from our respective first-personal perspectives.

3) **Respect** – as editors and authors we will respect the diversity of values and will be committed to working with such diversity that makes the principle of person centrality a unifying focus for practice.

   This principle means that the values of each individual and their communities must be the starting point and key determinant for all understandings and decisions by the editors and authors involved in the book.

The Principle of Respect has a number of other important implications for the way we develop this book

- A commitment to dialogue - we believe that the book must evidence our commitment to dialogue between professionals, service users and carers that recognizes the unique contributions each brings.
- Equality of citizenship - respect for diversity of values encompasses a number of specific policies and principles concerned with equality of citizenship and it is acknowledged it will be enacted with different levels and forms of interpersonal and collective power relations.
- Equality between peoples - We recognize that equality of citizenship may be constituted differently within different nations and cultures, and that. as this is an international publication, this will in itself introduce a range of ways of understanding the meanings and expectations of what equality is and of how respectful behavior is demonstrated.
- No go areas – We share the view that respect for diversity requires anti-discriminatory attitudes and behaviors because discrimination in all its forms is intolerant of diversity. Thus respect for diversity of values has the consequence that it is unacceptable to discriminate on grounds such as gender, sexual orientation, class, age, abilities, religion, race, culture or language.
- Our overall approach – In aiming to embody respect for diversity in developing this book we will:

Fig. 47.1 The modified NIMHE Values Framework adopted in developing the book

     o Be prepared to listen to and make the required effort to gain insight into how other people different from ourselves understand a given situation
     o Reflectively combine self-monitoring and self-management with positive self-regard
     o Believe it is possible to be respectful of our own individual humanity and vulnerability while at the same time, 1) recognizing that others may see things differently, and 2) accepting that others may hold views with which we disagree but nonetheless respect.
     o Recognize that working with values is relational and may evoke strong personal emotions.
     o We will give time and space to: 1) becoming aware of the different values at play; 2) being open, respectful and responsive to others values; and 3) balancing, where possible, the differing values to the best mutually constructive outcome.

Fig. 47.1 (continued)

47.3.1 Risks, Resources and Strengths

Although agreeing a Framework of Shared Values was a good start, there was considerably more to the process of co-writing the book. This required 'above and beyond' engagement from our contributors and an additional administrative load for Springer. There were multiple exchanges of drafts of individual chapters and of large sections of the book as a whole. Where differences arose, there were balancing compromises to find. These were important particularly in the light of the issues of Power and of Language Use/Communication that were extensively aired in both workshops. For example:

- *Speaker 6—equality between authors and editors means genuine two-way communication between people on an equal footing.*
- *Speaker 7—Is the book for psychiatrists or the general public? If the latter we must use language that anyone can understand.*
- *Speaker 6—we are the 'we' here—this is about what can 'we' do together—we are all stakeholders in the process.*
- *Speaker 2—I spend much of my time on projects where I feel the professionals present have no real idea what it means to be a psychiatric patient.*
- *Speaker 4—the point is to acknowledge and deal with the issues of power that come up—this is something that we can do something about—it is, literally, within our power.*
- *Speaker 1—yes, the power to work through the issues—that at least should be the intention of the editing process.*
- *Speaker 5—the issues of editorial power run both ways—the editors have to manage issues of academic power (such as peer review and citation ratings) as well as managing power relationships with authors.*
- *Speaker 1—the challenge is to have an impact—this requires successfully getting the book out and published but without compromising what we are trying to say.*

As editors, we thus had to rethink our role in the book, stepping back and relinquishing a part of the control we would normally have exercised. There were risks in this of course. We could have lost contributors (we did lose one). But such risks were more than compensated for by the many ways in which contributors supported the task of implementation. It was very helpful for a start that they were realistic about just how difficult this was likely to be:

- *Speaker 3—We know from experience that values-based practice isn't easy to implement.*
- *Speaker 1—a 2009 report from the Coalition Government puts service users first—but again it simply isn't happening—so if it doesn't happen with this book is it a con?*
- *Speaker 3—even here* [in co-writing the book] *we started with respect but when two people had different points of view everyone felt threatened—if we can't get it right in this room how can we expect to get service users' values acted on in the wider community.*

Notwithstanding the difficulties, however, contributors engaged positively with the process. Indeed, the dissensus[5] from which the book gradually emerged was managed as much by our co-writing contributors as by us as editors. In the first writing workshop, for example when emotionally distressing issues were raised, it was one of our contributors who brought the group together around our shared commitment to the mutual respect underpinning values-based practice. Contributors also came up with many practical ideas and assets:

- *Speaker 7—one way to have an impact is to build on the [VBP] Centre's and other resources established by different cultural groups—instead of giving us services, give us the money and control to set up our own services.*
- *Speaker 8—the learning from the book has to be structured to link up with what works—there are excellent cultural competency trainers (for example at the Steven Laurence Centre in London) and helpful publications (such as Robin Diangelo's "White Fragility", [2]) that really ring bells about the language that's used in psychiatry.*
- *Speaker 9—the engagement itself has to be sensitive to cultural values—for example there was a theatre project 20 years ago in London that involved a young director from the Brazilian favelas* [slums] *being asked to put on one of his productions—like most Brazilians his way of working included physical contact so he was devastated when in a break one of the theatre officials told him 'we invited you here to do your theatre but here we don't touch people'.*

Many further resources for implementation are included in the sources given in the Guides to Further Information at the ends of individual chapters.

---

[5] See Table 1.1 in the Introduction to Values-based Practice in chapter 1, "Surprised by Values: An Introduction to Values-Based Practice and the Use of Personal Narratives in this Book".

47.4   Why We Did It

Exceptional claims, as the familiar aphorism has it, require exceptional proofs. Our central claim in this book (that cultural values are a key factor in the causes, presentation and management of mental health issues), and the means by which we have chosen to establish that claim (by way of personal narratives), may seem to be, in the sense of the aphorism, 'exceptional'. At the very least it may be said, some justification is required for the extent to which the approach adopted diverges from the 'tried and tested' norms of contemporary scientific medicine.

47.4.1   Justifying Values?

We have offered the beginnings of the required justification in our opening chapter with our proposed inversion of the evidence hierarchy for values: personal narratives we argued may come at the bottom of the evidence hierarchy but they should come at the very top of the corresponding hierarchy for values (chapter 1, "Surprised by Values: An Introduction to Values-Based Practice and the Use of Personal Narratives in this Book", Fig. 1.3). This inversion we further argued, far from alienating values-based practice from evidence-based practice is an aspect of and directly reflects the partnership between them in clinical decision-making.

A full working out of this justification is beyond our scope here. Such working out might start with the history of ideas, looking at the (traditionally recognized) sources of contemporary understandings of mental health issues in the outputs from the Nineteenth Century *Methodonstreit*, and the influences of these sources on Karl Jaspers in developing his distinction between causal explanations and meaningful understanding of psychopathology. In the light of the contributions to this book, moreover, sources from the history of ideas should be extended beyond those traditionally cited to include, for example, work on the effects of colonization and slavery on norms of rationality, and, hence, how psychiatric diagnostic concepts are used in practice (see, for example, among other pertinent chapters in this book, chapters 11, "Madness, Mythopoetry and Medicine", 18, "Colonial Values and Asylum Care in Brazil: Reclaiming the Streets Through Carnival in Rio de Janeiro", 20, "Living at the Edge of Compromise: Balkan Pluralism as a Resource for Balanced Decision-Making" and Colin King's contribution to chapter 46, "Beyond the Color Bar: Sharing Narratives in Order to Promote a Clearer Understanding of Mental Health Issues Across Cultural and Racial Boundaries").

These sources might in turn lead to their counterparts in various areas of contemporary philosophy: to the philosophy of mind, for example, with work on levels of explanation and its applications across such areas as information theory, artificial intelligence and the neurosciences; to moral theory, notably in on-going debates about the logical relationship (the relationship of meaning) between assertions of fact and of value; and to cross-disciplinary work between the philosophy and sociology of science. Sources for all these and other relevant areas are given in the Guide to Further Information at the end of the chapter.

47.4.2 A Provisional Justification

The theoretical issues involved in grounding values-based practice on personal narratives are thus all too real. This is why as we noted in the introduction to Part II (chapter 6, "Theory First: An Introduction to Part II, Theory"), theory plays such a large role in values-based practice and in this book. For present purposes however, we believe our approach is at least provisionally justified by the diverse range and quality of the contributions to the book.

We return below to why we say 'provisionally justified' but a quick caste across the contents of the book is sufficient to show that its contributions are indeed nothing if not diverse. There is wide diversity in style and content. There is wide diversity of geographical regions and of cultural and ethnic representation. There is wide diversity of topics covering all the major forms of mental health issues and a range of treatment approaches (including self-management). There is, importantly, wide diversity of expertise including (with equal authority of voice) expertise by experience and expertise by training. Such diversity might suggest an inchoate storyline. But the contributions as we described in our introductory chapter 1 (Sect. 4), fell naturally into the established framework structure of values-based practice.

47.4.3 Why Diversity of Perspectives Is Important Clinically

The diversity of perspectives represented by the contributions to this book is important clinically. It is important across the board in the shared clinical decision-making that is the basis of contemporary person-centred clinical care. This is why values-based practice, offering as it does a way of engaging effectively with diverse value perspectives, is important across the board in health care (remember the story from orthopaedic surgery in chapter 1, "Surprised by Values: An Introduction to Values-Based Practice and the Use of Personal Narratives in this Book" about Mrs. Jones and her arthritic knee).

In mental health, this same diversity of perspectives has the further importance of providing a foil against abuse. Mental health interventions are notoriously vulnerable to being used abusively for purposes of political or personal control [3]. There are reasons (contested reasons to be sure) for believing that the vulnerability of mental health to abuse of this kind arises from the influence of unacknowledged values on judgements of rationality [4]. The influence of such values is evident in several chapters in this book: for example, in chapter 18, "Colonial Values and Asylum Care in Brazil: Reclaiming the Streets Through Carnival in Rio de Janeiro" with the impact on unacknowledged colonial values on attitudes to mental health in Brazil, chapter 27, "Nontraditional Religion, Hyper-religiosity, and Psychopathology: The Story of Ivan from Bulgaria" with the impact of unacknowledged values of rationality on the interpretation of DSM's 'criteria of clinical significance', and chapter 46, "Beyond the Colour Bar: Sharing Narratives in Order to

Promote a Clearer Understanding of Mental Health Issues Across Cultural and Racial Boundaries" with the impact of unacknowledged values of whiteness on racially disproportionate uses of involuntary psychiatric treatment in the UK. Other factors may be involved in abusive uses of psychiatry becoming institutionalized [5]. But it is in unacknowledged cultural values, so this line of reasoning goes, that the essential vulnerability of mental health to abuse has its origins.

In raising awareness of values, values-based practice thus has a role to play in mental health not only in promoting good practice (by supporting shared clinical decision making) but also in preventing bad practice (as a foil against abuse). But raising awareness of one's own values is difficult: recall our own surprise in chapter 1, at the extent to which our unacknowledged values of individualism had influenced the original development of values-based practice. Which is where the diversity of perspectives represented by the contributions to this book comes crucially into play. For just as in chapter 1, exposure to a diversity of value perspectives prompted insight into the way our own unacknowledged values had shaped values-based practice, so, too, may exposure to a diversity of value perspectives prompt similar insights into the ways unacknowledged values continue to shape approaches to mental health issues.

47.4.4 Why Diversity of Perspectives Has Been Important in This Book

As editors, we have had first-hand experience of the importance of diverse perspectives in illuminating values at a number of points in producing this book. As noted above, and as described in chapter 1, exposure to diversity of perspectives was important in the origins of the book. It was this that made us aware of the extent to which values-based practice itself had to that point been driven all unwittingly by values of individualism. We acknowledged our surprise at this illumination. The result, we said, is that the book owes its very existence to the diversity of perspectives on which it draws.

It is this same diversity operating now at the end of the book that was key to the outcomes we hope from the book. This is how this further illumination came about. As part of the process of co-writing we circulated drafts of the front and end matter for the book, including an earlier version of this concluding Chapter, to all authors for comment and input. Most, we were delighted to find, were well pleased. One contributor, however, Colin King (the lead author of chapter 46, "Beyond the Color Bar: Sharing Narratives in Order to Promote a Clearer Understanding of Mental Health Issues Across Cultural and Racial Boundaries"), made what at first came as a surprising observation. He pointed out that as editors we were *'speaking in the third person...'* but commenting *'... on first person accounts of the black and white cultural challenges...'* with the result that *'... your cultural values are absent.'*

In a subsequent conversation, Colin explained that he was drawing in this on Steven Gillard's observations (in chapter 46, "Beyond the Color Bar: Sharing Narratives in Order to Promote a Clearer Understanding of Mental Health Issues Across Cultural and Racial Boundaries") about personal pronoun use. Speaking in the third person about first personal experiences is a way of objectifying that experience while at the same time failing to 'see' our own values. In this case, Colin pointed out, we were at risk of failing to 'see' our own values as editors.

At one level, this might seem like old news. As we noted in the Forward to this book, it was our recognition that as editors (being all white, male and psychiatrists) we could not match the diversity of our contributors, that led to the book becoming a project in its own subject matter, values-based practice, operationalized through the co-writing procedures that in our writing workshops we went on to adopt. But this was precisely why Colin's observation was so important. For what his observation showed was that, notwithstanding the evident power of the values-based co-writing approach we had adopted, as evidenced by the quality of the contributions to the book, we as editors were still not able to 'see' our own values other than through the mirror of someone else's very different perspective. All of us are male. But as editors, we are white psychiatrists whereas Colin is a black writer and activist.

So there we have it. Generalizing Colin's observation takes us to the idea of an international open society of stakeholders in mental health as a key outcome from the book. As we describe below and in our Afterword,[6] an international open society of stakeholders serves as a 'hall of mirrors' through which we can come to mutual understanding of the values driving mental health practice. True, we had explored that idea previously. But it had been an idea in theory only. Colin's observation of our inability to 'see' our own values made it real.

47.4.5   Towards an 'Open Society' of Stakeholders in Mental Health

Exposure to diversity of values may operate at different levels, personal, professional, national or, as here, international. Internationally, exposure to diversity of values requires the development of what the social psychiatrist, Jim Birley, drawing on his experience countering political abuses of psychiatry as President of the Geneva Initiative for Psychiatry, called an 'open society' among mental health stakeholders [6]. Now, some 40 years on, it is in taking us a step towards Jim Birley's open society, that the diversity of contributions to this book is provisionally

---

[6] Bill Fulford and Colin King have developed this idea in more detail with the philosopher Anna Bergqvist in their '*Hall of Mirrors: Towards an open society of mental health stakeholders in safeguarding against political abuse*', (in English) in a special issue of the Polish journal of philosophy and psychiatry, Eidos, edited by Louis Sass. (Fulford, KWM., King, C., and Bergqvist, A., (2020) Eidos: a Journal for Philosophy of Culture. Volume 4, no 2, pps 23–38. https://doi.org/10.14394/eidos.jpc.2020.0014)

justified. Final justification will depend on Jim Birley's open society of mental health stakeholders becoming a reality. We return to how this is to be done in our Afterword.

47.5 Conclusions

In this chapter, we have described the values-based process we adopted in co-writing the book. This proved challenging emotionally and administratively. We addressed these challenges through two writing workshops and by way of many individual conversations and multiple exchanges of drafts. Although complex and difficult, we believe our co-writing approach to have been provisionally justified by the quality and range of narrative contributions this generated for the book. The diversity of perspectives represented by these contributions takes us an important step towards establishing the kind of open society among stakeholders that we have argued is required to support best practice in person-centred mental health care.

Which brings us, finally, to the 'mental health first' surprise we promised at the end of chapter 1. The surprise, to anticipate, is that in establishing in this way an open society among stakeholders, mental health will be first in leading the way in person-centred care for health care as a whole.

This follows from the Science Driven Principle of values-based practice. As we saw in the introduction to Part IV (chapter 24, "Linking Science with People: An Introduction to Part IV, Science"), this Principle arises from the way in which advances in medical science and technology impact on practice. Such advances as we described open up new choices and with choices go values. David Crepaz-Keay and co-authors (chapter 28, "Journey into Genes: Cultural Values and the (Near) Future of Genetic Counselling in Mental Health") provide a vivid illustration of the impact of this principle in psychiatric genetics with their 'Journey into Genes'. But it is the full import of this principle for mental health that brings with it our 'mental health first' surprise. For if cultural values are a key factor in linking science with people in mental health today, then, tomorrow, with future developments in medical science and technology, cultural values will become a key factor also in linking science with people across health care as a whole.

That mental health should be first in recognizing and responding to this key connection between values and evidence comes as a surprise when it is set against the 'mental health second' stereotype of Twentieth Century health care. According to this stereotype, mental health ran always behind and in second place to other areas of health care. The 'mental health first' surprise, then, arising from the full impact of the Science Driven Principle of values-based practice, is that in Twenty-First Century health care, mental health, in being the first to recognize the need for an international open society of stakeholders, and engaging in this open society through personal narratives of the kind presented in this book, is leading the way for health care as a whole. Mental health is thus first in the field in developing the resources to support a model of shared clinical decision-making, based equally on evidence and on values, that is at the heart of best practice in contemporary person-centred clinical care.

47.6 Guide to Further Information

For sources on the various areas of philosophy relevant to a full justification of the importance of a diversity of value perspectives in mental health (noted at the start of Sect. 4 in this chapter), please see *The Oxford Textbook of Philosophy and Psychiatry* [7]—chapters of this textbook together with key readings are available for free download from the new website of the *International Network for Philosophy and Psychiatry*.

For a detailed reading guide and many training and other resources for values-based practice, please see the website for the *Collaborating Centre for Values-based Practice in Health and Social Care* at St Catherine's College, Oxford at: values-basedpractice.org.

As described further in our Afterword, the Collaborating Centre is kindly supporting the authors and editors of this book in taking forward the development of an international open society of stakeholders in mental health.

References

1. National Institute for Mental Health England. The National Framework of Values for Mental Health. Originally published on-line on the NIMHE website. Available on the values-based practice website (https://valuesbasedpractice.org) or in hard copy in Woodbridge K, Fulford KWM. 'Whose values?' A workbook for values-based practice in mental health care. London: The Sainsbury Centre for Mental Health (or as a free download https://atvaluesbasedparctice.org); 2004.
2. Diangelo R. White fragility: why its so hard for white people to talk about racism. Boston: Beacon Press; 2018.
3. van Voren R, Keukens R. Ch 48: Political abuse of psychiatry. In: Sadler JZ, van Staden W, Fulford KWM, editors. The Oxford handbook of psychiatric ethics. Oxford: Oxford University Press; 2015.
4. Fulford KWM, Dewey S, King M. Values-based involuntary seclusion and treatment: value pluralism and the UK's Mental Health Act 2007. Ch 60. In: Sadler JZ, van Staden W, Fulford KWM, editors. The Oxford handbook of psychiatric ethics. Oxford: Oxford University Press; 2015.
5. Fulford KWM, Smirnov AYU, Snow E. Concepts of disease and the abuse of psychiatry in the USSR. Br J Psychiatry. 1993;162:801–10.
6. Birley J. Psychiatric ethics: an International Open Society. Chapter 11. In: Dickenson D, Fulford KWM, editors. In two minds: a casebook of psychiatric ethics. Oxford: Oxford University Press; 2000. p. 327–35.

7. Fulford KWM, Thornton T, Graham G. Progress in five parts. Chapter 1. In: Fulford KWM, Thornton T, Graham G, editors. The Oxford textbook of philosophy and psychiatry. Oxford: Oxford University Press; 2006. This book togeher with its associated readings will be available on open access and with free download on the new INPP Website that will be launched in early 2021.

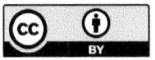

After Word: Where Next with the Book

Bill Fulford

How often do books hit the streets with ambitious agendas that all too quickly dissipate? This may be our fate with this book. But in our case, we have an asset on which to build in the community of thought and practice already established between us through our shared co-writing experience.

In our concluding chapter, we gave what amounted to a promissory note on next steps. Acknowledging the ambitious agenda with which we launched the book, we argued that this had been provisionally justified by its outcomes: by the diversity of perspectives our ambitious approach had produced and by the coherent organisation of these diverse perspectives across the book as a whole within the framework of values-based practice. These outcomes as we indicated took us a step towards what we called (borrowing from Jim Birley) an international 'open society' of stakeholders that, in linking science with people, would support shared clinical decision-making as the basis of person-centred clinical care. Final justification of our approach we concluded would depend on that open society becoming a reality.

This is where our plan bites for taking the work of the book forward. Our plan in essence is to build on and extend our established co-writing community into an international 'open society' of stakeholders consistent with Jim Birley's vision for the field.

Simple to state, we are well aware of the many roadblocks—theoretical, practical and political—in the way of implementing this plan. Our shared experience to date leaves us in no doubt on this point. Just how we tackle these roadblocks will depend in part on the resources available. Here we are delighted to have the confirmed support of the Collaborating Centre for Values-Based Practice in Oxford. The Centre as its name suggests is the focus for a growing number of collaborations in the theory and implementation of values-based practice (working of course always in partnership with evidence-based practice) across a wide range of areas of health care. As

Authors
The editors with input from all contributors.

B. Fulford (✉)
St Catherine's College, University of Oxford, Oxford, UK

D. Stoyanov et al. (eds.), *International Perspectives in Values-Based Mental Health Practice*, https://doi.org/10.1007/978-3-030-47852-0

such it is in a sense already an open society. Being primarily web-based, further-more, it is uniquely well placed to support international developments in the field.

1.1 Back to the Future

JL Austin, from whose version of ordinary language philosophy values-based prac-tice was originally derived (chapter 1, "Surprised by Values: An Introduction to Values-Based Practice and the Use of Personal Narratives in this Book"), would we believe have welcomed these plans as embodying yet a further important feature of his ideas about how to make progress in philosophy.

As a member of the British Intelligence Services in the Second World War, Austin had been much impressed by the power of teamwork for solving complex problems. Drawing on this experience, he argued for a similar teamwork approach in philosophy. The standard approach in philosophy, then as now, was what might be called 'the lone trader' model—a model in which 'the philosopher', working solo, interacts (usually competitively) within a narrowly defined group of similarly inclined peers. In his Saturday Morning Seminars in Oxford, Austin, as reported by his intellectual biographer, GJ Warnock ([1]), encouraged philosophers to break out of their self-imposed isolation and to work collaboratively with each other and with other disciplines, which is essentially what we plan to do. It is through collabora-tions of just the kind advocated by Austin that we plan to overcome the many road-blocks standing in the way of creating an open society of stakeholders to support the development of a culturally enriched form of values-based practice. All of which, given the power of ordinary language philosophy in the early development of the field and the range of additional resources available to a culturally enriched model of values-based practice, augurs well for the future of person-centred care in mental health and, thereby, in other areas of health care as well.

1.2 The Future

Just what success in person-centred mental health care will look like is itself a key question to be addressed. It involves after all a methodological conundrum—how are values to be validly evaluated?

As to tangible outcomes, we have helpful suggestions in hand from our contribu-tors. Kim Woodbridge-Dodd (chapter 44, "Reflections on the Impact of Mental Health Ward Staff Training in Race Equality and Values-Based Practice"), for example, suggests our aim should be *that professionals, service users and carers are enabled to engage in mutually meaningful discussions and effective decisions regarding well-being through robust arguments and examples of the relevance and implications of the diverse values at play in any given moment of care.* This is ambi-tious, certainly. But as one of the key figures in the early days of values-based practice, Kim is well placed to ensure that in our hopes for the future, as in our work together in the past, our gene for ambition will be once again effectively expressed.

Contact Us

To learn more and/or to join the collaboration, please go to: valuesbasedpractice.org and use the 'CONTACT US' button that appears on every page of the website.

Reference

1. Warnock GJ. J.L. Austin. Oxford: Oxford University Press; 1989.

Index

TO PACE OR NOT TO PACE